Fatigue Management

Amir Sharafkhaneh
Max Hirshkowitz

Editors

Fatigue Management

Principles and Practices for Improving Workplace Safety

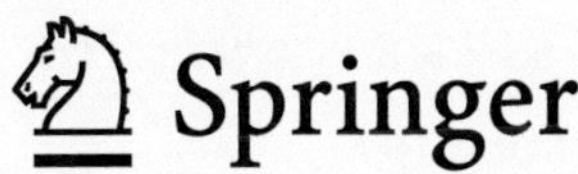 Springer

Editors
Amir Sharafkhaneh, MD, PhD
Department of Medicine
Baylor College of Medicine
Houston, TX
USA

Medical Care Line, Michael E. DeBakey
VA Medical Center
Houston, TX
USA

Max Hirshkowitz, PhD
Division of Public Mental Health and
Population Sciences
School of Medicine
Stanford University
Stanford, CA
USA

Department of Medicine
Baylor College of Medicine
Houston, TX
USA

ISBN 978-1-4939-9341-3   ISBN 978-1-4939-8607-1   (eBook)
https://doi.org/10.1007/978-1-4939-8607-1

This Springer imprint is published by the registered company Springer Science+Business Media, LLC part of Springer Nature.
The registered company address is: 233 Spring Street, New York, NY 10013, U.S.A.

Preface

In humans, sleepiness and fatigue represent two intertwined phenomena. While we recognize their differences, the terms are often used interchangeably. Living and working in a modern industrialized society involves engaging in many attention-intensive tasks. Some of these tasks demand sustained effort and lapses confer risk to the individual, coworkers, and/or the public. To help mitigate such risks, fatigue risk management procedures and occupational sleep medicine programs have evolved.

In this book, we discuss various factors including medical, neurological, psychiatric, and psychological factors underlying fatigue and sleepiness. Additionally, the authors review current fatigue and sleep management approaches.

The book begins with an overview of the concepts and definitions of fatigue. In Chap. 1, the editors provide a historical perspective on sleepiness and fatigue. Dr. Rose discusses the definitions and classifications of fatigue in Chap. 2. In the next two chapters, major authors in this field discuss assessments of fatigue in the laboratory (Drs. Bonnet and Arand in Chap. 3), in the field (Dr. Rose in Chap. 4), and in the clinical settings.

The book continues by exploring medical causes of fatigue. Drs. Primeau and Kushida discuss sleep disorders and fatigue in detail. Drs. Hirschowitz and Sharafkhaneh discuss how fatigue can be assessed in the clinical context. Drs. Ahmed and Thorpy discuss medical, neurological, and psychiatric conditions linked with fatigue. Drs. Sharafkhaneh, Rose, and Hirshkowitz then focus on medication and recreational agents that may result in fatigue. Chapter 9 by Drs. Won, Mohsenin, and Kryger explore treatment of sleep-related breathing disorders and how it may affect fatigue. Sleep disorders and fatigue continue in Chap. 10 by Drs. Masri, Jain, and Guilleminault with discussions about treating narcolepsy and hypersomnia. Dr. Herman discusses in more depth various aspects of sleep including circadian rhythm and fatigue. Drs. Maoghtader, Kanbar-agha, and Sharafhkaneh discuss the treatment of heart failure and improvement in fatigue. Finally, Drs. Bird and Alapat discuss management of fatigue in hospitalized patients. In Chap. 14, Drs. Alemohammad and Sadeghniiat-Haghighi discuss the issue of fatigue in the workplace. The final chapter provides an overall approach to the management of fatigue by Drs. Hirshkowitz and Sharafkhaneh.

It is our hope that this book will prove useful to practitioners involved in fatigue management. We strive to include information concerning a comprehensive approach to the issues involved. This approach attempts to augment and supplement existing paradigms for fatigue management and occupational sleep medicine programs. Ultimately, we anticipate that the information communicated in the book will benefit our patients struggling against fatigue and sleepiness to live more productive and better quality lives.

<table>
<tr><td>Houston, TX, USA</td><td>Amir Sharafkhaneh, MD, PhD</td></tr>
<tr><td>Stanford, CA, USA</td><td>Max Hirshkowitz, PhD</td></tr>
<tr><td>Houston, TX, USA</td><td></td></tr>
</table>

Contents

Contributors

Imran Ahmed, MD Department of Neurology, Sleep-Wake Disorders Center, Montefiore Medical Center, Bronx, NY, USA

Department of Neurology, Albert Einstein College of Medicine, Bronx, NY, USA

Philip Alapat, MD Department of Medicine – Pulmonary/Critical Care/Sleep, Baylor College of Medicine, Houston, TX, USA

Zahra Banafsheh Alemohammad, MD Occupational Sleep Research Center, Baharloo Hospital, Tehran University of Medical Sciences, Tehran, Iran

Donna L. Arand, PhD Kettering Health Network, Dayton, OH, USA

Garrett Bird, MD, CM Department of Pulmonary, Critical Care, Sleep, Steward Health Care, West Jordan, UT, USA

Michael H. Bonnet, PhD Wright State University Boonshoft School of Medicine, Kettering Sycamore Sleep Disorders Center, Miamisburg, OH, USA

Christian Guilleminault, MD, D Bio Stanford University Division of Sleep Medicine, Redwood City, CA, USA

John Herman, PhD, FAASM UT Southwestern Medical Center, Dallas, TX, USA

Max Hirshkowitz, PhD Division of Public Mental Health and Population Sciences, School of Medicine, Stanford University, Stanford, CA, USA

Department of Medicine, Baylor College of Medicine, Houston, TX, USA

Vikas Jain, MD, FAASM, CCSH Stanford University Division of Sleep Medicine, Redwood City, CA, USA

Faisal Kanbar-Agha, MD Sleep Disorders and Research Center, Michael E. DeBakey VA Medical Center, Houston, TX, USA

Meir Kryger, MD Yale University School of Medicine, Section of Pulmonary and Critical Care Medicine, New Haven, CT, USA

Veterans Affairs Connecticut Health Care System, West Haven, CT, USA

Clete Kushida, MD, PhD, RPSGT Stanford Sleep Medicine Center, Redwood City, CA, USA

Tony J. Masri, MD Stanford University Division of Sleep Medicine, Redwood City, CA, USA

Shahram Moghtader, MD Section of Pulmonary and Critical Care and Sleep Medicine, Baylor College of Medicine, Houston, TX, USA

Sleep Disorders and Research Center, Michael E. DeBakey VA Medical Center, Houston, TX, USA

Vahid Mohsenin, MD Yale University School of Medicine, Section of Pulmonary and Critical Care Medicine, New Haven, CT, USA

Michelle Primeau, MD Stanford Sleep Medicine Center, Redwood City, CA, USA

Mary Rose, PsyD Department of Medicine, Pulmonary, Critical Care and Sleep Section, Baylor College of Medicine and The Michael E. DeBakey Veterans Administration Hospital, Houston, TX, USA

Khosro Sadeghniiat-Haghighi, MD Occupational Sleep Research Center, Baharloo Hospital, Tehran University of Medical Sciences, Tehran, Iran

Amir Sharafkhaneh, MD, PhD Department of Medicine, Baylor College of Medicine, Houston, TX, USA

Medical Care Line, Michael E. DeBakey VA Medical Center, Houston, TX, USA

Michael Thorpy, MD Department of Neurology, Sleep-Wake Disorders Center, Montefiore Medical Center, Bronx, NY, USA

Department of Neurology, Albert Einstein College of Medicine, Bronx, NY, USA

Christine H. Won, MD, MS Yale University School of Medicine, Section of Pulmonary and Critical Care Medicine, New Haven, CT, USA

Veterans Affairs Connecticut Health Care System, West Haven, CT, USA

Chapter 1
Historical Perspective on Sleepiness and Fatigue-Related Accidents

Max Hirshkowitz and Amir Sharafkhaneh

Sleepiness and Fatigue

Sleepiness and fatigue go hand in hand, so much so that the terms are often incorrectly used interchangeably. Nonetheless, sleepiness is arguably the most important factor contributing to what are called "fatigue-related accidents." In material sciences, fatigue is the factor producing performance failure. In human studies, all stressors contribute to performance failure, and sleepiness is typically the predominant stressor.

Industrial Psychology, Human Factors, and Ergonomics

After World War II, fatigue in the workplace caught the eye of some in the nascent field of *industrial psychology*. The focus on practical applications at that time gave rise to a scientific assessment and modification of the workplace setting to increase efficiency. According to *The American Heritage Dictionary of the English Language, Fifth Edition* [1], industrial psychology is defined as "The branch of applied psychology that is concerned with efficient management of an industrial labor force and especially with problems encountered by workers in a mechanized environment." The *Collins English Dictionary* [2] maintains that industrial psychology is

M. Hirshkowitz, PhD
Division of Public Mental Health and Population Sciences,
School of Medicine, Stanford University, Stanford, CA, USA

Department of Medicine, Baylor College of Medicine, Houston, TX, USA

A. Sharafkhaneh, MD, PhD (✉)
Department of Medicine, Baylor College of Medicine, Houston, TX, USA

Medical Care Line, Michael E. DeBakey VA Medical Center, Houston, TX, USA
e-mail: amirs@bcm.edu

© Springer Science+Business Media, LLC, part of Springer Nature 2018
A. Sharafkhaneh, M. Hirshkowitz (eds.), *Fatigue Management*,
https://doi.org/10.1007/978-1-4939-8607-1_1

"the scientific study of human behaviour and cognitive processes in relation to the working environment." As the field developed, a specific area focused on *human factors*. The emphasis shifted from finding a human to fit a machine to designing a machine to fit a human. A great emphasis was placed on improving comfort, optimizing control mechanisms, and removing hazards posed by poorly thought-out designs. As the computer age approached, this area of study morphed into what we might now call ergonomics.

The resulting reengineered cockpits, control panels, and workstations certainly reduced physical stressors, discomfort, and other problems. Today's ergonomically designed office task chair is much more comfortable than those commonplace four decades ago (albeit, maybe making it too easy to sit at a desk for hours in front of a computer). However, intrinsically, this approach to a great extent externalizes the problems of sleepiness's contribution to fatigue. Thinking that the problem is "out there" can be seen in myths such as "highway hypnosis." The highway does not hypnotize the driver; however, it may be boring and non-stimulating. An alert driver will be bored; a sleep-deprived driver might fall asleep. Factors such as darkness, quiet, warmth, comfort, and recently having eaten do not produce sleepiness, but they will unmask already-existing sleepiness.

Improving the position of screens, dials, and switches on a control panel and making the operator more comfortable do not improve alertness. The graveyard shift operator facing an upstream battle against their circadian propensity to sleep is more likely to experience performance failure if they are comfortable and minimally stimulated. Inadvertently, standing desks that have recently become popular for improving workers' longer-term health actually help offset fatigue. Standing stimulates the central nervous system and improves wakefulness. That is why soldiers "stand watch" on guard duty at night. Many self-devised sleepiness countermeasures actually involve stimulating the nervous system. Splashing cold water on one's face, turning the air conditioner on high, turning up the radio's volume while driving, listening to talk radio rather than music when trying to stay awake, chewing gum, and drinking caffeinated beverages all increase sympathetic activation of the central nervous system. As such factors are studied in greater depth, better designs will evolve.

This is not to argue that industrial psychology, human factors, and ergonomics have not helped. Certainly spring-loaded throttles, dead man switches, audible and visual alarms, and proper positioning to improve monitoring have undoubtedly prevented many accidents and disasters. I've reviewed many accident cases in which the engineered countermeasures were intentionally defeated by the operators much to their own chagrin after the fact.

Defeating and/or ignoring countermeasures established to reduce sleep-related mishaps should not be a surprise to anyone. Industries in which public safety is involved had either self-imposed or government agency-mandated "hours of service (HOS)" regulations. For example, current (as of March 2017) HOS regulations for property-carrying and passenger-carrying drivers allow driving a maximum of 11 h after 10 consecutive hours off duty. Alternatively, drivers may drive a maximum of 10 h after eight consecutive hours off duty. My experience in accident review is that HOS regulations are commonly violated which sadly enough serves to verify their validity.

Physiology

In 1971, Ernst Simonson compiled and edited a volume entitled *Physiology of Work Capacity and Fatigue*. The contributors to this work discuss accumulation of metabolites and depletion of "energy-yielding" substances and hormones. They review what was known at the time about fatigue-related changes in electrolytes, permeability, colloid chemicals, muscle, heart, peripheral nerves, central nervous system, and body chemistry both in terms of substrate and regulation. An entire section is devoted to internal and external environmental stress and how it contributes to fatigue and influences work capacity.

Within the next decade, we began to appreciate more and more the role that physiological factors have on human performance.

In the following year, Robert Y. Moore published his findings that the suprachiasmatic nucleus was the master clock governing the circadian rhythm of sleep and wakefulness. Integration of our understanding of physiological mechanisms underlying sleepiness and fatigue began to accelerate. As a result we began to better understand the real culprits behind fatigue-related accidents.

The Real Culprits

By the mid-1970s, sleep research and sleep medicine expanded geometrically. In addition to more precise quantitative models of the effects of sleep deprivation (inadequate sleep), sleep medicine emerged as a medical subspecialty. Diagnostics and treatments for sleeping and waking disorders steadily advanced over the next three decades. Sleep-related breathing disorders as a major cause of sleepiness were recognized; pharmacological and behavioral treatments for insomnia were developed and validated with evidence-based medicine methodologies; positive airway pressure therapy for sleep apnea became widespread; new sleep disorders were discovered; and the genetics underlying narcolepsy were revealed.

In 1993 *Wake up America: A National Sleep Alert: Report of the National Commission on Sleep Disorders Research* was published. This landmark report summarized the findings of 2 years of work designed to determine the cost to the USA taken by sleep deprivation, sleep disorders, and sleep-related accidents. The toll was enormous.

National Commission and Its Report

Leger [3] summarized the National Commission report in a paper published in the journal *Sleep*. Accidents (in 1987) were the fourth leading cause of death in the USA, and motor vehicle accidents (MVAs) were the leading cause within that category. In 1988, MVAs accounted for 51% (49,000) of accidental deaths. When age is considered, MVAs are the number one leading cause of death among individuals age 1–37 years. Fifty-four percent of MVAs occur at night and most are single-vehicle accidents. Sleepiness is suspected in the majority of these cases. The resulting estimated cost for just sleepiness-related MVAs was between 29.2 and 37.9 billion dollars in 1988.

The aforementioned statistics beg the question "why wasn't this realized earlier?" One explanation is that the accidents are spread out in both time and space. There might be 75 highway fatalities related to sleepiness on any given day, but they are seldom reported beyond the local news. Furthermore, no formal systematic inquiry about the driver's recent sleep schedule or sleep health is universally mandated; consequently, statistics are difficult to compile. By contrast, if an event occurred in which there were 75 fatalities all in one place at one time, it would be national news. Furthermore, that news would remain in the public consciousness over a long period of time. Airline crashes can serve as an example. The location Lockerbie remains an immediate association for airliner crash for millions of people even after three decades. The concentration of carnage gets and holds our attention. The public would never endure 75 people being killed in a plane crash daily, the airline industry would be in ruins, and enormous pressure would be brought to bear to make air travel safer.

The work of the national commission detailed some of the major disasters in which sleepiness played an important role. These include the Exxon Valdez oil spill, the Space Shuttle Challenger launch, the Bhopal disaster, and the Three Mile Island nuclear power plant meltdown. The report also reviewed less sensational but very costly rail accidents, including the 1984 accident in Wiggins, CO, that left five dead and cost $3.8 million; the 1984 accident in Motley, MN, that left two dead and cost $1.3 million; the 1988 accident in Thompson, PA, that left four dead and cost $4.0 million; the 1989 accident in Corona, CA, that left four dead and cost $2.0 million; and the 1990 accident in Barstow, CA, that left three dead and cost $4.4 million, to mention a few.

Much credit goes to Dr. William C. Dement who tirelessly chaired the commission and his staff. Ultimately, the commission led to the creation of the "Sleep Institute" in the National Institute of Health's (NIH) National Heart, Lung, and Blood Institute (NHLBI).

Current Events and the Road Ahead

Drowsy driving continues notwithstanding efforts to raise public awareness. Nonetheless, progress has been made. The immediate past administrator of the National Highway Traffic Safety Administration (NHTSA), Mark Rosekind, helped raise awareness of fatigue's involvement in MVAs. Prior to that, Rosekind served on the National Transportation Safety Board (NTSB) between 2010 and 2014.

Twenty percent of all car crashes in the USA are thought by experts to result from drowsy driving. In the 2003 Staten Island Ferry crash that killed 11 and injured 71, the pilot lost consciousness after taking sedating medicines (tramadol and

Tylenol PM). Additionally, the relationship between driving, being sedentary, and obesity (especially for men) has now been connected to risk for undiagnosed sleep apnea. The commuter train crash in September 2017 and two other crashes within as many years all involve engineers with sleep apnea. A battle between regulatory authorities and labor will undoubtedly ensue. This political sticky wicket is a classic hot potato.

Engineering will ultimately circumvent the fatigue-related transportation accident problems. Expect to see such in the next decade or two. Rapidly advancing artificial intelligence and robotics will pilot vehicles for us. Self-driving cars are already being tested on the public streets. The technology currently available in production model cars can detect lane deviation and brake automatically for crash avoidance. These applications represent overture steps toward driverless vehicles. However, even when the technology becomes fully capable, societal adjustments must precede its adoption. Automated interstate highway trucking represents a very doable early application, but social, labor-relation, political, and liability issues need frank and honest discussion. Driverless conveyances of every sort will quickly follow once societal and economic issues reach resolution.

References

1. American Heritage Dictionary of the English Language, 5th ed. American Heritage Dictionary Editor. Boston: Houghton Mifflin; 2016.
2. Collins English Dictionary, 12th Edition. Collins Dictionary Authors. United Kingdom: Collins; 2014.
3. Leger D. The cost of sleep-related accidents: a report for the National Commission on Sleep Disorders Research. Sleep. 1994;17(1):84–93.

Chapter 2
Fatigue: Definitions and Classifications

Mary Rose

The evaluation and classification of fatigue in the workplace is a complicated and onerous task for a multitude of reasons. Fatigue is not only a common and significant complaint in many medical conditions but a significant burden in the occupational field. One major concern for defining and classifying work-related *fatigue* is that it is often used interchangeably with *sleepiness*. One challenge to defining fatigue is determining the weight to ascribe to subjective versus objective ways in which fatigue is manifested. The subspecialty area of sleep medicine, *occupational sleep medicine*, has developed in recent years in order to focus on these issues and to gain better awareness of the markers for fatigue and possible counter-fatigue measures that may be implemented to improve vigilance.

The purpose of this chapter is to describe definitions and classifications of fatigue in the workplace. This task requires us to look at the data on those factors which appear to be cited as influential in both subjective experiences of fatigue and objective data on those factors contributing to performance deficit and accidents. The cause of fatigue-related accidents is often referred to as lapses in vigilance or judgment (further defined in terms of the severity of, or time lapse of, inattentiveness [1]). This concept demonstrates the somewhat nebulous features of defining fatigue in the workplace, such that the origin and nature of such a lapse could be extremely broad and multifaceted. However, as will be discussed, they appear to originate primarily from sleep disturbance.

For the purposes of this chapter, the industries which are considered include primarily health care and transportation (trucking, aviation, nautical). Though the nature of the tasks being performed in each of these differs, each has been identified as major industries in which fatigue has serious consequences on the public safety.

Most workplace-related fatigue research has grown from the emerging field of occupational sleep medicine, which has only recently come into conception.

M. Rose, PsyD
Physical Medicine & Rehabilitation, Baylor College of Medicine, Dept of Neuropsychology,
TIRR Memorial Rehabilitation Network, Houston, TX, USA

© Springer Science+Business Media, LLC, part of Springer Nature 2018
A. Sharafkhaneh, M. Hirshkowitz (eds.), *Fatigue Management*,
https://doi.org/10.1007/978-1-4939-8607-1_2

Largely, lapses of attention are typically not attributed to mental or physical fatigue but rather to primary misalignment of sleep timing or to inadequate sleep prior to the fatigue-related incident. Belenky and Akerstedt define occupational sleep medicine as being concerned with "performance, productivity, safety, health and well being in the workplace or operational environment as effected by sleep restriction, circadian rhythm phase, and work load" [2]. It is herein that the emphasis on sleep is abundantly clear, with only *workload* mediating the total sum of the factors driving how work-related fatigue is defined. Despite the many types of physiological fatigue evaluated and treated in general medicine (muscular, mental, and psychomotor), these are rarely cited as the cause of major disasters in the workplace, and when they are, it is usually mental workload (not physical workload) in combination with total sleep time and/or circadian misalignment that is the cause of fatigue.

Despite this, incorporation of non-sleep-related fatigue into the definitions of worker fatigue would likely be beneficial in devising a more comprehensive model of these concepts as it does appear that individual characteristics and possibly issues such as novelty of task may also play a role in mediating fatigue. A likely reason why physical fatigue is very rarely a source of accidents is likely because, as an industrialized society, we have few jobs that rely upon human physical strength. The need for human mental focus and fine motor skills, however, has yet to be replaced by artificial means and remains an area of importance to understanding fatigue prognosticators. The ways in which this focus is affected by sleep disruption have been evaluated in several industries, such as aviation, trucking, and health care, and will be further discussed in other chapters of this book.

Belenky and Akerstedt have been two of the most influential researchers in clarifying fatigue in the workplace as a sleep- and workload-related concept. Fatigue has been defined subjectively by self-report but objectively as degraded performance [2, 3]. This is a crucial component to defining fatigue as it reinforces that the consequences of deficits caused by sleep loss, or misalignment of sleep, may not be *subjectively* identified by the fatigued worker. Most studies identify fatigue as a multifaceted combination of time awake and time of day (circadian rhythm). Workload variables (task complexity, task intensity, and time on the task) [2] lend further definition to how fatigue is identified in specific areas of transportation, health care, and hazardous materials management.

Several corresponding industries have launched extensive inquiry into identifying sources of fatigue and their mediators. The National Transportation Safety Board (NTSB) is responsible to highway, rail, aviation, marine, pipeline, as well as hazardous materials transportation [4]. The ways in which fatigue is defined by NTSB are possibly most evident in the structure of their recommendations for scheduling policies and practices which involve the hours of work focused on total hours of work, opportunity of uninterrupted sleep, and shift schedules. Guidelines and strategies also address evaluation and treatment of sleep apnea [4] further emphasizing the defining character of fatigue as a sleep-related problem.

Currently, there is no consistent strategy for classification of types of work-related fatigue into larger definitive concepts that would enable us to strategize causes and possible intervention strategies for management. Occupational sleep medicine incorporates definitions of both mental and physical weariness (a more classic definition of fatigue in medical populations) with sleepiness, the latter of which is concretely defined as the urge for or tendency toward sleep [5]. Overwhelmingly, nearly all studies of fatigue-related accidents, particularly those which are fatality based and/or economically catastrophic, involve sleep-related lapses in judgment.

The management of work-related accidents and injuries consequent to fatigue remains a serious and daunting task. One of the greatest challenges is differentiation between sleep- and fatigue-related issues, differentially defined above, which hinder productivity and decrease safety in the workplace. The National Transportation Industry has focused heavily on shift work, total sleep time, and untreated disorders such as sleep apnea [4], suggesting that sleep loss and inappropriate sleep timing are in fact at the heart of defining fatigue in the workplace.

The objective of classifying fatigue appears to center around four major goals: reduction of accidents, reduction of costs, improvement of overall quality of life/ health, and increased productivity in the workplace [6]. Determining an algorithm that may help to identify not only the level of fatigue but the severity of the consequences of such lapses even when mild is also under investigation [7] and is an area discussed in other chapters of this book.

Dawson et al. note that attempts have been made to better quantify fatigue in the workplace in order to develop a model for better identification and management via a biomathematical model of fatigue (BMMF). Their hope in design of this is as a model to facilitate the prediction of fatigue with a pattern of work and to compare it with varying shift patterns. The goal of this model would be to identify likelihood of fatigue with different patterns of work and facilitate strategies to manage risk due to fatigue [8].

Several models currently exist that attempt to predict risk. All of these appear to weigh total sleep time and circadian rhythm almost exclusively, again suggesting an actual sleep vs. fatigue definition of causes for worker lapses in judgment. Akerstedt's three-process model encapsulates the focus much of this work has taken, using a circadian and a homeostatic algorithm to predict alertness [9].

Several psychosocial factors have consistently been examined as playing a role in resistance to sleep loss/fatigue and are discussed in detail throughout this chapter. However, in general, age, sex, health issues, task novelty, and circadian alignment all appear to be influential in determining the course of fatigue.

Very few models of worker fatigue incorporate the influence that psychosocial factors play in the sleep-wake schedules of workers. Those who do night-shift work are known to maintain shorter total sleep times compared with their day-shift counterparts. Factors which contribute to decision-making for these schedules may influence fatigability and/or sleep drive differentially. It is likely that these models do not make use of these individual variations because the overriding identified variable of sleep loss has been consistently identified as a persistent aggravator of error in the trucking [7], aviation [10], nautical transportation, and health-care industries [11]. It has also been implicated in several notorious power plant industry disasters including the Three Mile Island, Bhopal, and Exxon Valdez [12]. Shift work and/or time of day were also concluded to negatively impact the disaster in Chernobyl, though the degree to which this was a causative factor was not certain to the NTSB [12].

The type of performance decrements and severity of decrements experienced by a worker may be understood in terms of the level of sleep loss they experience. If one breaks down categories of fatigue into levels of sleepiness, the type and severity of decrements are more easily described. Even mild sleep loss (7 h in bed per night for 7 days) results in decrements in performance and appears to be dose dependent to the severity of the sleep restriction [13]. It is notable that by this definition of mild sleep deprivation, then it is likely that many night workers could be classified as sleep deprived. In one of the largest studies of work schedules on total sleep duration and motor vehicle accidents in nurses, night-shift workers were found to sleep an average duration of only 6.5 h [14].

Executive functioning may be more sensitive to sleep loss, though the data on this is mixed and may suggest that specific components of executive functioning are more vulnerable to sleep loss [15]. Individual differences in executive functioning may also be protective against performance decrements under conditions of sleep loss [16]. Tasks in which executive functioning is essential may break down more rapidly under conditions of sleep loss or sleep misalignment. Thus, it may be that specific categories or levels of fatigue pose either differing levels of threat to performance decrements and accidents or that there is a critical point at which fatigue presents a tipping point for performance of some tasks to break down.

Akerstedt et al. found that in a sample of workers in Stockholm, fatigue was predicted by a combination of disturbed sleep, heavy work immersion, high work demands, social support, being female, being older, and being in a supervisory role [17]. Interestingly, total work hours and shift work were not significant predictors until they controlled for high work demands, which revealed total work hours as a significant variable. Their finding on age contradicted their 2002 findings that age *below* 49 years predicted fatigue. This finding was supported in the 2004 study that indicated that being female and having more work or hectic work (high work demands) were associated with fatigue. It is intriguing, however, that age was indicated as having a contradictory effect on fatigue vs. sleepiness in this study, with older age (which is well established) being associated with sleep disturbance.

In the future occupational medicine may focus on strategies to defining fatigue with regard to how individual variables such as age, sex, and individual factors such as general vigilance level, as well as novelty of tasks, may impact identified performance decrements. Fatigue in the workplace remains an area of investigation on the basic level of defining what constitutes fatigue. These inquiries almost always focus on more sleep-related aspects of consciousness. One of the greatest challenges to making changes in the workplace is not only education but training both workers and those who set policy to be aware of healthy and optimal conditions for sleep.

References

1. Miller JC. CRISP report: fatigue effects and countermeasures in 24/7 security operations. Alexandria, VA: ASIS International; 2010. Ref Type: Report.
2. Belenky G, Akerstedt T. Occupational sleep medicine. In: Kryger M, Roth T, Dement WC, editors. Principles and practice of sleep medicine. 5th ed. St Louis: Elsevier; 2012. p. 734–7.
3. Barker LM, Nussbaum MA. Fatigue, performance and the work environment: a survey of registered nurses. J Adv Nurs. 2011;67:1370–82.
4. Rosekind MR. Enhancing transportation safety: the importance of managing fatigue. Fatigue in transit operations. Transportation Research Board; Oct 12, 2011. Washington, DC: National Transportation Safety Board; 2011.
5. Dement WC, Carskadon MA. Current perspectives on daytime sleepiness: the issues. Sleep. 1982;5(Suppl 2):S56–66.
6. Rosekind MR, Gander PH, Gregory KB, et al. Managing fatigue in operational settings 2: an integrated approach. Hosp Top. 1997;75:31–5.
7. Moore-Ede M, Heitmann A, Guttkuhn R, Trutschel U, Aguirre A, Croke D. Circadian alertness simulator for fatigue risk assessment in transportation: application to reduce frequency and severity of truck accidents. Aviat Space Environ Med. 2004;75:A107–18.
8. Dawson D, Ian NY, Harma M, Akerstedt T, Belenky G. Modelling fatigue and the use of fatigue models in work settings. Accid Anal Prev. 2011;43:549–64.
9. Akerstedt T, Folkard S, Portin C. Predictions from the three-process model of alertness. Aviat Space Environ Med. 2004;75:A75–83.
10. Goode JH. Are pilots at risk of accidents due to fatigue? J Saf Res. 2003;34:309–13.
11. West CP, Tan AD, Habermann TM, Sloan JA, Shanafelt TD. Association of resident fatigue and distress with perceived medical errors. JAMA. 2009;302:1294–300.
12. Mitler MM, Carskadon MA, Czeisler CA, Dement WC, Dinges DF, Graeber RC. Catastrophes, sleep, and public policy: consensus report. Sleep. 1988;11:100–9.
13. Belenky G, Wesensten NJ, Thorne DR, et al. Patterns of performance degradation and restoration during sleep restriction and subsequent recovery: a sleep dose-response study. J Sleep Res. 2003;12:1–12.
14. Scott LD, Hwang WT, Rogers AE, Nysse T, Dean GE, Dinges DF. The relationship between nurse work schedules, sleep duration, and drowsy driving. Sleep. 2007;30:1801–7.
15. Tucker AM, Whitney P, Belenky G, Hinson JM, Van Dongen HP. Effects of sleep deprivation on dissociated components of executive functioning. Sleep. 2010;33:47–57.
16. Killgore WD, Grugle NL, Reichardt RM, Killgore DB, Balkin TJ. Executive functions and the ability to sustain vigilance during sleep loss. Aviat Space Environ Med. 2009;80:81–7.
17. Akerstedt T, Knutsson A, Westerholm P, Theorell T, Alfredsson L, Kecklund G. Mental fatigue, work and sleep. J Psychosom Res. 2004;57:427–33.

Chapter 3
Studies of Fatigue and Human Performance in the Laboratory

Michael H. Bonnet and Donna L. Arand

A Brief History

Systematic observations of fatigue and human performance date to the 1896 Patrick and Gilbert study [1] where three subjects were shown to have deficits in reaction time, memory, and voluntary motor ability during a period of 88–90 h of sleep deprivation. In the 1930s, Nathaniel Kleitman used a variety of performance measures including card dealing speed, multiplication speed, code transcription speed, and mirror drawing to show similar characteristic changes in performance and oral temperature across the 16-h period of wakefulness [2]. Kleitman also showed a strong correlation between simple reaction time and body temperature across the day and demonstrated that simple reaction time varied with body temperature when subjects either stood up or laid down for an hour [2]. Kleitman and Jackson later used a naval rotating duty schedule to observe changes in oral temperature and color naming across the entire 24 h with relative control for prior sleep to demonstrate both the 24-h circadian temperature rhythm and the strong inverse correlation of that rhythm with the time required to name a group of colors [2].

In the 1950s, extensive tests of performance during varying periods of sleep deprivation were performed at the Walter Reed Army Institute of Research. In a 1958 study [3], a strong relationship between oral temperature and fatigue ratings across 98 h of sleep deprivation was shown. The data demonstrated both changes related to circadian time and also a progressive increase in fatigue ratings and decreases in the oral temperature curve with each additional day of sleep loss. In addition, it was found that sleepy individuals started to have brief periods where

M. H. Bonnet, PhD (✉)
Wright State University Boonshoft School of Medicine, Kettering Sycamore Sleep Disorders Center, Miamisburg, OH, USA

D. L. Arand, PhD
Kettering Health Network, Dayton, OH, USA

© Springer Science+Business Media, LLC, part of Springer Nature 2018
A. Sharafkhaneh, M. Hirshkowitz (eds.), *Fatigue Management*,
https://doi.org/10.1007/978-1-4939-8607-1_3

they stopped responding completely [4]. These periods were found to be accompanied by a decline in EEG alpha amplitude and were called lapses.

As the measurement of sleep using EEG became more common, the relationship between sleep amounts, circadian time, and performance became more well defined. Yet, despite the development of objective measures of sleep; fatigue and sleepiness were still tracked by subjective measures such as the Stanford Sleepiness Scale. However, in 1977, an experiment that divided the 24-h day into 16 "90-min days" suggested that repeated polygraphic measurement of sleep onsets across the day could be an objective measure of fatigue [5]. The first formal use of the EEG to track sleepiness was a 1979 experiment that measured sleep latency during repeated brief nap attempts. The prominent circadian effects that were seen in sleep latencies during the baseline period were followed by rapid decreases in sleep latency during sleep deprivation and recovery to normal values following two nights of recovery sleep [6]. Other studies quickly validated the impact of sleep restriction, medication hangover, and circadian time on periodically measured sleep latency. It was found that latency to sleep after awakenings during nighttime sleep could also track sleepiness and medication effects during the sleep period [7]. These and many other observations led to rapid adaptation of the multiple sleep latency test (MSLT) as an objective measure of sleepiness. The MSLT has become the gold standard to measure sleepiness both in research and as a clinical test.

Since EEG and sleep latency testing is rather cumbersome and performance measures are sensitive to the circadian rhythm and sleep loss, it seems reasonable that psychomotor performance itself should provide a simple means to monitor fatigue. Unfortunately, there are large individual differences in psychomotor performance secondary to intelligence, age, disease, and training that have precluded the use of these tests as direct measures of sleepiness. However, one test, the OSLER, was developed in 1997 [8] to avoid some of these problems by using failure of response rather than level of performance to define sleepiness. Although this measure avoided problems associated with test performance and EEG monitoring, it allowed the possibility that patients could manipulate their "sleepiness" simply by deciding not to respond and, therefore, has not been widely used.

Current Conceptualization

Research in the area of fatigue and performance, like many areas, is a continuing replication of basic information imbued with new methodology and more sophisticated measures. It is now known that the basic controllers of sleepiness and performance include prior sleep amount and distribution, length of time awake, and the circadian time. Experiments usually try to control prior sleep by requiring "normal" nights of sleep before initiation of a sleep loss episode. Data from multiple regression analyses of behavioral and EEG data during sleep loss [9, 10] suggest that time awake accounts for 25–30% of the variance in alertness in 64 h of sleep loss, while circadian time accounts for about 6% of the variance. Figure 3.1 displays the effects

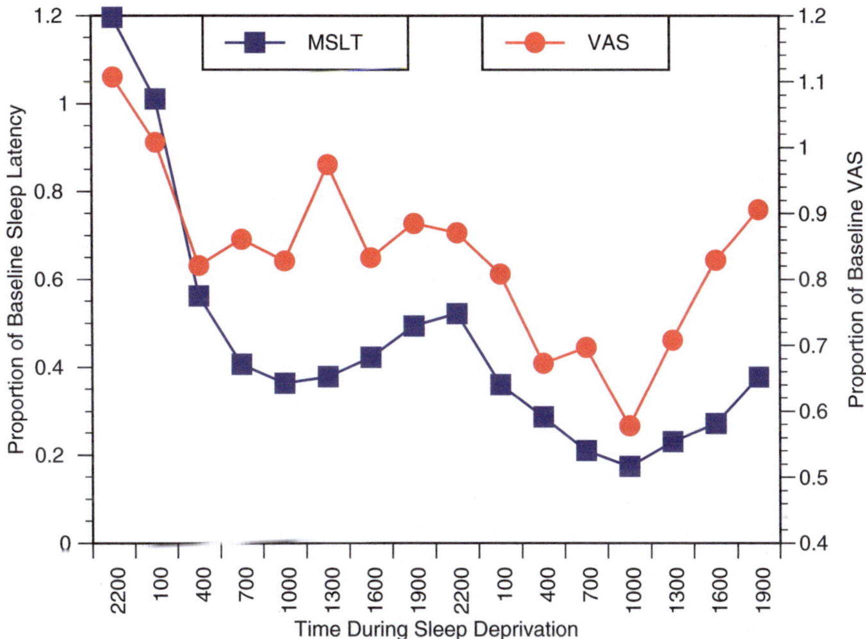

Fig. 3.1 MSLT and Visual Activation Scale across 64 h of total sleep deprivation. Data are observed value divided by baseline value. Data from Bonnet et al., 1995 [46]

of time awake and the circadian rhythm on objective alertness as measured by the MSLT and a Visual Activation Scale (VAS) measure of alertness/fatigue (very alert to very sleepy on a Likert scale) over 64 h of sleep loss. The data from both tests were controlled by dividing each observation by the respective prestudy baseline observation value. It can be seen from the figure that there is a clear circadian effect in each measure over each of the two nights and days of the study. The overlay of sleep deprivation can be seen in the comparison of the second night and day to the first night and day.

The performance and sleepiness effects associated with the circadian rhythm and sleep deprivation appear to be independent, and experimental techniques have been developed to evaluate the contributions of each. In one technique called a constant routine, subjects remain in bed for an extended period of time without time or social cues and are fed small amounts on an hourly basis to limit external influences on alertness and performance. In another technique called forced desynchrony, subjects are isolated in an environment with no time cues and placed on a 28-h day so that sleep and wake episodes occur at many different times in relation to the underlying circadian curve that is usually tracked by measurement of body temperature. In the constant routine technique, performance on a calculations task and alertness measured with a VAS scale were both found to decrease with rectal temperature across the night with a lag of about 4 h (i.e., body temperature minimum around 4 am with alertness and performance minimum around 8 am) and increase with body temperature across the day [11]. During forced desynchrony, the minimum in alertness occurred at the minimum of the rectal temperature rhythm, and the minimum of calculations performance occurred just past the minimum of body temperature as rectal temperature was starting to increase [11]. In general, alertness and performance were still maximal when prior wakefulness was short and body temperature was high and worst when prior wakefulness was longest and body temperature was low. A study that specifically examined cognitive task complexity in a constant routine design showed that tasks and levels of complexity within tasks had similar circadian curves for performance with matching trough placement [12].

Models have been constructed to predict sleep or performance based upon length of time awake, circadian time, and residual sleepiness at awakening (sleep inertia). A major goal of such modeling is to be able to predict fatigue and performance based upon various work schedules and timing factors. While a review of these models is beyond the scope of this chapter, good reviews are available [13]. One model published in free access [14] shows the use of circadian time, accumulating wake time (homeostatic sleep response) and grogginess at awakening (sleep inertia) to predict adaptation to shifts in sleep time. An example shows the impact of a 12-h shift (flight from New York to Hong Kong) on performance on a serial addition task with adaptation over 15 days. It also shows the impact of bright light intervention to improve adjustment in addition task performance that results in a more rapid return to baseline alertness.

However, such models have lacked some predictive accuracy because they have not incorporated information about individual differences or sources of arousal. Recent research has focused specifically on individual differences by looking at genetic relationships to sensitivity to sleep deprivation [15]. It has been reported that individuals with a PER3$^{5/5}$ genotype had greater nocturnal decrements on a number of performance tasks, particularly on tasks involving executive function [15].

Other studies have begun to explore the relationship between the arousal system and performance overall and in relation to sleep deprivation. For example, it has been known for many years that there is a high correlation between heart rate, used here to infer level of arousal, and sleep latency. This relationship predicts that young adults with higher heart rate should take longer to fall asleep in an MSLT than young adults with lower heart rates even with normal preceding sleep amounts, and this was found when young adults were selected to have either long or short MSLT latencies [16]. Current work has extended this arousal hypothesis by showing a strong correlation ($r = 0.67$) between heart rate variability and lapses in a simple reaction time task during 40 h of total sleep loss [17]. This was similar to the correlation of $r = 0.59$ between a VAS scale and lapses in the same study. The correlation of core body temperature with lapses ($r = 0.30$) was somewhat lower.

The use of total sleep deprivation to operationally produce graded levels of fatigue has produced a large literature describing sensitive measures and ameliorating factors. These will be described in the following sections.

Types of Performance Measures Most Sensitive to Fatigue

There are specific types of test that are impacted more significantly by sleepiness, and there are also test attributes such as length of testing that influence the sensitivity of each broad test type. The grouping by test type that follows was suggested by Lim and Dinges [18] in their meta-analysis of 65 studies that provided sufficient data to calculate effect size (a large effect size (ES) is a value of 0.8, a medium ES is 0.5, and a small ES is 0.2) from periods of sleep deprivation ranging from 24 to 48 h. The attributes that follow were initially suggested by Johnson in his review [19].

Test Types

Vigilance: Vigilance tests, which primarily involve monitoring the environment with occasional signal responses, are commonly used in studies. Either lapses or reaction time is measured. Lim and Dinges [18] calculated effect sizes for lapses and reaction times to be 0.76 and 0.73, respectively, from their pooled data. These effect sizes are somewhat smaller than those reported by Philibert in an earlier meta-analysis [20], probably because Philibert grouped studies into those ranging from 30 to 54 h of sleep loss with an effect size of 1.14 and those studies ranging from 24 to 30 h with an effect size of 0.55 (more studies fall into the shorter sleep deprivation length category).

Choice response: These tasks also involve monitoring but require monitoring multiple inputs and choosing a specific response (such as one light or letter in a 2×2 grid). Tests are often identified as choice reaction time, and a somewhat lower ES of 0.48 was reported for accuracy of responses during sleep loss [18].

Working memory: These tasks require a subject to maintain a set of items actively in memory for a brief time to make a decision and response. For example, on the N-back test, the subject must remember the position of a stimulus on the screen after one or more additional stimuli have been presented in different positions. The meta-analysis reported an ES of 0.56 for accuracy or response on these tests during sleep loss.

Short-term memory: Short-term memory tests typically involve presentation of a list of items that the subject writes down as presented, to provide evidence that the item has been understood, and then recalls after presentation of the last item. Impaired immediate recall for elements placed in short-term memory is a classic finding from early sleep deprivation studies. However, the Lim and Dinges analysis indicated an effect size of only 0.38 for short-term memory recall [18].

Processing speed: Processing speed measures the ability to repetitively perform simple cognitive tasks like serial addition or symbol translation on tasks like the Digit Symbol Substitution Test. The overall effect size for reaction time (i.e., number of items per period of time) for this type of task was also found to be moderate at 0.30.

Reasoning: Reasoning tasks like grammatical reasoning require the subject to judge the truth of logical statements and respond. In the meta-analysis from Lim and Dinges [18], overall reasoning accuracy was not statistically decreased during sleep loss (ES = 0.12).

Executive function: Prefrontal areas of the brain that are involved in novelty, divergent thinking, and temporal memory (planning, organization, and prioritization) are also impacted by sleep loss. Several studies have shown decrements in tasks involving these functions. Examples include decreased ability to make emotional judgments and a shift toward accepting short-term rewards (gambling tasks) even when long-term consequences were more adverse [21, 22] during sleep loss. These shifts toward risky decision making have been shown to be independent of reaction time measures [23]. However, another study that sought to break down executive function into component activities that could be evaluated separately suggested that non-executive components of cognition such as short-term memory were degraded during a sleep deprivation experiment, while "executive" functions like working memory scanning efficiency, resistance to proactive interference, or verbal fluency were not impacted [24]. This implies that changes in short-term memory or other more simple cognitive abilities might account for many executive function decrements.

Attributes that Modify Test Performance

Length of test: Individuals undergoing sleep loss can rally briefly to perform at baseline performance levels, but their ability to maintain that baseline level decreases as the length of the task increases. For example, subjects attempted significantly fewer addition problems compared with baseline after 10 min of testing following one night of sleep loss but reached the same criterion after 6 min of testing following the second night of sleep loss. It took 50 min of testing to show a significant decrease in percentage of correct problems after one night of sleep loss but only 10 min of testing to reach that criterion after the second night [25]. The implication is that longer performance tests are more likely to show decrements and that it is more difficult to show reliable differences during short-term sleep loss from tests <10 min in duration.

Knowledge of results: Immediate feedback of performance accuracy has been shown to improve performance during sleep deprivation [26, 27]. Simply not giving results to subjects with normal sleep doubled their number of very long responses (lapses) on a serial reaction time test [26]. One night of total sleep loss increased the number of lapses by 9.3 times the baseline level, but provision of immediate knowledge of results decreased the lapses to 2.3 times the baseline level. The 2.3 times baseline level was approximately the lapses seen after normal sleep when knowledge of results was not given [26].

Test pacing: Self-paced tasks are usually more resistant to sleep deprivation than tasks that are timed or in which items are presented externally. In a self-paced task, the participant can concentrate long enough to complete items correctly without penalty for lapses in attention that occur between items. When tasks are externally paced, errors occur if items are presented during lapses.

Proficiency level: Sleep loss probably affects new skills more than mastered skills. For example, a study of the effects of sleep loss on doctors in training showed significant performance loss in PGY 1 (first year) surgical residents but not in PGY 2–5 surgical residents [28].

Difficulty or complexity: Early research suggested that performance was worse on complex tasks during sleep loss. However, more recent studies suggest interactive effects. Ryman et al. [29] hypothesized that passively worded items on a logical reasoning task would be more difficult since reaction times to such items were longer before sleep deprivation. However, it was shown that subjects performed at baseline levels on passively constructed items while showing significant performance decline on the active constructions during sleep deprivation. Therefore, it was suggested that the passive items actually increased arousal level and that this was beneficial during sleep loss but not before sleep loss. Similarly, results showing better performance on a more complex cognitive task compared with a simpler version were attributed to increased frontal brain activation in the more complex task [30]. Another study which found larger decrements on vigilance tasks than complex tasks suggested that inherent interest helped to maintain performance on more complex tasks [31]. However, results differ if task difficulty is adjusted by increasing the speed at which work must be performed. When 1.25 s were allowed to complete mental arithmetic problems, a significant performance decline was found after two nights of sleep loss, but when the rate of presentation slowed to 2 s, a significant decline in performance decline was not found after sleep loss [32]. Similarly, in short-term memory tests, significant deficits may not be found after sleep loss when the memory load is low but may appear at higher memory loads [33]. The data imply that task variations that add an element of challenge may be more well preserved than those that just require increased production or effort.

Ameliorating Variables

As suggested above, environmental surroundings and emotional state can play a significant role in modifying fatigue. Such influences, which include activity, bright light, posture, naps, drugs, and motivation, are beginning to receive increased attention.

Activity: In one study [34], a 5-min walk immediately preceding MSLT evaluations increased MSLT values by about 6 min (on a maximum 20-min test). The arousal associated with the walk completely masked the impact of a 50% reduction of nocturnal sleep (about a 2-min impact on MSLT). Similarly, momentary arousal, such as indicating that 5 min remained on a task, was sufficient to reverse 75% of the decrement accumulated over 30 min of testing [27]. Other studies have shown that a period of exercise immediately before performing tasks provided transient reversal of some psychomotor and subjective [35] decrements secondary to sleep loss. However, more ambitious studies comparing high activity and low activity continuing over 40–64 h periods of sleep deprivation have shown no beneficial effects of exercise on overall performance [36] and no differential effects of the exercise on recovery sleep following sleep loss in humans [36]. These different results may arise because arousing stimuli act for a discrete period of time that may be <30 min [34] and the effect decreases with increased sleep loss. There may also be a trade-off between production of arousal and production of physical fatigue.

Bright light: Studies have shown improved night shift performance and objective alertness under bright light conditions [37, 38]. Bright light has also improved alertness and reaction time performance following two nights of 5-h sleep restriction [39]. However, bright light can also shift circadian rhythms. Therefore, it is not always clear whether bright light acts as a source of stimulation during sleep loss to help to maintain alertness or if the reported effects are based upon the shifting of underlying circadian rhythms.

Posture: One study has shown a significant 6.6-min increase in sleep latency when subjects were asked to fall asleep in the sitting position (60° angle) as opposed to lying down [40]. Such differences in alertness could be accounted for by increasing sympathetic nervous system activity, which occurs with these changes in posture [41]. Greater differences are associated with standing as compared with sitting [42].

Naps: Since performance decrements and sleepiness accumulate with increasing wakefulness, one would expect reversal of accumulating losses with periods of interjected sleep. Naps have been studied both in conjunction with sleep loss and also before sleep loss as a means of minimizing subsequent deficits. The interaction of naps, cognition, and performance have been reviewed in a recent paper [43]. Nap effects can be understood at the simplest level by viewing them as part of a split sleep schedule (i.e., partial sleep period at night and another partial sleep period or nap during the day). A number of laboratory studies have examined many possible parameters. A study by Nicholson et al. [44] and more recent studies that controlled for circadian time, prior wakefulness, and sleep inertia effects showed no significant performance differences on tasks such as reaction time, arithmetic tasks, or the DSST, when comparing split sleep schedules to normal nights [45, 44].

Of course, naps are often used as a supplemental sleep period. In this sense, a nap can be additional sleep prior to a period of sleep loss (often called a prophylactic nap) or can be used during sleep loss for partial benefit. Prophylactic naps have been shown to mediate the effects of total sleep deprivation periods that follow. The benefits seem to be directly related to the amount of additional sleep that is obtained even if the additional sleep is aided by sleeping medication [46]. These benefits to later performance and alertness were similar to that of caffeine given during sleep loss and additive with the beneficial effects of caffeine on psychomotor performance (see Drugs below).

Many studies have also looked at the potential beneficial effects of naps on alertness and performance when allowed during a period of sleep deprivation. The results of these studies are more complex because the impact of these naps is dependent upon circadian time, length of prior waking, length of nap, and how long after the nap that performance is measured. A major issue with using naps during periods of sleep loss is that naps longer than 30 min frequently result in subjects entering slow wave sleep. Awakenings from slow wave sleep are associated with sleep inertia, which can produce alertness and performance levels lower than those that would have occurred without the nap. Current laboratory studies suggest that naps as short as 10 min were more effective than longer naps because sleep inertia was avoided, and alertness and performance on reaction time and symbol substitution was improved [47]. However, naps are not recommended as the length of time awake increases or at the bottom of the circadian cycle [43].

Drugs: Many drugs have been studied in conjunction with sleep loss, but most studies have examined stimulants such as amphetamine, caffeine, methylphenidate, pemoline, and modafinil. A review of stimulant medications used in conjunction with sleep loss by the American Academy of Sleep Medicine was published in 2005 [48], and medication effects are reviewed in greater detail in a separate chapter in this text.

Very briefly, studies have shown that caffeine (doses of 200–600 mg), modafinil (doses of 100–400 mg), and amphetamine (doses of 5–20 mg) improved alertness as measured by the MSLT and performance for varying periods of time depending on dosage, half-life, and hours of total sleep deprivation. In a study of caffeine 600 mg and three doses of modafinil given during the first night of total sleep deprivation, both caffeine and modafinil (200 and 400 mg) were successful in maintaining response speed consistently above placebo levels for 12 h [49]. When caffeine 600 mg, modafinil 400 mg, or dextroamphetamine 20 mg were administered just prior to the second night of total sleep deprivation [50], caffeine and dextroamphetamine significantly improved response speed compared with placebo from midnight through 4:00 am while modafinil improved response speed through 10:00 am. Side effects were fewest after modafinil administration.

The effects of stimulant medication are decreased with increased sleep deprivation, but stimulant benefits can be improved when used in conjunction with naps or other types of arousal. The beneficial effect of caffeine 300 mg during sleep loss was approximately equivalent to a 3–4 h nap taken before the sleep loss period [51, 46]. Therefore, the combination of a 4-h prophylactic nap followed by 200 mg of caffeine at 01:30 and 07:30 resulted in significantly improved performance for 24 h (remaining at baseline levels) compared with the nap alone [52]. The combination of naps and caffeine appeared additive [52] and superior to 4 h of nocturnal naps [53]. The combination of 200 mg of caffeine at 22:00 and 02:00 and exposure to 2500-lux bright light had no impact above the effect of caffeine alone on a maintenance of wakefulness test but did provide significant benefit above caffeine alone on a vigilance task at three time points [54].

Studies have found that alcohol produced consistent decreases in alertness on the MSLT and performance measured by driving simulation [55]. Alcohol also interacted with sleep reduction so that the greatest sleepiness and all simulated driving "crashes" occurred in the condition that combined reduced sleep with alcohol. These results suggest that sleep loss and alcohol produce deficits of a similar magnitude and additive impacts on alertness.

One difficulty in assessing the degree of performance effects associated with sleepiness is the lack of a clear standard of pathology for most measures. However, well-known and accepted specific rules for blood alcohol content with respect to driving have led to the use of impairment associated with blood alcohol level as a standard reference for sleep loss effects and by inference fatigue. Three studies directly compared alcohol use with sleep deprivation and found similar results on different tasks. In one study [56], response speed was reduced by about half a second by 03:45 am (i.e., sleep loss) and to a similar extent by a blood alcohol content (BAC) of 0.1%. In another study [57], hand-eye coordination (in a visual tracking task) declined in a linear fashion during sleep loss and similarly with increasing BAC such that performance was equivalent at 03:00 to a blood alcohol level of 0.05% and equivalent at 08:00 (i.e., a full night of sleep loss) to a blood alcohol level of 0.1%. In a third study [58], subjects averaged one off-road (i.e. vehicle driving off of the road) incident every 5 min in a driving simulator after one night of sleep deprivation (at 7:30 am). Similar performance occurred with a BAC of 0.08%. These studies suggest that changes in response speed, visual tracking, and driving commonly found during the first night of total sleep deprivation are equivalent to changes associated with legal intoxication. The availability of such a metric shows that performance changes associated with fatigue produced by small amounts of sleep loss can be associated with significant consequences. These data serve as a justification for drowsy driving laws such as Maggie's law passed in New Jersey in 2003 that classified driving without having slept for more than 24 h as reckless driving.

Motivation: Motivation has been most frequently measured by the provision of cash incentives or by providing knowledge of results. In one study, monetary rewards for "hits" on a vigilance task and "fines" for false alarms [59] resulted in performance remaining at baseline levels for the first 36 h of sleep loss in a high-incentive group. Performance began to decline during the following 24 h but remained significantly better than in the "no incentive" group. However, the incentive was ineffective in maintaining performance at a higher level during the third day of sleep loss in comparison with the "no incentive" group. In another study, publication of daily test results was sufficient to remove the effects of one night of sleep loss [26]. In another variation, simply the knowledge that a prolonged episode of sleep deprivation was going to end in a few hours was sufficient incentive for performance to improve by 30% in a group of soldiers [60].

Partial Sleep Deprivation

Many of the early studies of the relationship between sleep amounts and performance were based on varying amounts of total sleep deprivation. However, the most common form of sleep loss is chronic partial sleep loss. A few large in laboratory studies have compared schedules of chronic partial sleep loss for up to 14 days. In these studies, participants were randomized to a sleep schedule allowing 3, 5, 7, or

9 h in bed each night [61] or 4, 6, or 8 h in bed each night [62], and performance was measured repeatedly across the day for several days. Results in these large studies were consistent. When subjects were allowed 8–9 h in bed, performance remained stable across the experimental periods. However, when sleep was chronically reduced, performance on psychomotor tasks such as reaction time (PVT) or memory (Digit Symbol Substitution) decreased as a function of amount of sleep allowed and number of nights of sleep restriction. Effects were large enough, for example, that performance, measured by lapses on the reaction time task, was as poor after 12–13 nights with 4 h allowed for sleep as it was after 66–84 h of total sleep deprivation [63].

Investigators have also examined the relationship between performance and objective and subjective sleepiness as a function of several schedules of partial sleep deprivation. One study analyze the relationship between MSLT data that had been recorded at baseline and over seven nights with time in bed reduced to 5 h per night [5] in relationship to lapses in a 10-min simple reaction time task (PVT) collected in a separate study [62] also at baseline and during seven nights with time in bed reduced to about 5 h per night. It was found that deficits in objective alertness and reaction time continued to accumulate consistently throughout the entire seven nights of sleep restriction without clear evidence for habituation or asymptote in effects. Also, there was a very high inverse correlation between the number of lapses on the performance task and sleepiness as measured with the MSLT ($r = -0.95$; $p < 0.0001$) [62].

In a more extensive study, Van Dongen et al. [63] examined changes in performance and subjective sleepiness during partial sleep deprivation with allowed sleep times of 4, 6, or 8 h per night in the laboratory over a 14-day period. Analogous data from simple reaction time lapses and the Stanford Sleepiness Scale are replotted in Fig. 3.2. The lapse data from an earlier partial sleep deprivation study [62] were replicated for nightly time in bed amounts of 4 and 6 h. It can be seen that performance continued to deteriorate in an approximate linear manner over the entire 14-day period. It is notable, however, that subjective ratings of sleepiness seemed to habituate and perhaps actually decrease after 5–7 nights despite increasing deficits in performance. The authors compared the results with changes in the same variables during studies of acute sleep deprivation. The increase in lapses after 14 days with 4 h in bed was similar to the increase in lapses seen after three nights and days of total sleep deprivation, while the increase in subjective sleepiness after 14 days with 4 h in bed was similar to the increase in subjective sleepiness seen after a single night of total sleep deprivation. These data suggest that chronic partial sleep deprivation is similar to total sleep deprivation for objectively measured sleepiness and performance lapses in that deficits accumulate in a relatively linear manner that is reduced in a dose-dependent manner by partial sleep on each night. However, the apparent habituation of subjective impression of sleepiness during chronic partial sleep deprivation appears to contrast with increasing subjective sleepiness during total sleep deprivation as seen in Fig. 3.1. This finding is relevant because it implies that individuals who become chronically partially sleep deprived may become unaware of their level of performance decrement and potential to fall asleep in a

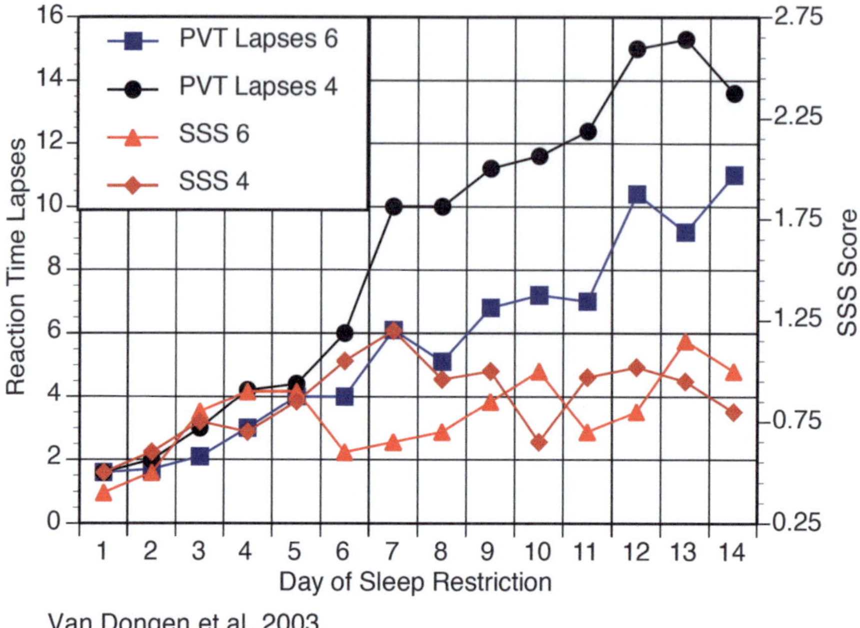

Fig. 3.2 Reaction time lapses and Stanford Sleepiness Scale scores across 14 nights with time in bed limited to either 4 or 6 h per night. Data are replotted from Van Dongen et al., 2003 [63]

catastrophic fashion. On a more theoretical level, this finding indicates that subjective and objective measurement of sleepiness can diverge.

When the Laws of Sleep and Alertness Break Down

The reported relationships between amount of prior sleep, hours of wakefulness, and circadian time have been generally robust. However, these relationships break down in several cases. As discussed in chapters that follow, patients with sleep disorders such as narcolepsy and sleep apnea may have significant sleepiness regardless of the length of their preceding sleep. The implication is that all sleep and perhaps all sleep systems are not the same. Patients with severe sleep apnea have a highly fragmented sleep pattern with periodic sleep disturbance associated with resumption of respiration. A number of studies have modeled similar patterns of disturbed sleep in laboratory studies with normal volunteers. These studies have indicated that periodic disturbance of sleep that occurs as frequently as once every 10 min or more often across the night without reduction in total sleep time will degrade the sleep process enough that, as in partial sleep deprivation, performance loss and increasing sleepiness will begin to accumulate [64]. Decrements in performance and alertness that have been associated with significantly fragmented sleep are similar to those that accumulate during sleep deprivation and probably interact with sleep loss. These studies challenge the idea that recovery of alertness and performance during sleep is simply a time-linked process. They suggest that there may be other means to alter the restorative process during sleep and that these other controllers could also have a measurable impact upon waking alertness and performance.

Acknowledgments This work was supported by the Wright State University Boonshoft School of Medicine and the Sleep-Wake Disorders Research Institute.

References

1. Patrick GTW, Gilbert JA. On the effect of loss of sleep. Psychol Rev 1896;3:469–83.
2. Kleitman N. Sleep and wakefulness. 2nd ed. Chicago: University of Chicago Press; 1963.
3. Murray E, Williams H, Lubin A. Body temperature and psychological ratings during sleep deprivation. J Exp Psychol. 1958;56:271–3.
4. Williams HL, Lubin A, Goodnow JJ. Impaired performance with sleep loss. Psychol Monogr. 1959;73(14):1–26.
5. Carskadon MA, Dement WC. Sleepiness and sleep state on a 90-min schedule. Psychophysiology. 1977;14:127–33.
6. Carskadon MA, Dement WC. Effects of total sleep loss on sleep tendency. Percept Mot Skills. 1979;48(2):495–506.
7. Bonnet MH, Webb WB. The return to sleep. Biol Psychol. 1979;8(3):225–33.
8. Bennett LS, Stradling JR, Davies RJ. A behavioural test to assess daytime sleepiness in obstructive sleep apnoea. J Sleep Res. 1997;6(2):142–5.
9. Rosa RR, Bonnet MH. Predicting nighttime alertness following prophylactic naps. Sleep Res. 1991;20:417.
10. Mikulincer M, Babkoff H, Caspy T, Sing H. The effects of 72 hours of sleep loss on psychological variables. Br J Psychol. 1989;80(Pt 2):145–62.
11. Dijk DJ, Duffy JF, Czeisler CA. Circadian and sleep/wake dependent aspects of subjective alertness and cognitive performance. J Sleep Res. 1992;1(2):112–7.
12. van Eekelen A, Kerkhof G. No interference of task complexity with circadian rhythmicity in a constant routine protocol. Ergonomics. 2003;48:1578–93.
13. Australian Civil Aviation Authority. Biomathematical fatigue modelling in civil aviation fatigue risk management application guidance. ed 1.0; 2010.
14. Dean DI, Forger D, Klerman EB. Taking the lag out of jet lag through model-based schedule design. PLoS Comput Biol. 2009;5(6):e1000418. https://doi.org/10.1371/journal.pcbi.1000418.
15. Dijk DJ, Archer SN. PERIOD3, circadian phenotypes, and sleep homeostasis. Sleep Med Rev. 2010;14(3):151–60.
16. Bonnet MH, Arand DL. Performance and cardiovascular measures in normals with extreme MSLT and subjective sleepiness levels. Sleep. 2005;28:681–9.
17. Chua E, Tan W, Yeo S, et al. Heart rate variability can be used to estimate sleepiness-related decrements in psychomotor vigilance during total sleep deprivation. Sleep. 2012;35:325–34.
18. Lim J, Dinges D. A meta-analysis of the impact of short-term sleep deprivation on cognitive variables. Psychol Bull. 2010;136:375–89.

19. Johnson LC. Sleep deprivation and performance. In: Webb WB, editor. Biological rhythms, sleep, and performance. New York: Wiley; 1982. p. 111–42.
20. Philibert I. Sleep loss and performance in residents and nonphysicians: a meta-analytic examination. Sleep. 2005;28:1392–402.
21. McKenna BS, Dicjinson DL, Orff HJ, Drummond SP. The effects of one night of sleep deprivation on known-risk and ambiguous-risk decisions. J Sleep Res. 2007;16(3):245–52.
22. Venkatraman V, Chuah YM, Huettel SA, Chee MW. Sleep deprivation elevates expectation of gains and attenuates response to losses following risky decisions. Sleep. 2007;30(5):603–9.
23. Venkatraman V, Huettel S, Chuah L, Payne J, Chee M. Sleep deprivation biases the neural mechanisms underlying economic preferences. J Neurosci. 2011;31:3712–8.
24. Tucker AM, Whitney P, Belenky G, Hinson JM, Van Dongen HP. Effects of sleep deprivation on dissociated components of executive functioning. Sleep. 2010;33(1):47–57.
25. Donnell JM. Performance decrement as a function of total sleep loss and task duration. Percept Mot Skills. 1969;29(3):711–4.
26. Wilkinson RT. Interaction of lack of sleep with knowledge of results, repeated testing, and individual differences. J Exp Psychol. 1961;62:263–71.
27. Steyvers FJJM, Gaillard AWK. The effects of sleep deprivation and incentives on human performance. Psychol Res. 1993;55:64–70.
28. Sturm L, Dawson D, Vaughan R, et al. Effects of fatigue on surgeon performance and surgical outcomes: a systematic review. ANZ J Surg. 2011;81:502–9.
29. Ryman DH, Naitoh P, Englund CE. Decrements in logical reasoning performance under conditions of sleep loss and physical exercise: the factor of sentence complexity. Percept Mot Skills. 1985;61(3 Pt 2):1179–88.
30. Chee MW, Choo WC. Functional imaging of working memory after 24 hr of total sleep deprivation. J Neurosci. 2004;24(19):4560–7.
31. Pilcher J, Band D, Odle-Dusseau H, Muth E. Human performance under sustained operations and acute sleep deprivation conditions: toward a model of controlled attention. Aviat Space Environ Med. 2007;78:B15–24.
32. Williams HL, Lubin A. Speeded addition and sleep loss. J Exp Psychol. 1967;73:313–7.
33. Babkoff H, Mikulincer M, Caspy T, Kempinski D, Sing H. The topology of performance curves during 72 hours of sleep loss: a memory and search task. Q J Exp Psychol A. 1988;40(4):737–56.
34. Bonnet MH, Arand DL. Sleepiness as measured by the MSLT varies as a function of preceding activity. Sleep. 1998;21(5):477–83.
35. Leproult R, Van Reeth O, Byrne MM, Sturis J, Van Cauter E. Sleepiness, performance, and neuroendocrine function during sleep deprivation: effects of exposure to bright light or exercise. J Biol Rhythms. 1997;12:245–58.
36. Webb WB, Agnew HWJ. Effects on performance of high and low energy-expenditure during sleep deprivation. Percept Mot Skills. 1973;37(2):511–4.
37. Dawson D, Encel N, Lushington K. Improving adaptation to simulated night shift: timed exposure to bright light versus daytime melatonin administration. Sleep. 1995;18:11–21.
38. Dijk D-J, Cajochen C, Borbely A. Effect of a single 3-hour exposure to bright light on core body temperature and sleep in humans. Neurosci Lett. 1991;121:59–62.
39. Phipps-Nelson J, Redman J, Schlangen L, Rajaratnam S. Blue light exposure reduces objective measures of sleepiness during prolonged nighttime performance testing. Chronobiol Int. 2009;26:891–913.
40. Bonnet MH, Arand DL. Arousal components which differentiate the MWT from the MSLT. Sleep. 2001;24:441–50.
41. Lindqvist A, Jalonen J, Parviainen P, Antila K, Laitinen LA. Effect of posture on spontaneous and thermally stimulated cardiovascular oscillations. Cardiovasc Res. 1990;24:373–80.
42. Bonnet MH, Arand DL. Level of arousal and the ability to maintain wakefulness. J Sleep Res. 1999;8:247–54.
43. Ficca G, Axelsson J, Mollicone D, Muto V, Vitiello M. Naps, cognition and performance. Sleep Med Rev. 2010;14:249–58.

44. Nicholson A, Pascoe P, Roehrs T, et al. Sustained performance with short evening and morning sleeps. Aviat Space Environ Med. 1985;56:105–14.
45. Mollicone D, Van Dongen H, Rogers N, Dinges D. Response surface mapping of neurobehavioral performance: testing the feasibility of split sleep schedules for space operations. Acta Astronaut. 2008;63:833–40.
46. Bonnet MH, Gomez S, Wirth O, Arand DL. The use of caffeine versus prophylactic naps in sustained performance. Sleep. 1995;18:97–104.
47. Brooks A, Lack L. A brief afternoon nap following nocturnal sleep restriction: which nap duration is most recuperative? Sleep. 2006;29:831–40.
48. Bonnet MH, Balkin TJ, Dinges DF, Roehrs T, Rogers NL, Wesensten NJ. The use of stimulants to modify performance during sleep loss: a review by the sleep deprivation and stimulant task force of the American Academy of Sleep Medicine. Sleep. 2005;28(9):1163–87.
49. Wesensten J, Belenky G, Kautz MA, Thorne DR, Reichardt RM, Balkin TJ. Maintaining alertness and performance during sleep deprivation: modafinil versus caffeine. Psychopharmacology (Berl). 2002;159:238–47.
50. Wesensten NJ, Killgore WD, Balkin TJ. Performance and alertness effects of caffeine, dextroamphetamine, and modafinil during sleep deprivation. J Sleep Res. 2005;14(3):255–66.
51. Walsh JK, Muehlbach MJ, Humm TM, Dickins QS, Sugerman JL, Schweitzer PK. Effect of caffeine on physiological sleep tendency and ability to sustain wakefulness at night. Psychopharmacology. 1990;101:271–3.
52. Bonnet MH, Arand DL. The use of prophylactic naps and caffeine to maintain performance during a continuous operation. Ergonomics. 1994;37(6):1009–20.
53. Bonnet MH, Arand DL. The impact of naps and caffeine on extended nocturnal performance. Physiol Behav. 1994;56(1):103–9.
54. Wright KP, Badia P, Myers BL, Plenzler SC. Combination of bright light and caffeine as a countermeasure for impaired alertness and performance during extended sleep deprivation. J Sleep Res. 1997;6:26–35.
55. Roehrs T, Beare D, Zorick F, Roth T. Sleepiness and ethanol effects on simulated driving. Alcohol Clin Exp Res. 1994;18:154–8.
56. Williamson AM, Feyer AM. Moderate sleep deprivation produces impairments in cognitive and motor performance equivalent to legally prescribed levels of alcohol intoxication. Occup Environ Med. 2000;57:649–55.
57. Dawson D, Reid K. Fatigue, alcohol and performance impairment. Nature. 1997;388:235. (letter).
58. Arnedt JT, Wilde GJ, Munt PW, MacLean AW. How do prolonged wakefulness and alcohol compare in the decrements they produce on a simulated driving task? Accid Anal Prev. 2001;33:337–44.
59. Horne JA, Pettitt AN. High incentive effects on vigilance performance during 72 hours of total sleep deprivation. Acta Psychol. 1985;58:123–39.
60. Haslam DR. The incentive effect and sleep deprivation. Sleep. 1983;6(4):362–8.
61. Belenky G, Wesensten NJ, Thorne DR, et al. Patterns of performance degradation and restoration during sleep restriction and subsequent recovery: a sleep dose-response study. J Sleep Res. 2003;12(1):1–12.
62. Dinges DF, Pack F, Williams K, et al. Cumulative sleepiness, mood disturbance, and psychomotor vigilance performance decrements during a week of sleep restricted to 4-5 hours per night. Sleep. 1997;20:267–77.
63. Van Dongen HPA, Maislin G, Mullington JM, Dinges DF. The cumulative cost of additional wakefulness: dose-response effects on neurobehavioral functions and sleep physiology from chronic sleep restriction and total sleep deprivation. Sleep. 2003;26:117–26.
64. Bonnet MH, Arand DL. Clinical effects of sleep fragmentation versus sleep deprivation. Sleep Med Rev. 2003;7:297–310.

Chapter 4
Studies of Fatigue and Human Performance in the Field

Mary Rose

Field vs. the Lab Studies

Inquiry into fatigue and human performance in the field explore the mechanisms through which performance declines in individuals and groups consequent to fatiguing influences. These include sleep loss and the circadian timing of sleep, as well as physical, emotional, and psychological exhaustion and strain. Akersteadt and Wright further discriminate between fatigue and sleepiness: "cognitive and muscle fatigue symptoms may be reduced by sedentary activity or rest without sleeping, whereas subjective sleepiness and the propensity for sleep are often exacerbated by sedentary activity or rest" [1]. Differentiating between the two general concepts of sleepiness and fatigue is essential so that we can determine strategies to understand and mitigate their course.

Field studies generally examine real-life changes in the industries of transportation and emergency work in order to determine how fatigue is manifested in those actively working in these environments. Studies in the field are important for several reasons. First they allow us to examine real-life causes of fatigue and sleepiness as well as strategies used by workers to allay fatigue. The latter may better guide us in understanding the subject experience of fatigue and sleepiness. Secondly, field studies allow us to examine what fatigue means to different industries, and the manner in which non-experimentally induced schedule preferences and individual fatigue management strategies are naturally used in these workplaces. Thirdly, field studies facilitate our recognition of how the subjective experiences of fatigue and sleepiness are mitigated by factors such as years of experience, sleep loss resilience, gender, burnout, comorbid depression, and coping strategies. In one study, variability between residents on a night off, on call, or on working emergency admissions

M. Rose, PsyD
Department of Neuropsychology, TIRR Memorial Hermann Rehabilitation Network, Physical Medicine and Rehabilitation, Baylor College of Medicine, Houston, TX, USA

© Springer Science+Business Media, LLC, part of Springer Nature 2018
A. Sharafkhaneh, M. Hirshkowitz (eds.), *Fatigue Management*,
https://doi.org/10.1007/978-1-4939-8607-1_4

appeared to be due to individual differences and not differences in the level of sleep deprivation [2].

The value of field studies is that they help us to better organize and design the schedule of workers with personal preference and proclivities in mind. They also facilitate identifying the most vulnerable times of the day to human error and weariness. Though several studies have established the impact of sleep loss and fatigue on performance, this has been well established and needs only select additional discussion here, to illuminate the specific problems in our population of focus.

One difficulty with field studies is that they lack the controls and manipulations of experimental lab studies and thus may have more unforeseen bias. Major design flaws in many of the lab, as well as field studies, have involved relatively small numbers of participants, selection bias, and measures that involve overlearned tasks or are not sensitive to sleep loss. Owens points out that self-report is an additional flaw in most of these studies [3]. However, alternatively, randomization and manipulation may also alter the behavior being observed, leading to bias. Field studies are more likely to expose natural behaviors of which the experimenter may have been unaware, and/or which may mitigate the sleepiness and fatigue. In addition to being more amenable to larger numbers of subjects who can be enrolled, field studies allow us to additionally observe how fatigue and sleepiness are experienced in natural environments and the strategies developed by individuals to compensate and adapt.

Field Studies in Specific Populations

Some of the major professional areas in which fatigue/sleepiness are of critical interest include health care, transportation, power plant, military, and law enforcement. One fascinating aspect of how fatigue is manifested in the field is the fact that it is defined differently in each of the abovementioned fields, and emphasis on what aspects of fatigue are important is variable. Studies of military, law enforcement, power plant, and transportation are focused heavily on physical reaction time, whereas studies of residents, medical students, and their attending physicians are largely focused on performance measures such as surgical outcome, decision-making, and procedures, though some emphasis has also been placed on mood and overall well-being [2, 4]. Studies of nursing professionals have an additional strong emphasis, rarely examined in field studies of physicians and physicians in training, of compassion and emotional fatigue.

Field Studies of Fatigue and Sleep Loss in Physicians

This chapter will review ways in which the effects of fatigue, one of the major mediators of which is sleepiness, sleep loss, and inappropriate timing of sleep, has been demonstrated *in the field* in physicians and physicians in training. There is no doubt that individuals with greater resilience to physical and emotional stress, as well as to sleep loss and/or circadian disruption, may self-select into fields where these more abrasive and challenging work schedules are anticipated. *However*, such individuals may also be less aware of or willing to acknowledge impairment. This is likely magnified by the bias in medical training to create a façade of health, even during significant times of distress, and to resist help-seeking behavior [5]. In fact, one study found that a vast majority of physicians report barriers to seeking help when their health suffers from stress or strain to include concern about letting colleagues down (70.6%) [5]. Fatigue, and possibly to a lesser degree sleepiness, may be affected not only by the total hours worked and the circadian timing of sleep but by other variables such as the work load demands, novelty, threat, risk, access to countermeasures, and breaks. Fragmentation of sleep and sleep inertia are also critical contributors to sleep-related performance errors. It may take several hours, with the first 15–30 being most vulnerable, to reach a fully alerted state upon waking from a high sleep pressure nap condition [6]. As residents are typically woken while on duty call to make immediate and sometimes critical decisions, this does not bode well for risk or medical error. In a study of 356 internal medicine residents, West et al. found that subjective medical errors were associated with subjective fatigue (self-defined) and sleepiness (Epworth) but that this relationship was mediated by levels of burnout and depression [7].

Types of Deficit Consequent to Sleep Loss and Fatigue

Health-care workers face a more specialized set of causes for fatigue than those in the transportation industry, consequent to the personalized nature of life or death situations that they face. Multiple field studies have been conducted with physicians and nurses to determine how emotional and psychological stress as well as work hours, timing of work, and patient loads affect performance. Deficits may come in the form of performance deficits (ability to carefully and accurately perform medical duties and to diagnose and treat properly), personal consequences to well-being (illness, mood disturbance, marital stress, lack of family time, increased risk for substance abuse, lack of self-enrichment time), and cognitive deficits (reaction time, ability to access divergent information, attention, concentration, and memory).

Performance Deficits

The most important studies to examine the contemporary effects of sleep loss on physicians in training are those studies conducted since the ACGME training guideline changes in 2003—which should provide a more representative contemporary sample of sleep and fatigue. One such study from 2012 indicated that of 27 orthopedic surgical residents, average total sleep time was 5.3 h [8]. In most experimental studies, significant deficits are seen when sleep consistently dips below 6 h of sleep, a dip which Horne refers to as violating the "core sleep" required to "repair the effects of wear and tear on the cerebrum" [9]. This would suggest a continued chronic state of neurocognitive harm to those in training. Post-call fatigue has been demonstrated to impair performance and poor surgical decision-making [10] and increased performance error during laparoscopic maneuvers [11]. Though short-duration reaction time test have not proven to show substantial deficit in sleep-deprived physicians [12], performance of more complex divergent thinking has been shown to be substantially impaired. Marcus and Loughlin (1996) found that 49% of house staff they interviewed noted falling asleep at the wheel within the past 3 years, 90% of which occurred post-call [13]. Hawkins found deficits in a number of areas including higher cognitive functioning in acutely sleep-deprived residents. Most interestingly, however, was that they were largely unaware of the extent of their impairment while sleep deprived [14]. Sawyer et al. examined the effects of call in residents taking call every second, third, or fourth night in relation to operating room participation and overall satisfaction. They found that on-call fatigue across groups was strongly related to the number of self-report errors. Increases of objective rates of error up to 20% in addition to slowed performance has also been found via repeated measures in surgical residents post-call compared with non-post-call status [15]. Arnedt found that the number of commission errors, driving simulator lane and speed variability, and psychomotor performance errors after 4 weeks of heavy call rotation (about 90 h per a week) was equivalent to a month of light call (~44 h duty per week) plus moderate alcohol intake 20 min before testing (~0.005 g% blood alcohol level) [16]. Given that the current ACGME guidelines allow for 88 h per week of call in specialty residencies, it does not require a leap of faith to imagine the likely impairment of residents under these conditions. However, this relationship is not always clearly linear. Barger et al. conducted a web-based survey of 2737 PGY1 critical care residents. Extended duration shifts were associated with a far greater incidence of preventable adverse events, medical errors, and attentional failures (falling asleep during surgery or while examining a patient). Residents were queried on their "belief that sleep deprivation or fatigue caused [them] to make a significant medical error" to determine the degree to which they *perceived* sleep loss and fatigue as responsible for errors. Extended duration of work shifts was associated with substantially more fatigue-related medical errors and fatality-related errors [17].

Call Status: the Chronicity of Sleep Loss, and the Trajectory of Recovery

Sleep deprivation research has often quantified sleep based upon the number of rested hours within a 24- or 36-h period [18, 19]. Such a strategy erroneously assumes that the effects of the deprivation are not cumulative. The effects of deprivation persist the day following rested sleep [20]. It is therefore important to control for the cumulative effects of sleep deprivation and to acknowledge that recovery may not be rapid post-call. The lack of positive findings in some studies may be due to the fact that the residents are assumed to be "rested" when not on call, despite that they are still sleep deprived, from the previous night call. Additionally, despite that residents and interns may have a prescribed time available to sleep, causes of sleep disruption that may further add to sleep difficulty are often under-recognized in studies. Richardson et al. found that total sleep time was often significantly impaired by the constant interruption of pages and difficulty returning to sleep [21]. Additionally, younger physicians may be less skilled at managing their personal time and in prioritizing their sleep and rest.

There is substantial evidence that house staff suffer significant impairment consequent to the acute sleep deprivation secondary to a day call. Friedman et al. found within subject differences between fatigued and non-fatigued residents in sustained attention tasks [22]. Hart et al. found that compared with non-sleep-deprived residents (those sleeping an average of 7.9 h in 24 h), sleep-deprived residents (those sleeping an average of 2.7 h in 24 h) were impaired on a number of vigilance and memory tasks [23]. Others have likewise found that performances on a variety of tests measuring reaction time, information processing, recall, sustained attention, and concentration were all impaired in residents post-call [24].

Some field studies examining the effects of post-call fatigue in physicians suggest a relatively rapid recovery (48 h) with regard to subjective mental fatigue and feelings of restedness [25]. The deficits in slow-wave sleep, sleep fragmentation, and sleep efficiency are significantly improved with protected sleep time and coverage [21]. However the impact of the mental fatigue and lack of restedness during the interim recovery work time is unknown. Schwartz et al. found that residents attributed their bleakest days more to lack of sleep than to any other queried factor, though other factors such as inadequate support, patient load, and peer competition also magnified their distress [26].

The Secondary Impact of ACGME Changes

The prominence of performance deficits as indicated via medical and diagnostic errors, as well as dangerous attentional lapses such as self-needle sticks and MVAs, has been well established in those on 24 h shift. At least for physicians in training, ACGME has set regulations restricting duty hours worked so that those in training in the USA at least no longer are subjected to the previously prolonged duty hours. In 2003 the ACGME restricted resident training hours to a maximum of 24 h shifts, and no more than 80 h per week. In 2011, these guidelines were further restricted to minimize PGY1 hours to 16 duty hours per shift and *recommend* strategic napping for other residents. Transfer of care hours was also restricted from 6 to 0 for PGY1 and 4 for PGY$\geq$2. Recommendations for length of time between shifts was also changed from "should have" language to "must have" depending upon PGY year and specialty.

This does not affect the hours regulated for attending physicians. In addition to an increase in attending staff work hours, Owens points out that the restriction on resident training hours has ironically likely led to an increase in working hours for nursing staff, as they are asked to cover an increasing number of nights, weekends, and extended shifts [27].

However, we should be cautious not to suggest that this means that the work load should be re-intensified for physicians in training but rather that hospitals need to increase staff to create reasonable work conditions. Studies of MVAs in nurses have shown that they are far more likely to report MVA after a rotating shift [28]. It is unclear if nursing staff have been working substantially longer since these changes. One study of 5317 self-report work shifts suggested that hospital staff nurses generally worked longer than scheduled daily, and generally worked more than 40 h per week. Half of the shifts worked exceeded ten and a half hours, and 39% of shifts were reported to include rotations of at least 12.5 consecutive hours of duty [29]. Rotating shift work and night shift have also been found to be associated with increased medication administration error by nursing staff [30].

Burnout and Compassion Fatigue

One area of fatigue discussed almost exclusively in the health-care field are burnout and compassion fatigue (the latter of which has been explored more in the nursing field). Burnout results from stress that arises from the clinician's interaction with the work environment [31], whereas compassion fatigue stems from the relationship between the clinician and the patient [9]. These types of fatigue are rarely discussed in non-emergency/health-care sectors and represent an additional layer of complexity to the more commonly evaluated and understood sleep- and circadian-related fatigue. Burnout and compassion fatigue likely magnify sleep-related fatigue as they are associated with greater dysphoria and likely sleep fragmentation. Sleep deprivation has been found a predictor of burnout in nursing in at least one study in nurses [32]. The concepts of compassion fatigue and burnout could be an instrumental dimension which has given greater depth to the impact of fatigue on health-care workers. Certainly, the associated dysphoria will magnify feelings of exhaustion, albeit not likely sleepiness. Therefore, theoretically we should see a clear relationship between burnout and compassion fatigue with generally low energy and lack of vigor but not sleep unless health-care staff suffering one of these simultaneously report comorbid insomnia.

Awareness and Self-Treatment

A valuable piece of evidence from the field that supports fatigue and sleepiness among medical student and health-care staff is the use of stimulant medication. A recent study shows that the use of stimulant prescription medication among medical students is disproportionately high [33]. It is unlikely that the field of medicine necessarily attracts such a disproportionate number of legitimately diagnosed adult attention deficit sufferers but rather that recognition of the benefits of stimulant use to performance is the driving force behind stimulant use. An anonymous self-report study of 9600 physicians suggested that they are less likely than age- and sex-matched counterparts to use illicit substances, but they are more likely to have used alcohol, opiates, and benzodiazepines [34]. Estimates on use of performance enhancers in physicians in practice have not been well established.

Chronic sleep deprivation degrades one's ability to recognize impairment [35]. As do physicians, nurses do not seem to acknowledge the serious role that fatigue plays in critical incidents. When intensive care and operating room nurses were questioned about error, approximately 60% agreed with the statement that, "Even when I am fatigued, I perform effectively during critical times" [36]. A reduction in size and number of synaptic connections (representing a renormalization) following sleep [37] represents a restoration of neurocognitive functioning; there is thus little doubt that neurocognitive functioning is impaired with prolonged sleep deprivation. However, failure to recognize deficit may also be a protective mechanism that fosters confidence and the ability to make life or death decisions without potentially catastrophic hesitancy.

Summary

Regulation of duty hours is driven by many factors. Those enduring the sleep loss consequent to prolonged and poorly timed hours of work are at least in part driving the current regulations. In medicine, support for modification to the duty hours has been apparently mixed. This is particularly disturbing as physicians in training tend to be young adults who may still have sleep drive needs that exceed that of their older counterparts. Additionally, younger caregivers are more prone to burnout and stress reactions [38].

So long as there is financial gain and low perception of personal risk, the battle to implement more carefully regulated duty hours is an uphill battle. Magnifying this is that perception of impaired functioning when one is sleep deprived is in itself impaired. The unfortunate misperception that the ability to endure sleep loss and excessive work hours is somehow a sign of academic virility and/or fitness has endured for many decades and is unlikely to subside without legislative enforcement as well as a change in the cultures perpetuating these beliefs. Owens points out that sleep deprivation during residency is likely to have the highest risks and stakes. Levine et al. did an extensive review of research on resident factors since the ACGME reduction of >16-hour work shifts and found not only the absence of adverse effect on resident education but also improvements in patient safety and resident quality of life in most of studies [39]. However, it is important to recognize that as Landrigan points out, with very few institution-based exceptions, no such restriction on duty hours exists for other health-care professionals such as nursing [40].

Areas which would benefit from greater examination in the field among health-care professionals include how sleep loss and fatigue impact overall perceived quality of life (harkening back to the Schwartz study of 1987 regarding *bleakness*), burnout and perceived self-efficacy, and its effects of more complex divergent thinking and problem solving. Additionally, though a somewhat dangerous area on which to tread, better understanding of individual resilience and optimal fit of individual to schedule would likely bring improvements to the field of health-care.

References

1. Akerstedt T, Wright KP Jr. Sleep loss and fatigue in shift work and shift work disorder. Sleep Med Clin. 2009;4:257–71.
2. Deary IJ, Tait R. Effects of sleep disruption on cognitive performance and mood in medical house officers. Br Med J (Clin Res Ed). 1987;295:1513–6.
3. Owens J. Medical resident/physician performance. In: Kushida C, editor. Sleep deprivation: clinical issues, pharmacology, and sleep loss effects. Monticello: Marcel Dekker; 2005. p. 335–62.
4. Rose M, Manser T, Ware JC. Effects of call on sleep and mood in internal medicine residents. Behav Sleep Med. 2008;6:75–88.
5. Adams EF, Lee AJ, Pritchard CW, White RJ. What stops us from healing the healers: a survey of help-seeking behaviour, stigmatisation and depression within the medical profession. Int J Soc Psychiatry. 2010;56:359–70.
6. Jewett ME, Wyatt JK, Ritz-De CA, Khalsa SB, Dijk DJ, Czeisler CA. Time course of sleep inertia dissipation in human performance and alertness. J Sleep Res. 1999;8:1–8.
7. West CP, Tan AD, Habermann TM, Sloan JA, Shanafelt TD. Association of resident fatigue and distress with perceived medical errors. JAMA. 2009;302:1294–300.
8. McCormick F, Kadzielski J, Landrigan CP, Evans B, Herndon JH, Rubash HE. Surgeon fatigue: a prospective analysis of the incidence, risk, and intervals of predicted fatigue-related impairment in residents. Arch Surg. 2012;147:430–5.
9. Horne JA. Why we sleep: the functions of sleep in humans and other mammals. Oxford: Oxford University Press; 1988.
10. Goldman LI, McDonough MT, Rosemond GP. Stresses affecting surgical performance and learning. I. Correlation of heart rate, electrocardiogram, and operation simultaneously recorded on videotapes. J Surg Res. 1972;12:83–6.
11. Taffinder NJ, McManus IC, Gul Y, Russell RC, Darzi A. Effect of sleep deprivation on surgeons' dexterity on laparoscopy simulator. Lancet. 1998;352:1191.
12. Samkoff JS, Jacques CH. A review of studies concerning effects of sleep deprivation and fatigue on residents' performance. Acad Med. 1991;66:687–93.
13. Marcus CL, Loughlin GM. Effect of sleep deprivation on driving safety in housestaff. Sleep. 1996;19:763–6.
14. Hawkins MR, Vichick DA, Silsby HD, Kruzich DJ, Butler R. Sleep and nutritional deprivation and performance of house officers. J Med Educ. 1985;60:530–5.
15. Sawyer RG, Tribble CG, Newberg DS, Pruett TL, Minasi JS. Intern call schedules and their relationship to sleep, operating room participation, stress, and satisfaction. Surgery. 1999;126:337–42.
16. Arnedt JT, Owens J, Crouch M, Stahl J, Carskadon MA. Neurobehavioral performance of residents after heavy night call vs after alcohol ingestion. JAMA. 2005;294:1025–33.
17. Barger LK, Ayas NT, Cade BE, et al. Impact of extended-duration shifts on medical errors, adverse events, and attentional failures. PLoS Med. 2006;3:e487.

18. McCall TB. The impact of long working hours on resident physicians. N Engl J Med. 1988;318:775–8.
19. Poulton EC, Hunt GM, Carpenter A, Edwards RS. The performance of junior hospital doctors following reduced sleep and long hours of work. Ergonomics. 1978;21:279–95.
20. Wilkinson RT. After effect of sleep deprivation. J Exp Psychol. 1990;66:439–42.
21. Richardson GS, Wyatt JK, Sullivan JP, et al. Objective assessment of sleep and alertness in medical house staff and the impact of protected time for sleep. Sleep. 1996;19:718–26.
22. Friedman RC, Bigger JT, Kornfeld DS. The intern and sleep loss. N Engl J Med. 1971;285:201–3.
23. Hart RP, Buchsbaum DG, Wade JB, Hamer RM, Kwentus JA. Effect of sleep deprivation on first-year residents' response times, memory, and mood. J Med Educ. 1987;62:940–2.
24. Lingenfelser T, Kaschel R, Weber A, Zaiser-Kaschel H, Jakober B, Kuper J. Young hospital doctors after night duty: their task-specific cognitive status and emotional condition. Med Educ. 1994;28:566–72.
25. Malmberg B, Kecklund G, Karlson B, Persson R, Flisberg P, Orbaek P. Sleep and recovery in physicians on night call: a longitudinal field study. BMC Health Serv Res. 2010;10:239.
26. Schwartz AJ, Black ER, Goldstein MG, Jozefowicz RF, Emmings FG. Levels and causes of stress among residents. J Med Educ. 1987;62:744–53.
27. Owens JA. Sleep loss and fatigue in healthcare professionals. J Perinat Neonatal Nurs. 2007;21:92–100.
28. Gold DR, Rogacz S, Bock N, et al. Rotating shift work, sleep, and accidents related to sleepiness in hospital nurses. Am J Public Health. 1992;82:1011–4.
29. Rogers DJ, Stark MM. Think drink, think drugs, think overdoses. J Clin Forensic Med. 1998;5:147–9.
30. Saleh AM, Awadalla NJ, El-masri YM, Sleem WF. Impacts of nurses' circadian rhythm sleep disorders, fatigue, and depression on medication administration errors. Egypt J Chest Dis Tuberc. 2013;63:145–53.
31. Ramirez AJ, Graham J, Richards MA, et al. Burnout and psychiatric disorder among cancer clinicians. Br J Cancer. 1995;71:1263–9.
32. Smart D, English A, James J, et al. Compassion fatigue and satisfaction: a cross-sectional survey among US healthcare workers. Nurs Health Sci. 2013;16(1):3–10.
33. Webb JR, Valasek MA, North CS. Prevalence of stimulant use in a sample of US medical students. Ann Clin Psychiatry. 2013;25:27–32.
34. Hughes PH, Brandenburg N, Baldwin DC Jr, et al. Prevalence of substance use among US physicians. JAMA. 1992;267:2333–9.
35. Van Dongen HP, Maislin G, Mullington JM, Dinges DF. The cumulative cost of additional wakefulness: dose-response effects on neurobehavioral functions and sleep physiology from chronic sleep restriction and total sleep deprivation. Sleep. 2003;26:117–26.
36. Sexton JB, Thomas EJ, Helmreich RL. Error, stress, and teamwork in medicine and aviation: cross sectional surveys. BMJ. 2000;320:745–9.
37. Bushey D, Tononi G, Cirelli C. Sleep and synaptic homeostasis: structural evidence in Drosophila. Science. 2011;332:1576–81.
38. Kuerer HM, Eberlein TJ, Pollock RE, et al. Career satisfaction, practice patterns and burnout among surgical oncologists: report on the quality of life of members of the Society of Surgical Oncology. Ann Surg Oncol. 2007;14:3043–53.
39. Levine AC, Adusumilli J, Landrigan CP. Effects of reducing or eliminating resident work shifts over 16 hours: a systematic review. Sleep. 2010;33:1043–53.
40. Landrigan CP, Czeisler CA, Barger LK, Ayas NT, Rothschild JM, Lockley SW. Effective implementation of work-hour limits and systemic improvements. Jt Comm J Qual Patient Saf. 2007;33:19–29.

Chapter 5
Studies of Fatigue and Human Performance in Patients with Sleep Disorders

Michelle Primeau and Clete Kushida

Clinically, fatigue can be attributed to a myriad of conditions. While multiple medical conditions (e.g., hypothyroidism, anemia, depression, cancer, HIV, etc.) are known to cause fatigue, this chapter will focus on sleep disorders that may cause fatigue and sleepiness by disrupting sleep and how disrupted sleep can impact performance. We will first discuss general information regarding sleep regulation and what changes may be seen in sleep physiology with a poor night's sleep. Then, studies of the effects of sleep deprivation on normal volunteers will be discussed, followed by performance studies in patients with obstructive sleep apnea (OSA), insomnia, circadian rhythm disorders, and narcolepsy.

Sleep Deprivation: Changes to Sleep Structure

It is readily apparent to anyone who has ever pulled an "all-nighter" that sleep deprivation increases one's tendency to sleep and that the longer one is awake, the greater the propensity for sleep. This accumulated need for sleep has been entitled "Process S" and is thought to be due to the accumulation of adenosine as a by-product of metabolism over the course of a given time period [1]. Quantitative measures of slow wave activity (SWA) using Fourier analysis to calculate spectral power in the delta frequency (0.5–5 Hz) have shown SWA to be a correlate of Process S, the homeostatic sleep drive, and can indicate the relative depth of sleep [2, 3]. After sleep deprivation, the body responds with an increased total duration of sleep as well as with greater "deep" sleep or slow wave sleep [2]. Over the course of the night, SWA declines, reflecting a dissipation of the homeostatic sleep drive.

M. Primeau, MD · C. Kushida, MD, PhD, RPSGT (⊠)
Stanford Sleep Medicine Center, Redwood City, CA, USA
e-mail: clete@stanford.edu

© Springer Science+Business Media, LLC, part of Springer Nature 2018
A. Sharafkhaneh, M. Hirshkowitz (eds.), *Fatigue Management*,
https://doi.org/10.1007/978-1-4939-8607-1_5

However, the homeostatic sleep drive is not the sole mechanism regulating the sleep-wake cycle; an intrinsic circadian process, "Process C," also acts throughout the day. Process C can be thought of as more of a wakefulness-promoting process, which balances Process S to allow for typical consolidation of wake and sleep periods [4]. Both processes work together to regulate vigilance, or ability to sustain attention [5], and subjective alertness and cognitive performance are highly correlated to the circadian phase [6].

After an "all-nighter," most college students will tell you that physically they don't feel well, and they may have changes to the way they sleep once they are able. These effects have been quantified. For example, it has been shown that individuals have increased sympathetic activity following a night of sleep deprivation [7]. Sleep deprivation also leads to diminished respiratory capacity (as measured by forced vital capacity, maximal voluntary ventilation, and hypercapnic ventilator response) and can worsen nocturnal respiration during recovery sleep, with longer obstructive events, low oxygen saturation, and greater peak negative inspiratory effort, seen with sleep-deprived animals [8, 9]. Furthermore, gastrointestinal and metabolic functions appear affected as well. Women with irritable bowel syndrome report worsening of symptoms after a poor night of sleep [10], and in rats, it has been demonstrated that sleep deprivation leads to increased energy expenditure [11].

But what does sleep deprivation do to change the structure of sleep? As mentioned above, during recovery sleep, there is an increase in SWA, which represents a discharging of the accumulated sleep debt. This sleep is perceived as "deeper," and indeed, it is more difficult to awaken someone in this kind of sleep [12]. There is a corresponding *decrease* in rapid eye movement (REM) sleep during the first recovery night, followed by an increase the following night, for no net change in REM sleep during the recovery period [3]. It appears that the body preferentially conserves NREM sleep, such that, as sleep deprivation extends, sleep drive accumulates, and NREM can enter into waking in the form of microsleeps and sleep-like neuronal synchronization in drowsy waking [13]. However, sleep propensity and the effects of recovery sleep are also under the control of Process C. If sleep deprivation ends at the beginning of the active period, when alerting signals are greater, recovery sleep tends to be fragmented [14].

Sleep Deprivation and Performance

Sleep deprivation negatively impacts performance, but the amount of decrement depends on the type of task, length of deprivation, and rate at which performed [15]. One meta-analysis found that, overall, sleep deprivation appears to have the greatest impact on mood, less so cognitive tasks, and the least amount of impact on motor tasks; furthermore, cognitive performance and mood are more effected by partial sleep deprivation (<5 h/24 h period) than by short- or long-term total sleep deprivation [15].

An individual's mood can be affected by sleep deprivation. Patients with total sleep deprivation become dysphoric and irritable [16], and tend to develop euphoria, talkativity, and increased activity from 4:30 to 6:30 am. With extended periods of sleep deprivation, patients have developed perceptual distortions, illusions, and paranoia [17]. Even without total sleep deprivation, but just disrupted sleep changes in mood have been noted. One study attempted to mimic the effects of OSA as applies to sleep fragmentation, by exposing subjects to a noise while they were sleeping every 2 min [18]. These patients experienced increased sleepiness, unhappiness, and unclear thinking, similar to a person who had experienced total sleep deprivation of 40–64 h.

Various tasks have been utilized in an attempt to quantify the cognitive effects of sleep deprivation. Attention encompasses alertness, the capacity to respond quickly to an unpredictable stimulus; sustained attention, the maintenance of attention for a long period of time; selective attention, ability to focus on one target; and divided attention, ability to deal with multiple types of information simultaneously. With total sleep deprivation, subjects show impaired performance on tests of alertness, sustained attention, and selective attention [19–22], and partial sleep deprivation over 5–7 nights also impaired performance [23, 24]. Likewise, memory is impaired by sleep deprivation. Total sleep deprivation leads to impairments in explicit, declarative (fact-related) memory and implicit, procedural (learned task-related), and working memory (short-term storage for immediate use), which may not even improve after two nights of recovery sleep [25–28]. Interestingly, with partial sleep deprivation, there appears to be different memory effects depending on the part of the night that is restricted. Plihal and Born demonstrated that preservation of early sleep appears to preserve explicit and declarative memory, while preservation of late sleep seems to preserve procedural and implicit memory [29, 30]. These authors further associate SWS with declarative (factual memory) and REM with implicit, non-declarative memory.

Effort and motivation are closely associated with outcome on any task and so have been studied in the contexts of performance in individuals with sleep deprivation and fatigue. It has been noted that sleep-deprived individuals appear to decrease their effort as they accumulate further sleep deprivation [31]; however, others have observed that sleep-deprived individuals actually *increase* effort when they realize they are performing inadequately [32]. It is thought that effort increases when an individual has increased motivation to complete a task, which researchers have done by either providing feedback on performance on a task [33] or providing a monetary reward [34], both of which have proven to improve performance.

Falling asleep while driving is a relatively common consequence of sleepiness [35]. One survey of individuals randomly selected at a freeway tollbooth demonstrated that many people driving long distances have significantly reduced their hours of sleep prior to driving a long distance [36], and one study of US truck drivers demonstrated a mean sleep duration of 4.78 h over 5 days and had electroencephalographic (EEG) evidence of microsleeps during the circadian night [37]. Sleepiness while driving increases the odds of having an accident 8.2 times that of people who are not sleepy, and there is a particular increased risk in individuals who have slept less than 5 h the night prior or who are driving in the early morning (2–5 am) hours [38].

OSA

Obstructive sleep apnea (OSA) occurs in up to 17% of the population and has been associated with increased mortality risk, particularly cardiovascular [39]. It is characterized as repetitive collapse of the airway during sleep, leading to hypoxia and sleep fragmentation. The gold standard for treatment remains continuous positive airway pressure (CPAP) which normalizes the sleep fragmentation and reduces hypoxic events. There has been increasing attention paid to the neurocognitive impairment incurred in OSA. The excessive sleepiness associated with OSA is linked to decreased motivation and activity, vigilance, and an increased risk of accidents while driving [40]. Mood is often noted to deteriorate first, with irritability, impatience, anxiety, and low mood potentially leading to disrupted relationships [40]. However, for patients who misperceive their daytime level of sleepiness, cognitive complaints may be the presenting symptom for OSA [40].

Patients with OSA have been found to have decreased ability to maintain attention, impaired executive functions, and impaired motor performance. The most consistent findings appear in tests of attention and vigilance. A meta-analysis of studies evaluating neuropsychological effects of obstructive sleep apnea found that while intelligence and verbal ability are not affected by OSA, vigilance is markedly impacted [41]. This is true of patients with severe OSA [42, 43], as well as in patients with milder OSA (RDI 10–30, [44]). This has led investigators to try to identify whether it is the fragmentation of sleep, or hypoxia, which is the cause of the problem. For example, in one study of sustained attention in individuals with OSA and matched controls, OSA patients had slower reaction times, as well as decreased cortical activation of centers known to participate in arousal and attention. Furthermore, the authors found a relationship with the arousal index (not hypoxia or the apnea hypopnea index, AHI) to be related to the delayed reaction time [45]. As such, attentional difficulties were thought to be due to sleep fragmentation, which other authors have corroborated [46], though hypoxia has been implicated as well [42].

Executive functioning is moderately effected by OSA [41]. Tests of executive functioning tend to evaluate performance on working memory, mental flexibility, planning, organizing, behavioral inhibition, and problem solving [41]. Some of the poor performance on measures of executive function may be exacerbated by decreased attention and vigilance as well [47]. Variable results have been found in tests of memory and learning. Individuals with variable severity of OSA were shown to perform worse on the Mini-Mental Status Exam, Brief Cognitive Screening Battery in memory and learning, and in verbal fluency, when compared to controls [48]. One study evaluating executive functioning, memory, and learning found minimal impairment of executive functioning and previously learned information but poorer recall of newly learned material [49]. Short-term verbal and visual memory has been demonstrated to be impaired in some studies [44, 49, 50], but not all [42].

The ability to maintain attention can have obvious impact on job performance and motor vehicle safety. Patients with OSA have an increased risk of falling asleep at the wheel [51]; one study of patients reporting subjective symptoms of OSA demonstrate 12× the risk of falling asleep while driving [52], and the risk of accidents may be particularly related to the severity of OSA [52, 53]. When adequately treated with CPAP, the risk of accidents in this population is reduced [54, 55].

As with the decreased risk of accidents seen with adequately treated OSA, similar improvements have been seen in regard to other neurocognitive measures. CPAP treatment reduces sleep fragmentation and hypoxia, and various groups have been studying the effect of CPAP treatment on cognitive measures. One review found that most commonly, improvements in attention and vigilance could be demonstrated, while improvements in executive functioning and memory were only seen in about half of the studies [56]. It also seems that adherence to PAP, for at least 6 h a night, is needed for optimal benefit [56]. As cognitive impairment in patients with OSA can potentially be reversed with adequate treatment of OSA, it was hypothesized that CPAP may help reduce some of the cognitive impairment seen in patients with Alzheimer's disease and comorbid mild to moderate OSA (AHI > 10) [57]. Not only does CPAP improve daytime sleepiness, it also showed either less deterioration or some improvement in cognitive functioning, particularly executive functioning and processing speed, that was sustained long term [57].

Insomnia

Insomnia typically is defined as difficulty falling asleep, staying asleep, or unrefreshing sleep; these symptoms affect 10–28% of people in the USA [58]. However, the current ICSD criteria also include a modifier for daytime impairment; when this is included, the prevalence drops to 9–15% of the population [58]. Patients with insomnia frequently report being sleepy but unable to fall asleep, less mentally sharp, more irritable, and less able to function at work [59], and there is an estimated $63.2 billion loss due to decreased productivity attributable to insomnia [60]. There have been many studies of cognitive function in insomnia that have tried to quantify the cognitive impairment seen in insomnia; however, inconsistent reports of deficits have led some to suggest that the cognitive complaints may be more of a reflection of individuals' selective attention to deficits in performance or that performance remains the same due to increased effort [59, 61]. A meta-analysis aiming to define the magnitude of cognitive differences in insomniacs pooled 24 studies evaluating general cognitive functioning, processing speed, attentional processes, various types of memory, and executive functioning [59]. Patients with insomnia had mild to moderate deficits in some measures of memory, reaction time, information processing, and selective attention, and while performance was maintained on simple tasks, it appeared to deteriorate on more complicated tasks [59, 62].

The outcome measures in insomniacs may be particularly sensitive to the sleep an individual had the night prior. One study demonstrated that patients with primary insomnia overall performed worse than controls on tests of reaction time, attention, and behavioral stability, and while there was some association with subjective report of wake after sleep onset (WASO), objectively confirmed WASO was the best predictor of performance, particularly when considered over the preceding three nights [63]. Other authors confirmed these findings with reaction time [64], executive function, processing speed, and short-term visual memory [65]. These recent studies have elucidated that the discrepancies in studies of cognitive functioning in insomniacs can be attributed to variations in total sleep time (TST), with those individuals shown to have abbreviated TST exhibited deficits similar to what is seen in partial chronic sleep deprivation.

As individuals with insomnia have evident cognitive impairment, one goal of treatment might be to show gains in those cognitive domains. However, one of the mainstays of treatment, benzodiazepines, are notorious for their next-day effects, including subjective report of cognitive dulling, impaired memory, and drowsiness [66]. Earlier reports proposed that improving the sleep of insomniacs would counteract the known cognitive effects observed in healthy volunteers [67]; however, even triazolam, a benzodiazepine with a short-half life (3 h), has been associated with objectively measured memory impairment [68], particularly at higher doses [69]. Newer agents, such as zolpidem, appear to preserve cognitive function the following day [70], unless administered in the middle of the night (4 am [71]).

As many patients wish to avoid the adverse effects of medications, behavioral treatments for insomnia have been developed and have been found to be very effective, both in primary insomnia and insomnia comorbid with other conditions [72]. A few studies have evaluated cognitive function after treatment with cognitive behavioral therapy for insomnia (CBT-I). In one, a group of insomniacs were compared to wait-list controls and individuals without insomnia on tasks of vigilance; both groups of insomniacs demonstrated a significantly faster response time on simple tasks of vigilance and a longer time on more complex tasks relative to controls, which normalized with CBT-I, and improvement was predicted by improved sleep efficiency [73]. Similarly, CBT-I was shown to be effective in a group of fibromyalgia patients with chronic insomnia at improving measures of executive functioning and attention [74].

Circadian Rhythm Sleep Disorders

Control of the sleep-wake cycle has been proposed to be control by two processes: accumulated sleep debt or homeostatic sleep drive (Process S) and the circadian rhythm (Process C), the biologically determined generator of alertness, and other biologic rhythms [75]. The circadian periodicity of alertness can impact performance on certain cognitive measures. Circadian rhythms of alertness and cognitive performance in humans were first demonstrated by Kleitman in the 1930s; he demonstrated that peak performance was associated with higher core body temperature [76] and has since been further described that decreased performance is correlated to increased melatonin levels [4, 77].

Circadian rhythm sleep disorders are characterized by consistent changes in the sleep-wake period that are misaligned with physical and social cues and can be separate into extrinsic (due to external cues, such as in jet lag or shift work disorder) or intrinsic (due to variable circadian rhythm, delayed or advanced sleep phase). There is limited direct study of cognition in these conditions, but as subjects with these disorders frequently have some sleep deprivation, impact can be extrapolated from other studies of sleep deprivation conditions. For example, teenagers tend to have a delayed sleep phase, going to bed later and naturally waking up later. However, during the week they frequently must go to school very early and potentially lose a significant number of hours of sleep, which can have impacts on mood, attention, reaction time, and memory, as above. Due to their natural inclination to sleep during that period, they may have functional impairment in the morning hours. While no direct studies of cognitive function in delayed sleep phase syndrome (DSPS), there have been studies evaluating the outcomes of treatment with either bright light therapy or melatonin and has shown a reduction in objective sleepiness and behavioral problems, respectively [75].

Similarly, patients with advanced sleep phase syndrome (ASPS) tend to go to bed early and awaken earlier than they would desire; due to trying to maintain socially acceptable, sleep-wake times can lead to sleep deprivation. Due to the shift in circadian alerting signals, it is suggested that patients with ASPS will experience increased sleepiness and diminished cognitive functioning in the evening [75]. Patients with free-running type circadian rhythm disorder tend to have a sleep-wake cycle which shifts about 1 h per day and is most commonly seen in blind individuals who are unable to use environmental cues to anchor their circadian rhythm [75]. These individuals tend to report cognitive impairment during their biologic night, when their alerting signals are at the nadir [75]. Irregular sleep-wake type varies from free-running in that there exists no evident pattern to sleep, which tends to occur in 1–4 h blocks throughout the day and is commonly seen in institutionalized elderly with cognitive impairment [75]. Fragmented sleep activity appears to be related to cognitive impairment [78], and improvement of the sleep-wake cycle can improve cognitive performance [79].

Shift work disorder (SWD) occurs when there exists a mismatch of the endogenous circadian rhythm and external sleep-wake signals, namely, occupational, with resultant difficulty falling asleep during allowed sleep period, excessive sleepiness during allowed wake period, and decreased functioning while at work [80]. Difficulties with functioning can be attributed to two main factors: sleep deprivation and being awake during circadian night. Shift workers tend to sleep 1–4 h less than individuals who work during the day, due to sleeping when alerting signals are high, meaning that these individuals are functioning with chronic partial sleep deprivation [81], which in combination with operating outside the circadian alert period can significantly impact cognitive performance.

The consequences of SWD can have wider societal impact, particularly in terms of certain professions, such as forms of transportation or medicine. The Federal Motor Carrier Safety Administration demonstrated that 32% of all fatal large truck accidents occurred at night, with 16.4% occurring between 12 and 6 am [82], and truck driver fatigue was found to contribute to 58% of accidents in one study [83]. Accidents have frequently been found to occur in early morning hours, when alerting signals are at their lowest, both in professionals involved in transportation [84, 85] and in those driving home at those hours [86, 87]. The performance deficits seen with 24-h sleep deprivation is comparable to a blood alcohol level of 0.10% [88]. While no studies have evaluated the direct impact of fatigue and medical errors in healthcare, surveys of physicians have documented fatigue-related errors. In one study of anesthesiologists, 90% reported fatigue-related errors [89]; in another survey of internal medicine residents, 41% reported fatigue to be the cause of their most significant medical mistake [90].

While there may be some self-selection in which individuals who experience less impairment are more likely to continue with shift work [75], long-term (10–20 years) shift work has been associated with cognitive impairment, even when compared for total sleep time, and required >4 years of schedule reversal to improve memory impairment [91]. One study comparing workers with SWD, without SWD, and day workers demonstrated that those with SWD experience deficits in memory and attention similar to what is seen in sleep deprivation and also noted that TST was shorter in individuals with SWD, primarily due to increased WASO [92], possibly due to individuals' alerting signals preventing from consolidating sleep during the day. Similar to other disorders discussed, cognitive impairment can also be inferred by results of treatment studies demonstrating improvement. Modafinil and armodafinil have been shown to improve performance on measures of reaction time, attention, and delayed recall [93, 94]. Like SWD, jet lag also can cause decrements in cognitive performance [95], which may be worse when traveling east [96]. Evidence also suggests that long-term (>4 years) exposure to jet lag is correlated to lower cognitive performance, higher cortisol levels, and brain atrophy [97, 98].

Narcolepsy

Narcolepsy is a disorder characterized by instability of sleep and wake with resultant sleep attacks, cataplexy, and evidence of REM intrusion (hallucinations, sleep paralysis). Patients with narcolepsy frequently report difficulties in attention, concentration, and memory, though research has not born out significant differences. It has been thought that those changes that are seen are likely attributable to the excessive sleepiness of the disorder, and not due to other changes in sleep architecture [99–101]. In one study of patients with narcolepsy with cataplexy (NC) on alerting medications versus healthy controls, patients demonstrated a longer reaction time with intact accuracy on tests of attention, indicating some slowing of information processing in the patient group [102]. This same study showed some mild deficits in verbal memory and significant impairments on tests of executive function; the authors felt that these results were attributable to a diminished capacity to maintain alertness during a given task [102].

Because of the role of hypocretin in processing of reward, some researchers have examined decision-making in NC [103]. Patients with NC tend to have reduced decision-making performance under ambiguous conditions, preferring high immediate reward with little concern for future negative consequences; furthermore, these findings were independent of their level of sleepiness [103]. The authors speculate that these patients have a blunting of emotional reactivity, which leads them to opt for the greater immediate response to compensate for their diminished reaction to a given stimuli. Others have confirmed the earlier findings of impaired executive functioning in NC and related the decision-making in tests of executive functioning to perception of reward [104]. Taken together, this suggests that earlier assumptions that impaired performance on measures of executive function being attributable to excessive sleepiness are inaccurate and instead may be directly related to hypocretin deficiency.

Stimulant medications are a cornerstone in the treatment of NC and have been examined for their potential impact on measures of cognitive function. While some studies have shown no difference on cognitive variables between medicated and unmedicated NC patients [102], others have shown an improvement in executive function in NC patients [105, 106].

Conclusions

Performance on various tasks of cognition varies not only with an individual's circadian rhythm but with the relative amount of sleep. Many studies have demonstrated impaired performance with sleep deprivation in normal volunteers. Sleep disorders such as obstructive sleep apnea, insomnia, and circadian rhythm disorders create situations equivalent to partial sleep deprivation, and as can be expected, performance deficits can be observed in each of these disorders; however, adequate treatment of each disorder appears to improve these cognitive deficits, underscoring the importance of identifying sleep disorders in the general population.

References

1. Porkka-Heiskanen T, Strecker RE, Thakkar M, Bjorkum AA, Greene RW, McCarley RW. Adenosine: a mediator of the sleep-inducing effects of prolonged wakefulness. Science. 1997;276:1265–8.
2. Achermann P, Dijk DJ, Brunner DP, Borbely A. A model of human sleep homeostasis based on EEG slow-wave activity: quantitative comparison of data and simulations. Brain Res Bull. 1993;31:97–113.
3. Borbely AA, Baumann F, Brandies D, Strauch I, Lehmann D. Sleep deprivation: effect on sleep stages and EEG power density in man. Electroencephalogr Clin Neurophysiol. 1981;51:483–93.

4. Dijk DJ, Czeiler CA. Paradoxical timing of the circadian rhythm of sleep propensity serves to consolidate sleep and wakefulness in humans. Neurosci Lett. 1994;166:63–8.

5. Akerstedt T, Folkard S. The three-process model of alertness and its extension to performance, sleep latency and sleep length. Chronobiol Int. 1997;14:115–23.

6. Dijk DJ, Duffy JF, Czeiler CA. Circadian and sleep/wake dependent aspects of subjective alertness and cognitive performance. J Sleep Res. 1992;1:112–7.

7. Lusardi P, Zoppi A, Preti P, Pesce RM, Piazza E, Forari R. Effects of insufficient sleep on blood pressure in hypertensive patients. Am J Hypertens. 1999;12:63–8.

8. Cooper KR, Phillips BA. Effect of short-term sleep loss on breathing. J Appl Physiol. 1982;53(4):855–8.

9. O'Donnell CP, King ED, Schwartz AR, Smith PL, Robotham JL. Effect of sleep deprivation on responses to airway obstruction in the sleeping dog. J Appl Physiol. 1994;77(4):1811–8.

10. Jarrett M, Heitkemper M, Cain KC, Burr RL, Hertig V. Sleep disturbance influences gastrointestinal symptoms in women with irritable bowel syndrome. Dig Dis Sci. 2000;45(5):952–9.

11. Bergmann BM, Everson CA, Kushida CA, Fang VS, Leitch C, Schoeller D, Refetoff S, Rechtschaffen A. Sleep deprivation in the rat: V. Energy use and mediation. Sleep. 1989;12(1):31–41.

12. Frederickson CJ, Rechtschaffen A. Effects of sleep deprivation on awakening thresholds and sensory evoked potentials in the rat. Sleep. 1978;1:69–82.

13. Borbely AA, Tobler I, Hanagasioglu M. Effect of sleep deprivation on sleep and EEG power spectra in the rat. Behav Brain Res. 1984;14:171–82.

14. Akerstedt T, Gillberg M. The circadian variation of experimentally displaced sleep. Sleep. 1981;4:159–69.

15. Pilcher JJ, Huffcutt AI. Effects of sleep deprivation on performance: a meta-analysis. Sleep. 1996;19(4):318–26.

16. Johnson LC. Physiological and psychological changes following total sleep deprivation. In: Kales A, editor. Sleep physiology and pathology. Philadelphia: JB Lippincott; 1969. p. 206–20.

17. Tyler DB. Psychological changes during experimental sleep deprivation. Dis Nerv Syst. 1955;16:293–9.

18. Bonnet MH. Effect of sleep disruption on sleep, performance and mood. Sleep. 1985;8(1):11–9.

19. Blagrove M, Alexander C, Horne JA. The effects of chronic sleep reduction on the performance of cognitive tasks sensitive to sleep deprivation. Appl Cognit Psychol. 1995;9:21–40.

20. Deaton M, Tobias JS, Wilkinson RT. The effect of sleep deprivation on signal detection parameters. Q J Exp Psychol. 1971;23:449–52.

21. Smith A, Maben A. Effects of sleep deprivation, lunch, and personality on performance, mood and cardiovascular function. Physiol Behav. 1993;54:967–72.

22. Norton R. The effect of acute sleep deprivation on selective attention. Br J Psychol. 1970;61:157–61.

23. Herscovitch J, Broughton R. Performance deficits following short-term partial sleep deprivation and subsequent recovery oversleeping. Can J Psychol. 1981;35:309–22.

24. Dinges DF, Pack F, Williams K, Gillen KA, Powell JW, Ott GE, Aptowich C, Pack AL. Cumulative sleepiness, mood disturbance, and psychomotor vigilance performance decrements during a week of sleep restricted to 4–5 hours per night. Sleep. 1997;20:267–77.

25. Polzella DJ. Effects of sleep deprivation on short-term recognition memory. J Exp Psychol. 1975;104:194–200.

26. Drummond PA, Brown GG, Wong EC, Gillin JC. Sleep deprivation-induced reduction in cortical functional response to serial subtraction. Neuroreport. 1999;10:3745–8.

27. Heuer H, Klein W. One night of total sleep deprivation impairs implicit learning in the serial reaction task, but not the behavioral expression of knowledge. Neuropsychology. 2003;17:507–16.

28. Stickgold R, James LT, Hobson JA. Visual discrimination learning requires sleep after training. Nat Neurosci. 2000;3:1237–8.

29. Plihal W, Born J. Effect of early and late nocturnal sleep on declarative and procedural memory. J Cogn Neurosci. 1997;9:534–47.
30. Plihal W, Born J. Effects of early and late nocturnal sleep on priming and spatial memory. Psychophysiology. 1999;36:571–82.
31. Meddis R. Cognitive dysfunction following loss of sleep. In: Burton A, editor. The pathology and psychology of cognition London: Methuen; 1982. p. 225–252.
32. Dorrian J, Lamond N, Dawson D. The ability to self-monitor performance when fatigued. J Sleep Res. 2000;9:137–44.
33. Steyvers FJJM, Gaillard AWK. The effects of sleep deprivation and incentives on human performance. Psychol Res. 1993;55:64–70.
34. Horne JA, Pettitt AN. High incentive on vigilance performance during 72 hours of total sleep deprivation. Acta Psychol. 1985;58:123–39.
35. Horne J, Reyner L. Vehicle accidents related to sleep: a review. Occup Environ Med. 1999;56(5):289–94.
36. Philip P, Taillard J, Guilleminault C, Quera Salva MA, Bioulac B, Ohayon M. Long distance driving and self-induced sleep deprivation among automobile drivers. Sleep. 1999;22:475–80.
37. Mitler MM, Miller JC, Lipsitz JJ, Walsh JK, Wylie CD. The sleep of long-haul truck drivers. N Engl J Med. 1997;337:755–61.
38. Connor J, Norton R, Ameratunga S, et al. Driver sleepiness and risk of serious injury to car occupants: population based case control study. BMJ. 2002;324:1125.
39. Young T, Finn L, Peppard PE, Szklo-Coxe M, Austin D, Nieto J, Stubbs R, Hla KM. Sleep disordered breathing and mortality: eighteen-year follow-up of the Wisconsin sleep cohort. Sleep. 2008;31(8):1071–8.
40. Jackson ML, Howard ME, Barnes M. Cognition and daytime functioning in sleep-related breathing disorders. Prog Brain Res. 2011;190:53–66.
41. Beebe DW, Groesz L, Wells C, Nichols A, McGee K. The neuropsychological effects of obstructive sleep apnea: a meta-analysis of norm-referenced and case-controlled data. Sleep. 2003;26:298–307.
42. Greenberg GD, Watson RK, Deptula D. Neuropsychological dysfunctions in sleep apnea. Sleep. 1987;10:254–62.
43. Kales A, Caldwell A, Candieux R, Velabueno A, Ruch L, Mayers S. Severe obstructive sleep apnea: II. Associated psychopathology and psychological consequences. J Chronic Dis. 1985;38:427–34.
44. Redline S, Strauss ME, Adams N, et al. Neuropsychological function in mild sleep disordered breathing. Sleep. 1997;20:160–7.
45. Ayalon L, Ancoli-Israel S, Aka AA, McKenna BS, Drummond SP. Relationship between obstructive sleep apnea severity and brain activation during a sustained attention task. Sleep. 2009;32(3):373–81.
46. Naismith S, Winter V, Gotsopoulos H, Hickie I, Cistulli P. Neurobehavioral functioning in obstructive sleep apnea: differential effects of sleep quality, hypoxemia and subjective sleepiness. J Clin Exp Neuropsychol. 2004;26(1):43–54.
47. Bedard MA, Montplaisir K, Richer F, Rouleau I, Malo J. Obstructive sleep apnea syndrome: pathogenesis of neuropsychological deficits. J Clin Exp Neuropsychol. 1991;1:950–64.
48. Bawden FC, Oliveira CA, Caramelli P. Impact of obstructive sleep apnea on cognitive performance. Arq Neuropsiquiatr. 2011;69(4):585–9.
49. Salorio CF, White DA, Piccirillo J, Duntley SP, Uhles ML. Learning, memory, and executive control in individuals with obstructive sleep apnea syndrome. J Clin Exp Neuropsychol. 2002;24:93–100.
50. Naegele B, Thouvard V, Pepin J, Levy P, Bonnet C, Perret J, et al. Deficits of cognitive executive functions in patients with sleep apnea syndrome. Sleep. 1995;18:43–52.
51. Findley LJ, Unverzagt ME, Suratt PM. Automobile accidents involving patients with obstructive sleep apnea. Am Rev Respir Dis. 1988;138:337–40.

52. Haraldsson PO, Carenfelt C, Diderichsen F, Nygren A, Tingvall C. Clinical symptoms of sleep apnea syndrome and automobile accidents. ORL J Otorhinolaryngol Relat Spec. 1990;52:57–62.
53. Wu H, Yan-Go F. Self-reported automobile accidents involving patients with obstructive sleep apnea. Neurology. 1996;46:1254–7.
54. George CF, Smiley A. Sleep apnea and automobile crashes. Sleep. 1999;22:790–5.
55. Antonopolous CN, Sergentanis TN, Daskalopoulou SS, Petridou ET. Nasal continuous positive airway pressure (nCPAP) treatment for obstructive sleep apnea, road traffic accidents and driving simulator performance: a meta-analysis. Sleep Med Rev. 2011;15(5):301–10.
56. Matthews EE, Aloia MS. Cognitive recovery following positive airway pressure (PAP) in sleep apnea. Prog Brain Res. 2011;190:70–83.
57. Cooke JR, Ayalon L, Palmer BW, Loredo JS, Corey-Bloom J, Natarajan L, Liu L, Ancoli-Isreal S. Sustained use of CPAP slows deterioration of cognition, sleep, and mood in patients with Alzheimer's disease and obstructive sleep apnea: a preliminary study. J Clin Sleep Med. 2009;5(4):305–9.
58. Ohayon MM. Epidemiology of insomnia: what we know and what we still need to learn. Sleep Med Rev. 2002;6(2):97–111.
59. Fortier-Brochu E, Beaulieu-Bonneau S, Ivers H, Morin CM. Insomnia and daytime cognitive performance: a meta-analysis. Sleep Med Rev. 2012;16:83–94.
60. Kessler RC, Berglund PA, Coulouvrat C, Hajak G, Roth T, Shahly V, Shillington AC, Stephenson JJ, Walsh JK. Insomnia and the performance of US workers: results from the America insomnia survey. Sleep. 2011;34(9):1161–71.
61. Orff HJ, Drummon SP, Nowakowski S, Perlis ML. Discrepancy between subjective symptomatology and objective neuropsychological performance in insomnia. Sleep. 2007;30(9):1205–11.
62. Covassin N, de Zambotti M, Sarlo M, de Min Tona G, Sarasso S, Stegagno L. Cognitive performance and cardiovascular markers of hyperarousal in primary insomnia. Int J Psychophysiol. 2011;80:79–86.
63. Edinger JD, Means MK, Carney CE, Krystal AD. Psychomotor performance deficits and their relation to prior nights' sleep among individuals with primary insomnia. Sleep. 2008;31(5):599–607.
64. Kronholm E, Sallinen M, Era P, Suutama T, Sulkava R, Partonen T. Psychomotor slowness is associated with self-reported sleep duration among the general population. J Sleep Res. 2011;20:288–97.
65. Fernandez-Mendoza J, Calhoun S, Bixler EO, et al. Insomnia with objective short sleep duration is associated with deficits in neuropsychological performance: a general population study. Sleep. 2010;33(4):459–65.
66. Holbrook AM, Crowther R, Lotter A, Cheng C, King D. Meta-analysis of benzodiazepine use in the treatment of insomnia. CMAJ. 2000;162(2):225–33.
67. Johnson LC, Chernik DA. Sedative-hypnotics and human performance. Psychopharmacology. 1982;76:101–13.
68. Bixler EO, Kales A, Manfredi RL, Vgontzas AN, Tyson KL, Kales JD. Next-day memory impairment with triazolam use. Lancet. 1991;337:827–31.
69. Nakra BRS, Gfeller JD, Hassan R. Triazolam on residual, daytime performance in elderly insomniacs. Int Psychogeriatr. 1992;4(1):45–53.
70. Dujardin K, Guieu JD, Leconte-Lambert C, Leconte P, Borderies P, de la Giclais B. Comparison of the effects of zolpidem and flunitrazepam on sleep structure and daytime cognitive functions. Pharmacopsychiatry. 1998;31:14–8.
71. Leufkens TRM, Lund JS, Vermeeren A. Highway driving performance and cognitive functioning the morning after bedtime and middle-of-the-night use of gaboxadol, zopiclone and zolpidem. J Sleep Res. 2009;18:387–96.
72. Morin CM, Bootzin RR, Buysee DJ, et al. Psychological and behavioral treatment of insomnia: update of the recent evidence (1998–2004). Sleep. 2004;29(11):1398–414.

73. Altena E, Van der Werf YD, Strijers RLM, Van Someren EJW. Sleep loss affects vigilance: effects of chronic insomnia and sleep therapy. J Sleep Res. 2008;17:335–43.
74. Miro E, Lupianez J, Martinez MP, Sanchez AI, Diaz-Piedra C, Guzman MA, Buela-Casal G. Cognitive-behavioral therapy for insomnia improves attentional function in fibromalgia syndrome: a pilot, randomized-controlled trial. J Health Psychol. 2011;16:770–82.
75. Reid KJ, McGee-Kock LL, Zee PC. Cognition in circadian rhythm disorders. Prog Brain Res. 2011;190:3–20.
76. Kleitman N. Sleep and wakefulness. Chicago: University of Chicago Press; 1963.
77. Cajochen C, Khalsa SB, Wyatt JK, Czeisler CA, Dijk DJ. EEG and ocular correlates of circadian melatonin phase and human performance decrements during sleep loss. Am J Physiol. 1999;277:R640–9.
78. Oosterman JM, van Someren EJ, Vogels RL, Van Harten B, Scherder EJ. Fragmentation of the rest-activity rhythm correlates with age-related cognitive deficits. J Sleep Res. 2009;18:129–35.
79. Riemersma-van der Lek RF, Swaab DF, Twisk J, Hol EM, Hoogendijk WJ, Van Someren EJ. Effect of bright light and melatonin on cognitive and noncognitive function in elderly residents of group care facilities: a randomized controlled trial. JAMA. 2008;299:2642–55.
80. ICSD-2. The international classification of sleep disorders: diagnostic and coding manual. Westchester: American Academy of Sleep Medicine; 2005.
81. Akerstedt T. Shift work and disturbed sleep/wakefulness. Occupational Med. 2003;53:89–94.
82. Federal Motor Carrier Safety Administration. Large truck crash facts. FMCSA-Ri02-003. 2002;34:29.
83. National Transportation Safety Board. Factors that affect fatigue in heavy truck accidents. Vol 1: Analysis. Safety Study NTSB/SS-95/01, Washington; 1995.
84. National Transportation Safety Board. Greyhound Run-off-the-road accident, Burnt Cabins, Pennsylvania, June 20, 1998. Highway Accident Report NTSB/HAR-00/01/Washington, DC/2000.
85. Cruz C, Della Rocco P. Investigation of sleep patterns among air traffic control specialists as a function of time off between shifts in rapidly rotating work schedules. In: Proceedings of the eighth international symposium on aviation psychology, vol. 2. Columbus: Ohio State University; 1995. p. 974–9.
86. Barger LK, Cade BE, Ayas NT, Cronin JW, Rosner B, Speizer FE, et al. Extended work shifts and the risk of motor vehicle crashes among interns. NEJM. 2005;352:125–34.
87. Rajaratnam SMW, Barger LK, Lockley SW, Shea SA, Wang W, Landrigan CP, O'Brien CS, Qadri S, Sullivan JP, Cade BE, Epstein LJ, White DP, Czeisler CA. Sleep disorders, health and safety in police officers. JAMA. 2011;306(23):2567–78.
88. Dawson D, Reid K. Fatigue, alcohol and performance impairment. Nature. 1997;388:235.
89. Gander PH, Merry A, Millar MM, Wellers J. Hours of work and fatigue-related error: a survey of New Zealand anaesthetists. Anaesth Intensive Care. 2000;28:178–83.
90. Wu AW, Folkman S, McPhee SJ, Lo B. Do house officers learn from their mistakes? JAMA. 1991;265(16):2089–94.
91. Rouch I, Wild P, Ansiau D, Marquie JC. Shiftwork experience, age and cognitive performance. Ergonomics. 2005;48:1282–93.
92. Gumenyuk V, Roth T, Korzyukov O, Jefferson C, Kick A, Spear L, et al. Shift work sleep disorder is associated with attenuated brain response of sensory memory and an increased brain response to novelty: an ERP study. Sleep. 2010;33:703–13.
93. Czeisler CA, Walsh JK, Roth T, Hughes RJ, Wright KP, Kingsbury L, et al. Modafinil for excessive sleepiness associated with shift-work disorder. NEJM. 2005;353:476–86.
94. Czeisler CA, Walsh JK, Wesnes KA, Arora S, Roth T. Armodafinil for treatment of excessive sleepiness associated with shift-work disorder: a randomized controlled trial. Mayo Clin Proc. 2009;84:958–72.
95. Beh HC, McLaughlin P. Effect of long flights on the cognitive performance of air crew. Percept Mot Skills. 1997;84:319–22.

96. Haughty GT. Individual differences in phase shifts of the human circadian system and performance deficit. Life Sci Space Res. 1967;5:135–47.
97. Cho K. Chronic 'jet lag' produces temporal lobe atrophy and spatial cognitive deficits. Nat Neurosci. 2001;4:567–8.
98. Cho K, Ennaceur A, Cole JC, Suh CK. Chronic jet lag produces cognitive deficits. J Neurosci. 2000;20:RC66.
99. Broughton R, Ghanem Q, Hishikawa Y, Sugita Y, Nevsimalova S, Roth B. Life effects of narcolepsy in 180 patients from North America, Asia and Europe compared to matched controls. Can J NeuroSci. 1981;8:299–304.
100. Rogers AE, Rosenberg RS. Tests of memory in narcoleptics. Sleep. 1990;13:42–52.
101. Aguirre M, Broughton R, Stuss D. Does memory impairment exist in narcolepsy-cataplexy? J Clin Exp Neuropsychol. 1985;7:14–24.
102. Naumann A, Bellebaum C, Daum I. Cognitive deficits in narcolepsy. J Sleep Res. 2006;15:329–38.
103. Bayard S, Abril B, Yu H, Scholz S, Carlander B, Dauvilliers Y. Decision making in narcolepsy with cataplexy. Sleep. 2011;34(1):99–104.
104. Delazer M, Hogl B, Zamarian L, Wenter J, Gschliesser V, Ehrmann L, Brandauer E, Cevikkol Z, Frauscher B. Executive functions, information sampling, and decision making in narcolepsy with cataplexy. Neuropsychology. 2011;25(4):477–87.
105. Becker PM, Schwartz JR, Feldman NT, Hughes RJ. Effect of modafinil on fatigue, mood and health-related quality of life in patients with narcolepsy. Psychopharmacology. 2004;171:133–9.
106. Schwartz JRL, Nelson MT, Schwartz ER, Hughes RJ. Effects of modafinil on wakefulness and executive function in patients with narcolepsy experiencing late-day sleepiness. Clin Neuropharmacol. 2004;27:74–9.

Chapter 6
Fatigue: Clinical and Laboratory Assessment

Max Hirshkowitz and Amir Sharafkhaneh

Definitions

To assess fatigue, one first must establish a working concept and operational definitions. Although details may vary, common elements for defining human fatigue include the following [1, 2]:

- Fatigue is perceived as a sense of tiredness, exhaustion, and/or lack of energy.
- Fatigue is often provoked by exceeding physical or mental capacity with increasing time-on-task, stress load, or both.
- Stress load increases may stem from external factors (work demand and poor workplace design) and/or internal factors (medical, neurological, and psychiatric illness; psychological stressors; and sleepiness).
- Fatigue increases the potential for performance failure.
- Sleepiness is one of the most important stressors provoking fatigue.

Fatigue can be non-pathological (i.e., part of the natural rest-activity cycle), or it can be pathological (evoked by a disease process). Non-pathological fatigue improves with rest.

M. Hirshkowitz, PhD (✉)
Division of Public Mental Health and Population Sciences, School of Medicine, Stanford University, Stanford, CA, USA

Department of Medicine, Baylor College of Medicine, Houston, TX, USA
e-mail: maxh@bcm.edu

A. Sharafkhaneh, MD, PhD
Department of Medicine, Baylor College of Medicine, Houston, TX, USA

Medical Care Line, Michael E. DeBakey VA Medical Center, Houston, TX, USA

© Springer Science+Business Media, LLC, part of Springer Nature 2018
A. Sharafkhaneh, M. Hirshkowitz (eds.), *Fatigue Management*,
https://doi.org/10.1007/978-1-4939-8607-1_6

Table 6.1 Causes and contributors to sleepiness

Physiological causes	Diseases and conditions
Insufficient sleep	Obstructive sleep apnea
Irregular sleep schedule	Narcolepsy and other hypersomnias
Environmentally disrupted sleep	Circadian rhythm disorder
Circadian mismatch	Brain injury
Stimulant withdrawal	Medical, endocrine, or infectious diseases
Sedating drug ingestion	Neurological conditions
	Psychiatric conditions
	Severe insomnia

The terms "fatigue" and "sleepiness" are often used interchangeably. For example, "fatigue-related accidents" usually involve performance decrement or lapses related to inadequate sleep, disrupted sleep, or poorly timed sleep. When fatigue-related accidents threaten public safety, regulatory agencies often impose hours-of-service rules. Also, the close link between sleepiness and fatigue makes sleep schedule and sleep-cycle review the logical starting point for post hoc accident investigations.

Factors Contributing to Human Fatigue

Many factors can contribute to fatigue. Some of these are enumerated in Table 6.1. During assessment, procedures designed to detect and assess potential contribution of these factors should be systematic and thorough.

Homeostatic Drive

Mandated hours-of-service rules aim to reduce sleep deprivation and thereby diminish the potential for fatigue-related accidents. Those industries in which accidents constitute a risk to public safety receive greater attention. Thus, transportation industries receive special scrutiny. When a commercial airliner crashes, few survive. For each truck driver killed in a crash, usually three or four other people also die. After more than six decades without change, the Department of Transportation's Federal Motor Carrier Safety Administration updated the hours-of-service rule. Also, the Accreditation Council for Graduate Medical Education adopted an hours-of-service policy for resident physicians. Both of these rules clearly target sleepiness and aim to reduce sleep deprivation.

Sleep deprivation, inadequate sleep schedule, and prolonged wakefulness all conceptually speak to sleep's homeostatic characteristics. As wakefulness continues beyond typical duration, physiological and biochemical processes increase the drive for sleep. This drive can manifest emotionally, physically, or both. Kleitman framed this as the "hypnotoxic theory" and posited that some substance built up during wakefulness and was removed during sleep [3]. The complimentary metaphor is that a substance is depleted during wakefulness and replaced during sleep. Research indicates both occur; however, no simple bodily fluid test exists to index sleep debt.

Prolonged episodes of wakefulness increase sleepiness and create stress, both of which can contribute to fatigue-impaired performance. Individuals may sense they are becoming fatigued; however, the performance failure, not the sensation, is what causes the failure. Much like a machine bolt undergoing metal fatigue, the metal has no awareness it is about to fail, but fail it does. In engineering, instruments and test processes can help alert observers to increasing failure probability. In human fatigue, such instruments do not exist; however, performance failure may result from response slowing, response lapsing, or actual sleep onset.

Unpaid Sleep Debt

Individuals who do not attain adequate amounts of sleep to restore their brain and bodily functions build up a sleep debt. Individuals who acutely or chronically restrict sleep add to their sleep debt. By contrast, compensatory sleep can decrease sleep debt. "Sleeping in" and napping represent common strategies people use to repay their debt. Individuals with unpaid sleep debt are prone to drowsiness, diminished performance, and performance errors. Whether or not sleep debt consequences become manifest depends largely on the individual's reserve capacity to perform, the duration of the task, the amount of sleep debt, and the intrinsic stimulation provided by the task. Obviously, whether the individual is taking stimulants also affects performance.

Circadian Rhythm

Sleep deprivation represents one piece of the fatigue and sleep puzzle. Another key piece involves the circadian rhythm regulation of sleepiness and alertness. The term circadian derives from circa meaning approximately and *dias* meaning day. The circadian rhythm refers to the daily rhythm of sleep and wakefulness. Thus, task performance after 20 continuous hours of prior wakefulness will likely differ when performed at 4:00 AM compared to 11:00 AM. Clearly homeostatic and circadian factors interact with respect to behavior and performance. Homeostatic regulation predicts increasing sleepiness as a function of prior wakefulness; however, during a typical day, we do not become increasingly sleepy as the day progresses. Usually, we are not sleepier at 7 PM than at noon or sleepier at noon than at 7 AM. Under normal circumstances, the circadian alerting process begins in the morning with increasing intensity over the course of the day. This arrangement allows the circadian alerting process to offset increasing homeostatic sleep drive. When this circadian alerting factor declines at night, the residual homeostatic drive is unleashed, and the individual becomes very sleepy.

Without delving into details concerning the underlying neurophysiology, it suffices to say that the human circadian sleep-wake rhythm responds to light and, in particular, the blue part of light's spectrum. An alerting center exists in the hypothalamic suprachiasmatic nucleus (SCN). SCN activity is suppressed by melatonin. Melatonin is released in darkness and is suppressed by light. Thus, darkness allows melatonin to suppress the brain's alerting center.

Shift Work

The risk of performance failure increases when an individual's sleep-wake schedule is out of synch with the circadian rhythm. Studies repeatedly reveal associations between the circadian trough and operational errors and accidents compared to the rhythm's peak. Because the circadian rhythm responds to light, night shift workers are particularly vulnerable. While it is possible to shift one's circadian rhythm with bright light and/or melatonin, staying shifted can be a challenge. Inadvertent light exposure and social pressures to temporarily adopt a daytime schedule (to participate in community, family, or peer group events) undermine attempts to stay shifted. Rotating shifts intentionally move the work period to a different phase in the circadian cycle, thereby destabilizing any progress toward stabilizing one's rhythm.

The night shift worker with a normal daytime entrained circadian rhythm faces an increasing homeostatic sleep drive throughout the work period. They must maintain performance without the hypothalamic alertness center's aid. If this combination of increasing sleep drive and loss of alerting counterbalance exceeds the individual's reserve capacity to perform, the stage is set for a fatigue-related mishap. If the person's reserve capacity is decreased by an "unpaid" sleep debt, the situation deteriorates further.

Shift workers, especially night shift workers, tend to accrue sleep debt due to insomnia. Realize, however, the type of insomnia experienced is rather unique. A typical scenario involves an exhausted individual returning home in the morning. After working all night, their homeostatic sleep drive is near maximum. The individual has no difficulty falling asleep even though their circadian alerting system has become activated (because light has suppressed melatonin release, thereby disinhibiting the alerting system). However, several hours later problems develop. After 4 h the majority of sleep debt is dissipated, but the alerting system has dramatically increased its output. The individuals awaken with difficulty returning to sleep. They may sleep on-and-off for a few more hours and ultimately give up trying to sleep. They get up and start their day, even though they had insufficient sleep. The following night shift work is more difficult because their unpaid sleep debt is taxing their reserve capacity to perform. This cycle tends to self-perpetuate and increases risk for fatigue-related performance decline and accidents.

Sleep Disturbances and Disorders

In the most global sense, sleep serves to restore the brain and body. Much like any system, resupply and waste disposal are needed to maintain function. For humans, some of the key elements occur during sleep. Therefore, several factors influence sleep's restorative capacity, including:

- Sleep time duration
- Sleep timing
- Sleep continuity
- Sleep depth
- Sleep quality

The most obvious and conceptually simplest factor is *sleep time duration*. That is simply the number of hours of sleep a person gets per day. While there is some variation in daily sleep need due to individual differences, most adults need 7–9 h per day. In addition to the amount of time, the *timing of sleep* within the circadian cycle makes a difference. With all other factors being equal, for humans, daytime sleep is less efficient than nocturnal sleep for functional restoration. The difficulties encountered by night shift workers described above speak to the importance of proper "sleep timing" to avoid adverse fatigue-related problems.

Sleep continuity, while less obvious, unarguably plays a key role. If an individual were awakened 90 times per night, but for only 10 s each time, the total sleep duration lost would be merely 15 min. However, the adverse effects of such disruption would be immense and could not be compensated for by 15 min of additional sleep. By contrast, *sleep depth* is hidden within the structure of sleep. Sleep is not a single process. Differences in brain, eye, and muscle activity suggest sleep can be separated into distinct stages. One stage in particular is characterized by high voltage, low frequency brain activity. Some sleep scientists and clinicians argue that this "slow wave sleep" represents deeper sleep, and it contributes preferentially to sleep's restorative function. Sleep research mostly supports this conceptualization. Furthermore, some individuals suffering from fatigue-related disorders have diminished or altered slow wave sleep.

Sleep quality, while conceptually attractive, is difficult to define or measure. Sleeping soundly is the common language descriptor for what is meant. Individuals who self-rate their sleep as poor quality may feel a need to sleep more or indicate they awaken unrefreshed. Quality may turn out to be a composite of all of the factors influencing sleep's restorative function. Nonetheless, we may need less sleep if it is high quality and more when it is low quality.

Sleep disorders can adversely affect sleep in several ways, including:

- Reducing sleep time
- Reducing sleep continuity
- Reducing sleep quality
- Directly altering the mechanisms controlling sleep and/or wakefulness

Specific sleep disorders can adversely affect sleep in any single or combination of the ways indicated above. An untreated sleep disorder can severely tax an individual's reserve capacity. The resulting unremitting stress from sleepiness increases the odds of fatigue-related performance failure or accident.

Some sleep disorders decrease overall sleep duration. An individual with sleep onset insomnia may have delayed sleep onset but nonetheless awaken at the same time each morning. Whether the delayed sleep onset is related to anxiety, depression, substance use, environmental factors (e.g., noise), medical condition (e.g., pain), or neurological condition, the end result is reduced sleep time.

Many sleep disorders, including those that primarily reduce sleep duration, also fragment sleep. Environmental factors (e.g., noise, temperature, and allergens), medical factors (e.g., pain), and work schedules producing chaotic sleep-wake cycles notoriously reduce sleep continuity. Obstructive sleep apnea can severely fragment sleep. Once the upper airway collapses during an obstructive apnea episode, a several second or longer awakening must occur to reopen the airway so breathing can resume. In severe cases, more than 400 such sleep disruptions may occur in a single night. Additionally, there may be blood oxygen desaturations and momentary wild swings in blood pressure. If untreated, the net result over time includes sleepiness, hypertension, and heart disease. Other sleep-related movement disorders (e.g., periodic limb movement disorder and sleep bruxism) may similarly fragment sleep thereby reducing sleep continuity.

Sleep quality, while a conceptually attractive concept, is somewhat elusive. As previously mentioned, it is difficult to quantify. However, sleep disorders research often involves recording brain, eye, muscle, breathing, leg movement, heart rhythm, blood oxygenation, and snoring sounds in the laboratory. These sleep study recordings are called polysomnograms and the recording process polysomnography. It is possible to grade an individual's polysomnograms for its approximation to the norm. A wide variety of measures can be tabulated, including (but not limited to) sleep efficiency, sleep stage percentages, latency to sleep onset, and sleep stability (based on the phenomenon cyclic alternating pattern). Such parameters can be used individually or combined to index sleep quality. Sleep researcher has reported many aberrations associated with sleep disorders, some generally sensitive and others quite specific. This research arena, however, is still mainly investigational.

Sleep disorders can also stem from pathophysiologies of the basic underlying neurological mechanism controlling sleep and wakefulness. In such cases, sleep duration, continuity, and quality may appear normal; however, the individual remains drowsy, excessively sleepy, and unable to perform. Such disorders can be debilitating but thankfully they are rare.

Medical, Neurological, and Psychological Factors

In addition to sleep disorders, many medical, neurological, psychological, and psychiatric conditions are associated with fatigue.

Medical Factors

Patients with chronic cardiorespiratory conditions commonly report fatigue. In patients with congestive heart failure, chronic obstructive pulmonary disease, and asthma, the fatigue is attributed to changes in muscle structure, deteriorated nutritional status, hypoxia, comorbid conditions, and medications. Sleep problems (e.g., insomnia) secondary to these diseases also contribute to fatigue. Fatigue is also associated with renal, hematological, and endocrine pathologies. Mechanisms underlying fatigue in chronic kidney disease are attributed to anemia, protein energy wasting, depression, uremia, and mineral and bone disorders. Endocrine disorder-related fatigue occurs in hypothyroidism, adrenal insufficiency, pituitary conditions, hypogonadism, diabetes, hypercalcemia, and parathyroid disorders. Anemia-related fatigue can arise from infections, malignancies, autoimmune diseases, otherwise benign hematological disorders, chronic kidney disease, and endocrine disorders. Cancer-related fatigue afflicts 70% or more of patients with cancer. It is persistent and distressing. Mood disorders, anemia, myeloid suspension, pain, and electrolyte disturbances play a role. Furthermore, cancer treatments are associated with fatigue, including radiation, chemotherapy, stem cell transplantation, hormonal regimens, and biological treatments.

Neurological Factors

Neurological conditions associated with fatigue are often divided according to whether the fatigue is central, peripheral, or both. Conditions mainly associated with central fatigue include stroke, cerebrovascular disease, demyelinating disease (e.g., multiple sclerosis), infectious disease (e.g., meningitis), sleep disorders, extrapyramidal disorders (e.g., Parkinson's disease), granulomatous disease (e.g., neurosarcoidosis), central nervous system vasculitis, and paraneoplastic disease. Peripheral fatigue accompanies spinal muscle atrophy, myopathies, and neuromuscular junction conditions (e.g., myasthenia gravis). Both central and peripheral fatigue present with post-polio syndrome, myotonic dystrophies, infectious diseases, mitochondrial diseases, amyotrophic lateral sclerosis, and post-Guillain Barre syndrome.

Psychological and Psychiatric Factors

Keeping in mind that any ongoing stressor can undermine performance, especially over time, any psychological and psychiatric conditions can potentially contribute to fatigue. Simple stressors relating to monetary, family, or social problems tax an individual's functional reserve. These same factors can contribute to disrupted sleep mediated by anxiety and worry. When psychological problems reach diagnostic psychiatric criteria, the contribution becomes more substantial. Anxiety disorders, depression, bipolar disorders, dementias, posttraumatic stress disorder, and seasonal affective disorder can contribute to fatigue-related performance failures. These psychiatric illnesses also notoriously disrupt sleep and are associated with chronic fatigue syndromes.

Substance Use

A wide assortment of medications and recreational drugs produce drowsiness, sleepiness, fatigue, and behavioral inertia and can reduce attentional capacity [4]. Medications include (but are not limited to) sedatives, sedative-hypnotics, antipsychotics, analgesics, anxiolytics, anticancer drugs, antihistamines, and certain antidepressants. Alcohol and some forms of cannabis can also produce sedation and fatigue. Additionally, it is important to note that withdrawal from stimulants (either prescribed, legal, or illicit) often produces profound sleepiness. Similarly, drugs meant for other purposes may contain stimulants and when discontinued, drowsiness occurs.

Assessment

Overview

In standard clinical practice, patients typically present seeking help. They have a problem, symptom, or impairment. During the clinical encounter, the patient provides information with self-interest to maintain or improve health. A patient may shape self-reported accounts during clinical interview due to personality type (e.g., minimizers vs. exaggerators), defense mechanisms (e.g., denial), embarrassment, or social concerns (e.g., infidelity). Nonetheless, the information obtained is mostly accurate. In stark contrast, when an individual needs evaluation for regulatory purposes, things dramatically change. The situation becomes very biased, and the individual often feels he or she is there to prove something.

Fatigue assessment can be difficult. Quantitatively, few indices provide guidance. Assessments conducted for regulatory purposes or compensation are complicated by each situation's demand characteristics, the individual's agenda, or both. When conducting a "fit for duty" evaluation, the person undergoing testing usually has a stake in the outcome. If he or she desires to go back to work, they will likely minimize or deny drowsiness, sleepiness, and fatigue. This holds even more so if the evaluation occurs in the wake of an accident or error. By contrast, individuals seeking compensation may exaggerate their problems. Consequently, clinicians realize any self-reported information will likely contain bias. Additionally, any tests demanding cooperation to achieve valid results also require careful scrutiny. For example, performance tests require "best effort," but a person seeking compensation may not try as hard in order to appear more impaired. The opposite agenda, that is, to appear less impaired on a sleep propensity test can also be strategically defeated. Sleep propensity instructs an individual to "relax and allow yourself to fall asleep," instructions roundly ignored if the individual's intention involves remaining awake.

From the standpoint of normal physiology, fatigue is considered weakness (or weariness) produced by repeated exertion or decreased cellular, tissues, or organ response after excessive stimulation (or activity). Normally, function recovers after rest. Stressors promote fatigue. In non-pathological mental fatigue, sleepiness is usually the primary stressor. Many forms of fatigue include both a physical and mental component. Therefore, it is understandable why fatigue and sleepiness are so often equated.

Individuals being evaluated for fatigue should have standard medical, neurological, and psychiatric assessments to determine if diseases or conditions previously described in Section IIF are present. It is beyond the scope of this chapter to discuss details of such evaluations; however, guidance can be found in other chapters in this book.

Sleep Schedule and Timing

Assessing an individual's sleep schedule and habits provides essential information when evaluating fatigue. Establishing sleep duration, sleep timing, and sleep quality are key elements. This serves both a priori assessment for establishing (or reestablishing) fitness-for-duty or a posteriori evaluation conducted in an accident's wake. A series of simple questions can characterize usual sleep duration, sleep schedule, sleep schedule variability, napping, and environmental factors potentially affecting sleep (see Table 6.2). However, because this information is self-reported, situational demand characteristics may diminish accuracy. For example, an individual may

Table 6.2 Sleep schedule questions

1. What time do you typically go to bed on work days (provide as a range, if it varies an hour or more)?		
2. What time do you typically awaken and get out of bed on work days (provide as a range, if it varies an hour or more)?		
3. What time do you typically go to bed on non-work days (provide as a range, if it varies an hour or more)?		
4. What time do you typically awaken and get out of bed on non-work days (provide as a range, if it varies an hour or more)?		
5. How many naps do you typically take per week?	_______ per week	
6. How long is one of your typical naps?	_______ minutes	
7. Are your naps refreshing (circle one)?	Yes	No

wish to minimize the apparent level of their sleep deprivation and thereby overreport their sleep schedule duration. In situations where obvious primary and secondary gains hinge on self-reported information, validation requires objective measures.

Usual bed times and arising times on work days provide a good starting point. These data establish whether the major sleep cycle occupies the daytime or nighttime. Sometimes, the schedule will partially overlap both day- and nighttime. Non-night sleep schedules on work days commonly indicate night shift work. Night shift workers not only have an increased vulnerability for fatigue but also to insomnia, absenteeism, and some medical problems. Workers on rotating shifts suffer similar problems.

Of course, usual bed and arising times allow calculation of approximate time in bed. It is a safe bet that time in bed will exceed total sleep time (unless sleep efficiency is 100%). Once work day bed times and arising times are established, they can be compared to bed and arising times on non-work days. Any change in schedule going from work to non-work days affords additional useful information. Is sleep on non-work days extended or reduced? Is the sleep period shifted to begin and end at later times than on work days (phase delayed)? Alternatively, on non-work days does the sleep period begin and end earlier (phase advanced)? Or… is duration and phase altered? Sometimes, the sleep schedule is too chaotic to reasonably characterize as extended, reduced, advance, or delayed; that in itself is telling.

Routinely extending the time in bed on non-work days often indicates inadequate sleep during work days. Chronic sleep deprivation increases potential for fatigue-related errors and performance failure.

Augmenting the sleep history with a 3–4 week sleep diary can provide additional insight and document night-to-night variability. For evaluations conducted for regulatory purposes, actigraphy should also be considered to objectively document the rest-activity cycle (see section below). Sleep diaries can track self-reported time taken to fall asleep; amount of time slept; number of awakenings; overall sleep quality; sleep satisfaction; caffeine use and timing; medication use and timing; napping; meals; work times; and exercise times, frequency, and strenuousness. The diary's usefulness depends on how diligently it is maintained. An accurate diary can identify factors adversely affecting sleep.

Additional Sleep-Related Testing

Sleep Disorders Screening Tests

Many psychometric instruments are available for evaluating sleep and fatigue. The three most commonly used are the STOP-BANG questionnaire [5], the Epworth sleepiness scale [6], and the brief fatigue inventory. In addition to these three, we also recommend administering a mood disorder screening instrument (e.g., Beck or Zung Depression Inventories), an anxiety disorder screening instrument (e.g., general anxiety disorder GAD-7 or Spielberger state-trait anxiety index), and a generalized sleep problems questionnaire (e.g., Pittsburgh Sleep Quality Index [PSQI], Sleep Disorders Questionnaire [SDQ], or Global Sleep Assessment Questionnaire (GSAQ). More specialized tests to detect insomnia (e.g., Brief Insomnia Questionnaire) and restless legs syndrome also exist (e.g., International Restless Legs Scale). If screening tests detect possible mood, anxiety, or sleep disorders, follow-up with a specialist would be prudent.

Individuals, especially men, who are overweight and work sedentary jobs are at risk for having sleep-disordered breathing. Sleep-disordered breathing often causes sleepiness. The STOP-BANG questionnaire has both high sensitivity and specificity. Affirming five of the eight items strongly suggests sleep-disordered breathing with three indicating possible risks. Questionnaire items are shown below:

1. Do you snore loudly (loud enough to be heard through closed doors)?
2. Are you tired, fatigued, or sleeping during the daytime?
3. Has anyone observed you stop breathing in your sleep?
4. Do you have or are you being treated for high blood pressure?
5. Is your BMI greater than 35 kg/m?
6. Are you over 50 years old?
7. Is your neck circumference greater than 40 cm?
8. Are you male?

The final four items are anthropometric and can either be measured and/or obtained from the medical record. Paper-and-pencil versions of the test provide a conversion table for neck circumference from collar size and a look-up table for BMI by height and weight. The Epworth sleepiness scale is also an eight-item questionnaire that asks the respondent to estimate their probability of dozing (never, slight, moderate, or high) in different situations. The following situations are included:

1. Sitting and reading
2. Watching TV
3. Sitting, inactive in a public place (e.g., a theater or a meeting)
4. As a passenger in a car for an hour without a break
5. Lying down to rest in the afternoon when circumstances permit
6. Sitting and talking to someone
7. Sitting quietly after lunch without alcohol
8. In a car, while stopped for a few minutes in traffic

The Brief Fatigue Inventory is useful to help differentiate some aspects more associated with fatigue compared to sleepiness. It was developed to assess fatigue severity in patients with cancer or patients who were undergoing cancer treatment. It focuses on fatigue's impairment of an individual's ability to function. This ten-question instrument has been well validated and is available in many different languages.

Table 6.3 Polysomnography recording channels

Channels	Activity	Purpose
Frontal, central, and occipital EEG	Brain activity	To classify sleep stages, to recognize sleep onset, and to identify CNS arousals
Left and right EOG	Eye movements	To classify sleep stages and help recognize sleep onset
Submentalis (chin) EMG	Skeletal muscle tone	To classify sleep stages and identify CNS arousals during REM sleep
Single channel ECG	Heart rhythm	To screen for arrhythmias
Nasal-oral thermistors and nasal pressure transducer	Airflow	To identify sleep apnea, hypopnea, and respiratory effort-related arousal events
Chest wall and abdominal movement and/or intercostal EMG	Respiratory effort	To differentiate central from obstructive SRBD events
Pulse oximeter (set to an averaging time of ≤3 s)	Oxygenation	To identify oxyhemoglobin desaturation events and score hypopnea events
Left and right anterior tibialis EMG	Leg movements	To identify activity associated with RLS and PLMD

EEG electroencephalography, *EOG* electrooculography, *EMG* electromyography, *ECG* electrocardiography, *CNS* central nervous system, *REM* rapid eye movement, *SRBD* sleep-related breathing disorder, *RLS* restless legs syndrome, *PLMD* periodic limb movement disorder

Polysomnography

- Polysomnography is a sleep test, usually performed in a laboratory. Its purpose is to diagnose several sleep disorders, specifically sleep-related breathing disorders, narcolepsy, a variety of parasomnias, nocturnal seizures, and other disorders associated with hypersomnolence [7–9]. The American Academy of Sleep Medicine (AASM) Scoring Manual [10] summarizes recommended procedures. In general, continuous bioelectrical and/or sensor recordings are made of brain, eye movement, breathing, heart rhythm, blood oxygen level, and leg movements. Table 6.3 summarizes these procedures. If possible, patients should maintain their usual sleep schedule, diet, and exercise habits; however, a large meal within 2 h of bedtime should be avoided. During the day and evening before testing, patients abstain from alcoholic beverages, naps, and caffeinated beverages.

Home Sleep Testing for Sleep-Disordered Breathing

Home sleep testing usually involves recording cardiopulmonary activity using a portable apparatus worn at night in the patient's home. The apparatus typically records airflow, respiratory effort, heart rate, snoring sounds, and oxyhemoglobin saturation. If a brain wave channel is recorded, central nervous system arousals can also be scored. These tests, especially when conducted for regulatory purposes, may be performed with an attendant present to assure chain of custody and rule out tampering. Clinically, home sleep testing is used to confirm sleep-disordered breathing. However, *home sleep testing cannot rule out sleep apnea* because it is intrinsically less sensitive than polysomnography [11].

Maintenance of Wakefulness Test

The maintenance of wakefulness testing provides an objective measure of an individual's volitional capability to remain awake [12]. Four, 40-min, daytime test sessions are scheduled 2 h apart.[1] The subject sits in a dimly lit room and *attempts to remain awake* while brain, eye movement, and chin muscle activity are recorded. Individuals with normal alertness can remain awake during testing sessions. Additionally, many individuals with mild sleepiness can successfully remain awake on all test sessions. Although the ability to remain awake on all test sessions does not guarantee safety, being unable to remain awake certainly raises concern and indicates significant risk.

Multiple Sleep Latency Test

The multiple sleep latency test is procedurally similar to the maintenance of wakefulness test; however, the subject is instructed to *not resist falling asleep* during test sessions [13]. The multiple sleep latency test objectively indexes sleep tendency. The test may involve four or five test sessions, depending on whether REM sleep occurs during test sessions. The first test session commences approximately 2 h after the subject arises from a prior night's laboratory polysomnography. The same bio-parameters are recorded as in the maintenance of wakefulness test. A mean sleep latency of 5 min (or less) indicates excessive sleepiness.

Actigraphy

An actigraph is a wristwatch-like device that records movement [7]. Often used to confirm self-reported diary information, actigraphy provides objective information about sleep schedule, rest-activity cycle, and circadian patterns. A clinical actigraph should not be confused with consumer electronic devices used for self-monitoring. At present, these consumer devices have not been validated to detecting sleep and wakefulness. Actigraphy shows demonstrated clinical utility [14]; however, we are not aware of any that can assure chain of custody for regulatory purposes.

---

[1] Some regulatory agencies require 60-min test sessions.

Dim Light Melatonin Onset

Melatonin strongly marks the circadian rhythm's placement in a 24-h time period. In the evening, the pineal gland releases melatonin at dusk, and it in turn inhibits a hypothalamic arousal system. Saliva or blood levels of melatonin taken in the evening under conditions of dim light will mark circadian phase. Dim light melatonin onset occurred approximately 2 h before bedtime and 14 h after wake [15] in young healthy normally entrained subjects. Determining dim light melatonin onset can provide information about a person's circadian rhythm.

Clinical Laboratory Testing

Bodily fluids (e.g., blood and urine) can provide useful information concerning possible sleep and fatigue issues. In regulatory and forensic situations, drug testing is usually required. Urinalysis and blood tests for sedating substances, analgesics, stimulants, antihistamines, anxiolytics, alcohol, and illegal substances are routine in the wake of accidents. It should be remembered that withdrawal from stimulants can produce profound sleepiness and fatigue, but detection may be difficult if a substance's half-life is short. Aside from drug testing, other medical drug panels can provide critical information. Thyroid function tests for individuals with fatigue, ferritin testing for restless legs syndrome, and HLA typing for narcolepsy should be considered if clinical suspicion is high.

Follow-Up

To understand fatigue, its causes and its severity, the clinician needs to integrate information obtained by interview, questionnaires, and assessments. A combination of factors often synergize producing fatigue as the end results. Each stressor, be it related to sleep inadequacy, sleep disruption, health problems, ongoing psychological issues, and/or work environment, adds to the problem. Specific problems related to sleep duration, sleep disruption, sleep quality, sleep timing, occult sleep disorders, and adequate time off frequently play a major role. Sometimes the clinician may need to proceed with further testing to explore such factors as indicated by results of initial evaluations. The work environment, work shift scheduling, health-related factors, and lifestyle all must be considered when formulating interventions to manage fatigue. No matter how a clinician proceeds, proper follow-up of the assessment data is needed to outline proper effective interventions.

References

1. Hirshkowitz M. Fatigue, sleepiness, and safety: definitions, assessment, methodology. Sleep Med Clin. 2013;8(2):183–9.
2. Lerman SE, Eskin E, Flower DJ, George EC, Gerson B, Hartenbaum N, Hursch SR, More-Ede M. Fatigue risk management in the workplace. JOEM. 2012;54(2):231–58.
3. Kleitman N. Sleep and wakefulness. Chicago: University of Chicago Press; 1939.
4. Hirshkowitz M, Rose MW, Sharafkhaneh A. Neurotransmitters, neurochemistry, and the clinical pharmacology of sleep. In: Chokroverty S, editor. Sleep disorders medicine. 3rd ed. Philadelphia: Saunders-Elsevier; 2009. p. 67–79.
5. Chung F, Yegneswaran B, Liao P, et al. STOP questionnaire a tool to screen obstructive sleep apnea. Anesthesiology. 2008;108:812–21.
6. Johns MW. A new method for measuring daytime sleepiness: the Epworth sleepiness scale. Sleep. 1991;14:540–5.
7. Hirshkowitz M. Introduction to sleep medicine diagnostics in adults. In: Barkoukis TJ, Matheson JK, Ferber R, Doghramji K, editors. Therapy in sleep medicine. Philadelphia: Elsevier; 2012. p. 28–40.
8. Standards of Practice Committee of the American Academy of Sleep Medicine. Practice parameters for the indications for polysomnography and related procedures: an update for 2005. Sleep. 2005;28:499–521.
9. Mahowald MW, Cramer-Bornemann MA. NREM sleep parasomnias. In: Kryger MH, Roth T, Dement WC, editors. Principles and practice of sleep medicine. Philadelphia: Elsevier/ Saunders; 2005. p. 889–96.
10. Iber C, Ancoli-Israel S, Chesson A, Quan SF for the American Academy of Sleep Medicine. The AASM manual for the scoring of sleep and associated events: rules, terminology and technical specifications. 1st ed. Westchester: American Academy of Sleep Medicine; 2007.
11. Hirshkowitz M, Sharafkhaneh A. Comparison of portable monitoring with laboratory polysomnography for diagnosing sleep-related breathing disorders: scoring and interpretation. Sleep Med Clin. 2011;6:283–92.
12. Mitler MM, Miller JC. Methods of testing for sleepiness. Behav Med. 1996;21:171–83.
13. Carskadon MA, Dement WC, Mitler MM, et al. Guidelines for the multiple sleep latency test (MSLT): a standard measure of sleepiness. Sleep. 1986;9:519–24.
14. Sadeh A. The role and validity of actigraphy in sleep medicine: an update. Sleep Med Rev. 2011;15(4):259–67.
15. Burgess HJ, Savic N, Sletten T, Roach G, Gilbert SS, Dawson D. The relationship between the dim light melatonin onset and sleep on a regular schedule in young healthy adults. Behav Sleep Med. 2003;1(2):102–14.

Chapter 7
Clinical Assessment of Medical, Neurological, and Psychiatric Conditions Associated with Fatigue

Imran Ahmed and Michael Thorpy

Introduction

The perception of fatigue is subjective and difficult to define; therefore, no exact definition has been made. Fatigue can be either physical, mental, or both and is described as an overwhelming sense of tiredness, lassitude, or lack of energy. It is characterized by a decreased ability to initiate or maintain activities and/or difficulty with concentration, memory, or emotional stability. Accordingly, it can affect an individual's ability to physically or mentally function at home or at work and may lead to medical leave or disability from employment. Physical fatigue typically occurs after vigorous muscle activity such as exercising, whereas mental fatigue can occur after intense concentration or frustrating mental tasks, and can result in impaired ability to concentrate, or other forms of impaired executive functioning.

However, the term "fatigue" can be used interchangeably with a phrase suggesting an increased tendency to fall asleep (sleepiness) such as "excessively sleepy," "somnolence," "sleepiness," or "drowsiness." The terms fatigue and sleepiness are used in different clinical or social contexts. Fatigue in sleep medicine is differentiated from sleepiness as a symptom that is not associated with an increased tendency to fall asleep as by definition there is no physiological drive for sleep, so on lying down, sleep does not occur, but instead wakefulness and rest ensues [1–3]. The patient who has significant sleepiness will fall asleep in situations that might otherwise not result in sleep, such as when sitting relaxed, in a lecture, in front of television, or when sitting quietly reading. Sleepiness during waking hours results in cognitive changes that can put the patient at risk of poor educational or work

I. Ahmed, MD (✉) · M. Thorpy, MD
Department of Neurology, Sleep-Wake Disorders Center, Montefiore Medical Center, Bronx, NY, USA

Department of Neurology, Albert Einstein College of Medicine, Bronx, NY, USA
e-mail: iahmed@montefiore.org; thorpy@aecom.yu.edu

© Springer Science+Business Media, LLC, part of Springer Nature 2018
A. Sharafkhaneh, M. Hirshkowitz (eds.), *Fatigue Management*,
https://doi.org/10.1007/978-1-4939-8607-1_7

performance and at risk for accidents, not only motor vehicle accidents but accidents at work or in the home [4]. In the 2008 National Sleep Foundation Poll of 1000 people, over a third of respondents reported falling asleep or dozing off while driving and about 2% of these individuals admitted to having a motor vehicle accident attributable to their sleepiness over the prior year.

Fatigue in nonclinical context, such as when the term is used by the governmental agencies, such as the National Transportation Safety Board (NTSB), or corporate entities, denotes mental or physical fatigue as well as sleepiness that results in impaired cognitive function and work or other activities. The Federal Aviation Administration defines fatigue as: "Fatigue is a condition characterized by increased discomfort with lessened capacity for work, reduced efficiency of accomplishment, loss of power or capacity to respond to stimulation, and is usually accompanied by a feeling of weariness and tiredness." (http://www.faa.gov/pilots/safety/pilotsafety-brochures/media/Fatigue_Aviation.pdf).

This chapter will primarily discuss the role of sleepiness in the clinical assessment of medical, neurological, and psychiatric conditions but will also address physical and mental fatigue that may occur concurrently with, or may be independent of, sleepiness.

Epidemiology

The exact prevalence of fatigue in society or in clinical conditions is difficult to ascertain, as the understanding of fatigue varies depending upon the researcher, or the person asked. Both physical and mental fatigue and sleepiness can occur in association with medical, neurologic, and psychiatric conditions. Subsequently, the prevalence can vary depending on the patient population studied. For instance, the prevalence of fatigue in cancer patients ranged from 37 to 100% [5, 6], for stroke patients it ranged from 40 to 70% [7], and for patients with inflammatory bowel disease, 40% reported fatigue [8]. In the community and primary care setting, fatigue seems to have a prevalence ranging between 7 and 45% [9, 10] and is suspected to be more common in women [11, 12]. In the workplace, about 55% of participants in one study involving 4188 employees were noted to have a sleep disorder and/or a sleep complaint; many of whom were also described as having fatigue [13].

Etiology

There are many possible causes of fatigue, some of which are listed in Table 7.1. Sleep disorders such as insomnia, behaviorally induced insufficient sleep syndrome, shift work sleep disorder, obstructive sleep apnea (OSA), restless legs syndrome, and

Table 7.1 Common causes of fatigue

Medical disorders
Addison's disease
Anemia, including iron deficiency anemia
Anorexia or other eating disorders or malnutrition
Arthritis, including rheumatic disease
Cancer
Congestive heart failure
Diabetes mellitus
Fibromyalgia
Hypercalcemia
Hypo- or hyperthyroidism
Infection (e.g., bacterial endocarditis, HIV/AIDS, cytomegalovirus, tuberculosis, and mononucleosis)
Kidney disease
Liver disease
Persistent pain
Systemic lupus erythematosus
Psychiatric disorders
Anxiety disorder
Depression
Somatization disorder
Alcohol or drugs (e.g., narcotics or cocaine) use
Medications
Antidepressants
Antihistamines
Antihypertensives
Diuretics
Sedatives, hypnotics
Steroids
Neurologic disorders
Multiple sclerosis
Parkinson's disease
Stroke
Sleep disorders
Behaviorally induced insufficient sleep syndrome
Circadian rhythm disorders, e.g., shift work type
Insomnia
Narcolepsy
Sleep apnea
Fatigue syndromes
Chronic fatigue syndrome: (CFS)
Idiopathic (or nonspecific) chronic fatigue

Table 7.2 Key questions in the clinical evaluation

• Can you describe what you mean by fatigue?
• How long have you had fatigue?
• Does your fatigue last all day or does it occur at a certain time of the day or after a certain activity?
• Does your fatigue worsen as the day progresses?
• Have you had fatigue in the past? If so, does it tend to occur in regular cycles?
• How many hours do you sleep each night?
• Do you have trouble falling asleep? Do you wake up during the night?
• Do you wake up in the morning feeling rested or fatigued?
• What is your sleep pattern during the week and on weekends or days off work?
• Do you snore or has anyone ever told you that you snore?
• Has anyone noticed that you have episodes where you stop breathing during sleep?
• Do you feel bored, stressed, unhappy, or disappointed?
• How are your relationships with friends, family, significant others, and/or co-workers?
• Has anyone close to you recently passed away?
• Have you had more activity (mental or physical) lately?
• Do you exercise regularly?
• What is your diet like? Do you eat at regular times during the day?
• Has your diet changed recently?
• Have you lost or gained weight?
• Do you have any other symptoms that are associated with the fatigue, e.g., headaches or nausea?
• Which medications (prescription or over-the-counter) or herbal supplements do you take, if any?

narcolepsy have all been associated with mental fatigue [13] or sleepiness [14]. When the fatigue is due to an underlying medical or psychiatric disorder, usually it is one of several presenting symptoms characteristic of the respective underlying disorder.

The pattern of fatigue and sleepiness may help physicians determine its cause. For instance, patients who awake in the morning feeling refreshed and then shortly afterward develop sleepiness with activity can suggest an underactive thyroid. On the other hand, patients who awake during the early morning hours feeling sleepy and then have a persistent low level of energy or a feeling of sleepiness for the rest of the day may be depressed or have behaviorally induced, insufficient sleep syndrome.

History

When a patient presents to a clinician with fatigue, further clarification may be necessary to better understand whether the complaint is one of insomnia, excessive daytime sleepiness, or sleep deprivation (due to work or personal obligations). When the fatigue is due to a medical illness, the patient typically associates it with activities they are unable to complete, and there are often other symptoms attributable to the medical illness. The etiology of the fatigue can occasionally remain unknown, especially when there are few other associated symptoms. Table 7.2, Key

Questions in the Evaluation of Fatigue, lists some questions that can assist in arriving at a diagnosis. A detailed sleep history coupled with a medical, psychiatric, social, and family history, appropriate questionnaires, and a physical examination are all important in creating a differential diagnosis.

Insomnia

A complaint of insomnia or sleep deprivation (i.e. any combination of difficulty in falling asleep, staying asleep, not sleeping long enough, or feeling unrested upon awakening) is often associated with a complaint of tiredness, fatigue, irritability, and other mood changes during waking hours. These patients can have difficulty carrying on their usual activities such as housework, or activities related to their occupation without a great increase in effort. Patients with insomnia can also complain of memory, concentration, and attention problems, as well as having an abnormal feeling of "fuzziness" or grogginess that occurs intermittently or continuously throughout the day. Chronic insomnias (such as psychophysiological insomnia) are 24-h a day problems so that there is difficulty in sleeping at night as well as difficulty in sleeping during the daytime. Accordingly, patients are often unable to take naps during the daytime [14]. This being said, occasionally, patients with psychophysiologic insomnia may find themselves falling asleep for brief periods when seated and relaxed in the early evening.

Many patients with chronic insomnia will worry about their insomnia during the daytime. Subsequently, as their bedtime approaches, this intense concern about the inability to sleep often results in a further delay in falling asleep at night. In addition, the patient may find that following a bad night of sleep, there is a tendency to stay in bed later the next morning. If fatigued or tired during the daytime, the tendency is to go to bed early to try to get more sleep. As a result, the sleep period often becomes erratic and spread out over a larger portion of the 24-h a day [15]. Any sleep that does occur, therefore, occurs within a 12-h window and at irregular times.

In addition to the patient's worrying about their poor sleep, other information about the patient's waking activities is also necessary. Behaviors when awake can influence sleep quality either positively or adversely. Obtaining information on exercise, exposure to bright light, caffeine or alcohol consumption, and other awake activities are all important aspects of the insomnia history. Daytime bright light exposure and daytime activity are important to strengthen circadian rhythms that ultimately improve sleep quality; however, bright light exposure or exercising (or increased physical activity) during the night (e.g., during a nocturnal awakening or close to bedtime) is counterproductive to good sleep. Conversely, decreased light exposure and inactivity during waking hours can also be detrimental to a good quality sleep.

Caffeine's stimulatory effects can have a negative effect on sleep. Since the half-life of caffeine ranges between 3 and 7 h, even a single serving of a caffeine containing drink in the morning can have adverse consequences on nocturnal sleep for some patients [16]. Alcohol initially has a sedative effect that can facilitate sleep onset; however, once metabolized, it can result in frequent awakenings during the second half of the night. Other activities such as eating large meals, drinking excessive amounts of fluid, smoking, eating stimulating foods (e.g., foods with high sugar or caffeine content), or performing other stimulating activities close to bedtime or during nocturnal awakenings may all be counterproductive.

Napping

A history of napping also provides useful information when evaluating mental fatigue. People typically have a biological inclination to nap during the afternoon or early evening. In fact, a 2008 study by Dautovich et al. found that, at least in older adults, napping during this time resulted in better quality sleep when compared to those who did not nap [17]. Nevertheless, people without a sleep disturbance should be able to remain awake throughout the day, if they desired. Patients with a sleep disturbance, on the other hand, are often unable to resist this midafternoon biological propensity and may feel an overwhelming urge to sleep at this time. Patients with insomnia frequently are in a hyperarousal state and are less likely to fall asleep during the daytime than normal sleepers; as mentioned earlier, these patients often manifest with feelings of irritability, mood changes, and/or fatigue and tiredness. Some patients with psychophysiological insomnia, on the other hand, will involuntarily nap when in a relaxed situation [14]. Additionally, frequent or prolonged napping during the day or napping close to bedtime can contribute to a patient's insomnia. Of note, any patient with a complaint of insomnia with frequent napping should direct the clinician to evaluate for the possibility of other sleep disturbances, such as insufficient sleep syndrome, OSA, or a circadian rhythm disorder.

Patients with a complaint of excessive sleepiness can unintentionally fall asleep (for a variable duration of time) at inappropriate times during waking hours. After the nap, the patient may awaken feeling refreshed or still feeling sleepy. Awakening feeling refreshed is a classic description of the naps that occur in narcolepsy patients [18] as opposed to awakening unrefreshed, which is typical of naps that occur in patients with disrupted nighttime sleep (e.g., due to OSA or idiopathic hypersomnia).

Excessive Daytime Sleepiness

An assessment of excessive sleepiness should attempt to better understand the severity of the patient's sleepiness. Since sleepiness is not always subjectively recognized, questions regarding falling asleep in everyday situations are often more revealing. It is important to find out if the patient tends to fall asleep easily when involved in sedentary activities such as watching television, using a computer, or when reading. It is equally, if not more, important to determine whether the patient

Table 7.3 Epworth sleepiness scale [21]

Situation	Chance of dozing			
Sitting and reading	0	1	2	3
Watching television	0	1	2	3
Sitting, inactive in a public place (e.g., theater or a meeting)	0	1	2	3
As a passenger in a car for an hour without a break	0	1	2	3
Lying down to rest in the afternoon when circumstances permit	0	1	2	3
Sitting and talking to someone	0	1	2	3
Sitting quietly after lunch without alcohol	0	1	2	3
In a car, while stopped for a few minutes in traffic	0	1	2	3

How likely are you to doze off or fall asleep in the situations described below, in contrast to just feeling tired?
0 = would never doze
1 = slight chance of dozing
2 = moderate chance of dozing
3 = high chance of dozing

is significantly sleepy at times when required to be active, especially while driving. It should be considered a medical emergency if a patient falls asleep while driving or even when they have a tendency to doze off while waiting at red traffic lights or when in slow moving traffic. In addition, features regarding narcolepsy (often a missed diagnosis) such as cataplexy, sleep paralysis, and hypnagogic hallucinations should be asked of any patient with sleepiness [18]. Droogleever et al. found that in addition to sleepiness, a majority of narcolepsy with cataplexy patients suffered from severe physical fatigue with subsequent severe functional impairment [19].

As mentioned above, some patients with significant sleepiness may not be aware that they are sleepy. A 2002 study on anesthesia residents by Howard et al. demonstrated that the residents did not perceive themselves to be asleep about half the time they had actually fallen asleep [20]. Accordingly, a history from a bed partner, caretaker, or close friend can be very helpful for collaborating or refuting the patient's statements on sleepiness.

Additionally, questionnaires have been developed to formalize the assessment of a patient's subjective sleepiness. Some of these subjective questionnaires include the Epworth sleepiness scale (ESS), the Karolinska sleepiness scale (KSS), sleep logs, and the visual analog scale (VAS). The ESS is commonly performed on each patient at the initial evaluation, no matter what the sleep complaint, and is often also performed at follow-up visits to measure any change in sleepiness over a 2-week period [21] (Table 7.3). The patient rates their sleepiness severity in eight typical scenarios with a resultant score that ranges from 0 to 24. Patients with a score of ten or higher should be considered to have an abnormal level of daytime sleepiness, and those with a score over 15 have severe daytime sleepiness. Objective measures of a patient's sleepiness and performance are also available and include the multiple sleep latency test (MSLT), the maintenance of wakefulness test (MWT), and the psychomotor vigilance test (PVT). Actigraphy can also be utilized to assess sleepiness; it can give information on the patient's sleep-wake cycle, including sleep duration. The MSLT, however, is the most commonly used objective test of sleepiness. These tests have various applications in different clinical situations and will be discussed later in this chapter.

There are many questionnaires available to subjectively measure fatigue in general (i.e., both physical and mental fatigue). Some are applicable in only research settings; others can be used clinically. The fatigue questionnaire, the fatigue severity scale, the multidimensional assessment of fatigue, and the SF-36-version 1 vitality (energy/fatigue) subscale of the short form health survey are fatigue questionnaires that have all demonstrated excellent internal consistency/reliability and good to excellent validity [22].

Behaviorally Induced Insufficient Sleep Syndrome

Occasionally, when evaluating mental fatigue, the history will reveal the presence of behaviorally induced insufficient sleep syndrome. Behaviorally induced insufficient sleep syndrome is classified under the hypersomnias of central origin category in the ICSD-3. This disorder occurs when patients intentionally deprive themselves of sleep because of some social or work commitments with the end result of obtaining less than their genetically predetermined sleep requirement. Not uncommonly, patients' occupations "unofficially" require them to work extended hours, subsequently limiting the time for personal obligations and leaving only a few hours, if any, for mental/physical relaxation; the part of the patient's life that is frequently sacrificed is their sleep time. The consequences of insufficient sleep (or sleepiness) have been demonstrated in multiple studies. An individual's ability to adapt to chronic sleep deprivation, albeit usually not completely, varies between individuals and is believed to be genetically linked. The period gene PER and the allele HLA DQB1O602 have been proposed as potential biomarkers of interindividual differences in sleepiness, physiological sleep, and fatigue to chronic partial sleep deprivation [23]. Goel et al. have also found that catechol-O-methyltransferase Val158Met polymorphism predicts individual differences in sleep physiology resulting from sleep loss, but not cognitive or executive functioning [24]. Nonetheless, outcomes such as behavioral lapses of attention, needing increased time to complete tasks, impaired cognitive speed, decreased accuracy, learning and recall deficits, and other impaired executive functions have all been noted by various researchers as resulting from insufficient sleep [25–28]. These symptoms should also be included when taking a history.

Circadian Rhythm Disorders

In addition to assessing the severity of sleepiness and its consequences, further questioning should try to elicit the cause of the sleepiness and/or the disrupted sleep. Some patients with a complaint of sleepiness and/or insomnia will have a circadian rhythm sleep disorder that can be determined by obtaining a history of either difficulty in falling asleep or early morning awakening in the presence of sleep episodes that are relatively free of awakenings [14]. Bedtime and wake times are important to determine, not only during the work week but also on weekends or days off work. Similarly, the patient's work schedule should be identified as it may be the major contributor to the patient's poor sleep and subsequent fatigue, typical of shift work sleep disorder. The elderly with a complaint of early morning awakening should be particularly evaluated for advanced sleep phase syndrome and a young adult with a complaint of sleep onset difficulties evaluated for delayed sleep phase syndrome. A sleep log or diary to show the daily sleep pattern is most important in these evaluations; actigraphy testing can serve as a useful adjunct to the sleep diary, especially when the sleep diary is not entirely reliable (e.g., when a caregiver that does not sleep in the same room as the patient is completing the diary for the patient).

Obstructive Sleep Apnea

Obstructive sleep apnea involves repetitive episodes of cessation of breathing (apneas) or partial upper airway obstruction (hypopneas) that is often associated with reduced blood oxygen saturation, snoring, and sleep disruption. Excessive daytime sleepiness, snoring, daytime fatigue, and/or insomnia are not uncommon as the presenting clinical complaint [29–31]. The patient may not report episodes of apnea or gasping or choking; however, the bed partner may observe these events; thus, interviewing the bed partner about the patient's sleep behaviors, as mentioned above, is often helpful.

Aside from the symptoms of snoring, episodes of choking or gasping for air, and witnessed apneic events, other symptoms such as nocturia or if the person is a mouth breather should be identified by history. Romero et al. reported that the symptom of nocturia identified sleep apnea in patients with a sensitivity, specificity, positive predictive value (PPV), and negative predictive value (NPV) of 84.8%, 22.4%, 80.0%, and 27.9%, respectively. He also found that the symptom of nocturia appeared to be comparable to snoring as an initial screen to help identify OSA patients in certain clinic populations [32].

Restless Legs Syndrome

Some patients may have difficulty falling asleep due to pain or leg discomfort that urges them to move their legs in bed, suggesting restless legs syndrome (RLS). This delay in falling asleep can shorten total sleep duration and contribute to daytime symptoms of fatigue. RLS is characterized by a complaint of a nearly irresistible urge to move the legs. This urge tends to have a circadian pattern, usually occurring more frequently in the evening or during the night. It is also worse when at rest and relieved with walking or moving the legs.

Medical Illness

There are many medical illnesses that are directly or indirectly associated with fatigue (Table 7.1). A careful review of systems, including questions screening for pain disorders, thyroid dysfunction, heart failure, diabetes, infections (e.g., HIV, endocarditis, infectious mononucleosis, etc.), connective tissue diseases, or a possible malignancy can often identify the source of fatigue. There are also neurologic disorders, such as Parkinson's disease or multiple sclerosis, which can be identified as the source of fatigue.

Medical and neurologic disorders can disrupt a patient's sleep through pain or discomfort and subsequently result in sleepiness during waking hours. Other disorders directly affect the wake promoting areas of the brain, resulting in sleepiness. Cerebrovascular disease, for example, can disrupt a patient's sleep as there is an increased prevalence of sleep apnea in stroke patients [33, 34]. Metabolic disorders, such as thyroid disease or diabetes, can manifest as excessive sleepiness or disrupt nocturnal sleep [35–39]. Additionally, a review of the patient's medications both prescribed and over-the-counter is necessary when evaluating fatigue.

Psychological and Psychiatric Illnesses

The history should also include questions that attempt to identify certain psychiatric or psychologic disorders. A 2003 study by Darbishire et al. found that about half of their patients with chronic fatigue attributed their symptom to psychological causes [40]. Psychiatric disorders, such as depression or anxiety, chronic fatigue syndrome, and fibromyalgia, are all associated with fatigue.

Mood disorders, such as major depressive disorder, can clinically manifest with excessive daytime sleepiness [14, 41–43]. This sleepiness is believed to be either a manifestation of anergic depression (which also involves lack of interest, withdrawal, deceased energy, or psychomotor retardation) [44] or may be a nonspecific homeostatic coping response to the depressive disorder [45]. Questioning the patient about symptoms of reduced appetite, tearfulness, depressive affect, or suicidal ideation can help identify depression. Standard validated questionnaires are also available as depression screening tools, e.g., the patient health questionnaire (PHQ9) [46] (Table 7.4). In contrast to depressive disorders, excessive sleepiness in anxiety disorders such as nocturnal panic attacks are often due to disrupted nocturnal sleep [47]. If a patient is suspected of having an anxiety disorder, the generalized anxiety disorder assessment questionnaire (GAD-7) can be helpful [47] (Table 7.5).

Conversion disorders can also manifest excessive sleepiness or fatigue. An Australian pediatric study by Kozlowska et al. found fatigue was a common

Table 7.4 The patient health questionnaire (PHQ-9) [46, 84]

	Not at all	Several days	More than half the days	Nearly every day
1. Little interest or pleasure in doing things				
2. Feeling down, depressed, or hopeless				
3. Trouble falling or staying asleep, or sleeping too much				
4. Feeling tired or having little energy				
5. Poor appetite or overeating				
6. Feeling bad about yourself—or that you are a failure or have let yourself or your family down				
7. Trouble concentrating on things, such as reading the newspaper or watching television				
8. Moving or speaking so slowly that other people could have noticed? Or the opposite—being so fidgety or restless that you have been moving around a lot more than usual?				
9. Thoughts that you would be better off dead or hurting yourself in some way?				

Over the last 2 weeks, how often have you been bothered by any of the following problems? (check one in each row)

Table 7.5 Generalized anxiety disorder assessment questionnaire (GAD-7) [47, 85, 86]

	Not at all	Several days	More than half the days	Nearly every day
1. Feeling nervous, anxious, or on edge				
2. Not being able to stop or control worrying				
3. Worrying too much about different things				
4. Trouble relaxing				
5. Being so restless that it is hard to sit still				
6. Becoming easily annoyed or irritable				
7. Feeling afraid as if something awful might happen				

Over the last 2 weeks, how often have you been bothered by the following problems? (check one in each row) complaint in these patients [48]. Additionally, Hicks and Shapiro described a conversion disorder case of narcolepsy with resolution of symptoms after disclosure of severe psychological stress [49]. Furthermore, as with any medical disorder, the clinician must consider the possibility of factitious disorders or malingering [50, 51]; therefore, careful questioning about the patient's psychosocial circumstances is important. Patients have feigned sleepiness and fatigue to procure stimulant medication from physicians.

Family/Social History

Fatigue itself is not known to be hereditary; however, some causes of fatigue, such as diabetes mellitus or anemia, can have a genetic predisposition. Some sleep disorders including sleep apnea syndrome, narcolepsy, and restless legs syndrome also have a familial tendency [14]. Accordingly, appropriate inquiries about the patient's family history need to be made.

Exploring relationships with other family members, determining if there is any financial, personal, or social stressors that may contribute to the patient's sleep disturbance, is a vital part of the social history. Additionally, a history about a patient's recreational drug use and alcohol habits, as well as the level of physical activity, should be investigated.

Physical Exam

The physical examination should complement the history to identify the source of the mental fatigue. The examination should always include determination of the patient's blood pressure and vital signs. Height, weight, body mass index, and neck circumference should all be obtained as well as a determination of the distribution of body fat (e.g., abdominal, neck, etc.) as these can show a patient's predisposition toward sleep-related breathing disorders. Noting the patient's level of alertness, grooming, and the presence of psychomotor agitation or retardation can provide a window to the patient's psychiatric status and/or severity of sleepiness. Thyroid size may prove relevant as thyroid enlargement can contribute to airway obstruction [52–56]. Further evidence of thyroid disease, e.g., goiter, thyroid nodules, ophthalmologic changes, may suggest hypothyroidism as the cause of fatigue. The presence of lymphadenopathy advocates for the possibility of an infectious or malignant etiology to the patient's fatigue. The upper airway evaluation should include determination of airway size, the presence and size of tonsillar tissue, tongue size, and the size and shape of the soft palate and uvula. A cardiopulmonary examination to look for signs of heart or lung disease is necessary as well.

A neurological and vascular evaluation of the extremities may indicate a vascular problem, neuropathy, or a radiculopathy which could be a possible source of nocturnal sleep disruption. Appropriate EMG and nerve conduction studies may be needed for further assessment of possible nerve lesions, while a lower extremity ultrasound or other studies may be required to assess vascular disorders. A neurological examination can also be revealing when evaluating fatigue due to multiple sclerosis, strokes, Parkinson's disease, narcolepsy, idiopathic hypersomnia, or REM sleep behavior disorder.

Laboratory Evaluations

Almost undoubtedly, certain laboratory studies would be required to supplement or confirm any positive information obtained by the history and physical exam; however, in a patient with fatigue, extensive testing is usually of little diagnostic value in the absence of any revealing findings (on history or exam). A 1990 prospective study by Lane et al. on a hundred adults with at least 1 month of fatigue found that laboratory investigations explicated the etiology of the fatigue in only about 5% of patients [57].

Blood Work

Nevertheless, some basic laboratory screening tests are warranted. These may include a complete blood count with differential to look for anemia or an infection, a comprehensive metabolic panel to look for any electrolyte abnormalities or renal disease, liver function tests to assess liver function, and a thyroid-stimulating hormone level to evaluate for thyroid disease. Tests, such as an erythrocyte sedimentation rate, urinalysis, or a hemoglobin A1c test, can also be useful screens. Other studies, such as Lyme titer level, HIV testing, serum and urine toxicology, or a rheumatoid factor test, should also be done on selected patients if there is clinical suspicion [58]. Vitamin D deficiency has also been associated with fatigue and excessive sleepiness and can be assessed if clinically suspected [59, 60].

Patients with clinical suspicion of RLS also require biochemical screening to ensure that there is no evidence of renal impairment or other chemical abnormality. A serum ferritin level and iron studies should be determined [61]. A serum ferritin level of less than 50 μg/L or an iron saturation of less than 16% indicates a need for iron replacement therapy in a patient with RLS [61]. The serum ferritin level is more often used as a measure of cerebral iron stores than the percent iron saturation.

Electroencephalogram (EEG)

Other studies can be tailored to the suspected etiology of the fatigue. For instance, an EEG can be done if sleep-related seizures or subclinical seizures are suspected. A routine EEG with sleep, hyperventilation, and photic stimulation can turn out normal even in patients known to have seizures. This is especially common in patients with mesial frontal lobe seizures [62]. If the EEG is nondiagnostic, then it should be repeated after sleep deprivation. After about three consecutive unrevealing EEGs, a prolonged daytime EEG or long-term video-EEG monitoring for 24 h or longer may be needed if seizures are still clinically suspected. In some severe cases, invasive intracranial recording may be necessary.

Other Studies

An endoscopic evaluation by an otolaryngologist to better define the airway anatomy in suspected OSA patients can be useful in selected patients. It can help determine the location of the obstruction, whether or not it is due to enlarged turbinates, a small nasal choanae, enlarged adenoids or tonsils, or a prolapsing epiglottis. Additionally, cephalometric X-rays on patients who have mandibular abnormalities (e.g., micrognathia or retrognathia) can provide information that is helpful if upper airway surgery is being considered.

Other tests, such as EMG and NCV studies, may be required for better evaluation of a neuropathy or a radiculopathy that is mimicking RLS symptoms. Pulmonary function tests can help identify and determine the severity of pulmonary disorders that may be responsible for the fatigue. A 12-lead EKG, 24-h Holter monitoring, and/or an echocardiogram can help identify cardiac sources of the sleepiness.

Neuroimaging

To date, definitive neuroimaging markers have not been identified for fatigue. Neuroimaging, however, can help determine if a neurologic illness is associated with the fatigue. A MRI of the brain, for instance, can help identify strokes, multiple sclerosis, or seizure foci that can cause the sleepiness. It may also identify other lesions, such as a third ventricle tumor (e.g., colloid cyst), that can cause intermittent episodes of lethargy [63].

Recently, neuroimaging studies evaluating fatigue have identified anatomical changes in the brain. Pellicano and Riccitelli found atrophy of the areas of the parietal cortex in multiple sclerosis patients with fatigue [64, 65]. In another study on chronic fatigue syndrome, de Lange found that the lateral prefrontal cortex was atrophied in these patients, and this atrophy was at least partially reversible with treatment of the fatigue [66].

Polysomnography

In order to better understand the cause of the patient's fatigue, objective evaluation with polysomnographic monitoring may be necessary, especially when disturbed nocturnal sleep is suspected. A polysomnogram is ideally performed for the duration of the patient's major sleep period. Standard placement of electrodes and other sensors measures the various parameters of sleep, including sleep stages, cardiac rhythm, respiratory and muscle activity, as well as oxygen saturation. Videos of patients are also typically recorded throughout the study to identify any abnormal sleep behaviors. Other measures such as end-tidal carbon dioxide concentration, or gastroesophageal pH, body position, or sounds of snoring can also be determined.

Sleep studies are generally not indicated if insomnia is believed to be the cause of the fatigue [67]; however, in some patients, particularly older patients, OSA or other disruptive nocturnal events may underlie the insomnia, and therefore polysomnography may be necessary. In narcolepsy, polysomnography should document the absence of other causes of excessive sleepiness, such as a sleep-related breathing disorder, and is then followed by a multiple sleep latency test (MSLT). If other causes of sleepiness are identified on the polysomnogram, they need to be appropriately treated before a diagnosis of narcolepsy can be confirmed.

Multiple Sleep Latency Test (MSLT)

The severity of sleepiness, regardless of cause, can be objectively assessed with the MSLT. This study, however, is more often utilized to confirm the diagnosis of narcolepsy [68]. It is performed immediately following a polysomnogram that demonstrates at least 7 h of sleep and rules out other causes of the sleepiness, e.g., OSA. The MSLT consists of four or five 20-min nap opportunities that are scheduled at 2-h intervals throughout the day with the first nap occurring approximately 1.5–3 h after awakening from the major sleep period. If the MSLT shows two or more sleep onset REM periods with a mean sleep latency of 8 min or less, it is consistent with a diagnosis of narcolepsy.

Studies defining which mean sleep latency values on MSLT studies are indicative of mild, moderate, or severe sleepiness are limited; however, some studies do offer good approximations of normal values in certain populations [69]. Levine, Roehrs et al. [70], and later John [71] collected and tabulated MSLT data from 176 normal sleepers and determined the MSL to be between 11.1 min (in subjects aged 18–29) and 12.5 min (in subjects age 30–60) with an overall MSL of 11.5 ± 5.1 min. Other smaller studies also calculated the normal MSL to be close to this value [72]. On the other hand, Richardson et al. found severe sleepiness can be identified in patients with a mean sleep latency of 5 min or less over the four or five nap opportunities [73].

REM sleep can occur during any one nap of a MSLT study and still be considered within the normal range. Patients who achieve REM sleep over two or more naps, however, are likely to have a sleep pathology [68, 74–76]. If the patient has a normal amount and percentage of REM sleep at night and two or more sleep onset REM periods occur during the day, then this is highly suggestive of narcolepsy [77]. Alternatively, if a patient has a REM period that occurs within 15 minutes during the preceding baseline polysomnogram and then only has at least one REM period during the MSLT study, this is also suggestive of narcolepsy.

Maintenance of Wakefulness Test (MWT)

The maintenance of wakefulness test (MWT) [78] is similar to the MSLT in that it is performed in much the same way, typically 1.5–3 h after the major sleep period, and consists of "napping" opportunities at 2-h intervals. However, in the MWT, the patient is placed in a semi-reclining position in street clothes and asked to try to remain awake during the four 40-min nap opportunities. The time from lights out to the onset of sleep (defined as three consecutive epochs of stage N1 sleep or any one epoch of stage N2, N3, or REM sleep) for each nap is recorded.

Studies reporting normative MWT values [79] are scarcer than those for MSLTs. A total of 97.5% of the 64 normal subjects studied had a mean sleep latency of >8.0 min, and 59% of normal subjects remained awake for the entire 40 min across each of four nap opportunities. Accordingly, a mean sleep latency <8.0 min on the 40-min MWT is considered abnormal; values greater than this but less than 40 min are of uncertain significance [69, 80]. The ability to remain awake for the entire 40 min over each of the four naps strongly supports a patient's ability to remain awake in other more alerting situations (i.e., a MSL of 40 min) [69, 80].

The MWT is indicated to assess treatment response in patients with excessive sleepiness or for determining patients' ability to stay awake during employment [79]. For example, a patient who has been placed on modafinil or other alerting medication or an OSA patient treated with CPAP therapy may undergo an MWT to demonstrate their ability to remain awake when desired. The test is also required annually by the Federal Aviation Administration (FAA) to determine fitness for work in pilots (www.faa.gov). Some employers require episodic MWT testing of OSA patients who are on CPAP to ensure daytime alertness.

Psychomotor Vigilance Test (PVT)

The PVT is not routinely used in clinical practice and currently serves mostly as a research tool; however, its usefulness to assess the behavioral consequences of mental fatigue is evident. The PVT measures a patient's ability to sustain attention by using the reaction time to successive stimuli to measure deficits in attention and performance [80]. In a study comparing two versions of the PVT on 21 patients, both versions demonstrated an increase in reaction time with increasing hours of wakefulness [81].

Actigraphy

Actigraphs are monitors that measure rest and activity and work in a similar way as pedometers. For sleep purposes, the actigraphs are typically worn on the wrist, similar to a watch, on the non-dominant hand. Patients wear the unit for at least a week to aid in the assessment of their sleep disorder, namely, insomnia, circadian rhythm

Table 7.6 Diagnostic criteria: chronic fatigue syndrome [www.cdc.gov]

Both criteria should be met
1. New-onset, unexplained, persistent fatigue not due to exertion and unrelieved by rest that results in a significant reduction in premorbid activity
2. At least four of the below symptoms are present for 6 months or more:
(a) *Arthralgia* (in multiple joints)
(b) New-onset *headaches* or exacerbation of prior headache
(c) Tender cervical or axillary *lymphadenopathy*
(d) Prominent *malaise* following physical or mental activity
(e) *Memory or concentration* disturbance
(f) *Myalgias*
(g) *Pharyngitis* that is frequent or recurring
(h) *Sleep disturbance* (namely, nonrestorative sleep)

sleep disorders, or excessive sleepiness (when an MSLT cannot be performed). The sleep actigraph works on the basic premise that people move more when they are awake than when they are asleep. This activity variance is typically plotted in a graphic format for interpretation.

Fatigue Syndromes

Often a comprehensive evaluation of the fatigue may still not make the diagnosis any clearer. At this point, a clinician should consider the fatigue syndromes, namely, chronic fatigue syndrome (CFS) and idiopathic chronic fatigue (ICF). These syndromes are typically diagnoses of exclusion. CFS manifests as unexplained fatigue that lasts for at least 6 months and is usually associated with flu-like symptoms, neuropsychological complaints (e.g., excessive irritability, confusion, difficulty thinking), and/or a sleep disturbance [58]. If the fatigue is debilitating and persists for over 6 months and does not meet the Center for Disease Control (CDC) criteria for CFC (Table 7.6), it is then termed idiopathic chronic fatigue. ICF may represent a variant of CFS; however, the CDC criteria for CFS was intentionally made restrictive as to allow for better selection of a more uniform population for research purposes [82].

Treatment

Multiple pharmaceutical and behavioral therapies are available for the management of fatigue; specific treatments are tailored to the patient depending upon the etiology. A patient with hypothyroidism as the cause of fatigue, for example, would be best managed with thyroxine supplementation, while a patient with fatigue due to insufficient sleep would be optimally treated by increasing their total sleep time. A detailed

Table 7.7 Behavioral strategies for improving fatigue

1. Observe proper sleep hygiene, including getting sufficient amount of sleep per night
2. Eat a healthy balance diet with at least eight 8-ounce glasses of fluid a day
3. Keep active; exercise regularly
4. Perform relaxation techniques regularly
5. Avoid excessive amounts of stress in your personal and professional life
6. Avoid alcohol, tobacco, or recreational drug use
7. Avoid excessive caffeine use; judicious use of caffeine may be appropriate

discussion regarding management of the individual disorders that cause fatigue is beyond the scope of this chapter and will be addressed elsewhere in this book.

Some basic behavioral therapies regardless of etiology will help at least partially improve fatigue (Table 7.7). Exercising, good sleep hygiene, and getting sufficient amount of sleep at night are paramount. The average adult requires 7.5–8 h of sleep per night; however, the average adult actually gets only about 7 h of sleep during the weekday with about 25% acknowledging that they are not getting enough sleep [National Sleep Foundation: 2011 Sleep in America Poll]. Maintaining a regular sleep-wake schedule and allowing sufficient time for sleep (it's that important that it needed to be mentioned again) are recommended. Avoiding sedating medications (if possible) or changing the timing of these medications (e.g., taking sedating medications at bedtime instead of during the day) may prove beneficial. Avoiding recreational drugs or alcohol will help minimize fatigue. Alcohol may be helpful to fall asleep at night but then usually causes sleep to become disrupted in the second half of the night, and it is best avoided [83]. Judicious caffeine use may help combat sleepiness; however, excessive use may lead to a withdrawal phenomenon or its use close to bedtime can actually exacerbate the symptom.

Occasionally, pharmaceutical assistance is required to help alleviate the symptom of excessive sleepiness, even when the underlying disorder is being treated (e.g., residual sleepiness in OSA patients being treated with CPAP or persistent insomnia in patients being treated with cognitive behavioral therapy). Medications can be prescribed to optimize nocturnal sleep when sleep is disrupted with subsequent improvement in daytime sleepiness (e.g., zolpidem, anxiolytics, sedating antidepressants, sodium oxybate, etc.) or to maintain wakefulness during the waking hours (e.g., modafinil, armodafinil, amphetamines, etc.)

Summary

When evaluating mental fatigue or sleepiness, it is very important to obtain a sleep history including information about the patient's bedtime, time it takes to fall asleep, number and duration of nocturnal awakenings, activity during the awakenings, final wake time, and time it takes to get out of bed after the final awakening. It is also just as important to obtain information about the patient's activities during waking hours, including information on naps. Inquiries should also be directed to identify the etiology of the fatigue, including medical, neurologic, and psychiatric disorders as well as sleep disorders. Often interviewing the patient's bed partner or caregiver about the patient's symptoms proves valuable.

Sleep disorders such as insomnia, obstructive sleep apnea, restless legs syndrome, circadian rhythm disorders, insufficient sleep syndrome, or narcolepsy have all been associated with excessive sleepiness. After an appropriate history is taken, a comprehensive exam should complement the evaluation. Serologic investigations are typically of low yield in the workup of fatigue, unless other associated clinical symptoms are suggestive of a diagnosis. Other laboratory investigations are also performed if clinical suspicion warrants.

Polysomnographic monitoring, including MSLTs and MWTs, are invaluable when evaluating sleepiness. They can either make or confirm a diagnosis and can also assess the severity of the sleepiness. Actigraphy can be used to determine sleep duration as well as an individual's circadian sleep-wake cycle, while PVT studies measure a behavioral consequence of mental fatigue.

Treatment of sleepiness should be targeted at the underlying etiology. However, symptomatic treatment is occasionally necessary, especially, if the cause is found to be a central nervous system hypersomnia, a circadian rhythm sleep disorder, such as shift work disorder, or residual sleepiness after treatment of obstructive sleep apnea syndrome.

References

1. Lerdal A. Energy, fatigue, and perceived illness in individuals with multiple sclerosis: a multimethod approach. Doctoral Dissertation. Oslo: Department of Behavioral Science in Medicine, University of Oslo, Unipub AS; 2005.
2. Lerdal A, Bakken LN, Kouwenhoven SE, et al. Poststroke fatigue—a review. J Pain Symptom Manag. 2009;38(6):928–49.
3. Lee KA, Lentz MJ, Taylor DL, et al. Fatigue as a response to environmental demands in women's lives. Image J Nurs Sch. 1994;26(2):149–54.
4. Mitler M, Carskadon MA, Czeisler CA, et al. Catastrophes, sleep, and public policy: concensus report. Sleep. 1988;11:100–9.
5. Cavalli Kluthcovsky AC, Urbanetz AA, de Carvalho DS, et al. Fatigue after treatment in breast cancer survivors: prevalence, determinants and impact on health-related quality of life. Support Care Cancer. 2011;13:1901–9.
6. Weis J. Cancer-related fatigue: prevalence, assessment and treatment strategies. Expert Rev Pharmacoecon Outcomes Res. 2011;11(4):441–6.
7. Kirkevold M, Christensen D, Andersen G, et al. Fatigue after stroke: manifestations and strategies. Disabil Rehabil. 2011;13:665–70.
8. Römkens TE, van Vugt-van Pinxteren MW, Nagengast FM, et al. High prevalence of fatigue in inflammatory bowel disease: a case control study. J Crohns Colitis. 2011;5(4):332–7.
9. Kant IJ, Bültmann U, Schröer KA, et al. An epidemiological approach to study fatigue in the working population: the Maastricht Cohort Study. Occup Environ Med. 2003;60(Suppl 1):i32–9.

10. Lewis G, Wessely S. The epidemiology of fatigue: more questions than answers. J Epidemiol Community Health. 1992;46(2):92–7.
11. Fuhrer R, Wessely S. The epidemiology of fatigue and depression: a French primary-care study. Psychol Med. 1995;25(5):895–905.
12. Ridsdale L, Evans A, Jerrett W, et al. Patients with fatigue in general practice: a prospective study. BMJ. 1993;307(6896):103–6.
13. Rosekind MR, Gregory KB, Mallis MM, et al. The cost of poor sleep: workplace productivity loss and associated costs. J Occup Environ Med. 2010;52(1):91–8.
14. ICSD-2. International classification of sleep disorders. 2nd ed. Chicago: American Academy of Sleep Medicine; 2005.
15. Spielman AJ, Saskin P, Thorpy MJ. Treatment of chronic insomnia by restriction of time in bed. Sleep. 1987;10(1):45–56.
16. Tiffin P, Ashton H, Marsh R, et al. Pharmacokinetic and pharmacodynamic responses to caffeine in poor and normal sleepers. Psychopharmacology. 1995;121(4):494–502.
17. Dautovich ND, McCrae CS, Rowe M. Subjective and objective napping and sleep in older adults: are evening naps "bad" for nighttime sleep? J Am Geriatr Soc. 2008;56(9):1681–6.
18. Thorpy M. Current concepts in the etiology, diagnosis and treatment of narcolepsy. Sleep Med. 2001;2(1):5–17.
19. Droogleever Fortuyn HA, Fronczek R, Smitshoek M, et al. Severe fatigue in narcolepsy with cataplexy. J Sleep Res. 2011;21(2):163–9.
20. Howard SK, Gaba DM, Rosekind MR, et al. The risks and implications of excessive daytime sleepiness in resident physicians. Acad Med. 2002;77(10):1019–25.
21. Johns MW. A new method for measuring daytime sleepiness: the Epworth sleepiness scale. Sleep. 1991;14(6):540–5.
22. Neuberger GB. Measures of fatigue. Arthritis and Rheum (Arthritis Care Res). 2003;49(5S):S175–83.
23. Goel N, Dinges DF. Behavioral and genetic markers of sleepiness. J Clin Sleep Med. 2011;7(5 Suppl):S19–21.
24. Goel N, Banks S, Lin L, et al. Catechol-O-methyltransferase Val158Met polymorphism associates with individual difference in sleep physiologic responses to chronic sleep loss. PLoS One. 2011;6(12):e29283.
25. Olson EJ, Drage LA, Auger RR. Sleep deprivation, physician performance, and patient safety. Chest. 2009;136(5):1389–96.
26. Lee JH, Wang W, Silva EJ, et al. Neurobehavioral performance in young adults living on a 28-h day for 6 weeks. Sleep. 2009;32(7):905–13.
27. Franzen PL, Siegle GJ, Buysse DJ. Relationships between affect, vigilance, and sleepiness following sleep deprivation. J Sleep Res. 2008;17(1):34–41.
28. Banks S, Dinges DF. Behavioral and physiological consequence of sleep restriction. J Clin Sleep Med. 2007;3(5):519–28.
29. McNicholas WT, Ryan S. Obstructive sleep apnoea syndrome: translating science to clinical practice. Respirology. 2006;11(2):136–44.
30. White DP. Sleep apnea. Proc Am Thorac Soc. 2006;3(1):124–8.
31. Ancoli-Israel S, Ayalon L. Diagnosis and treatment of sleep disorders in older adults. Am J Geriatr Psychiatry. 2006;14(2):95–103.
32. Romero E, Krakow B, Haynes P, et al. Nocturia and snoring: predictive symptoms for obstructive sleep apnea. Sleep Breath. 2010;14(4):337–43.
33. Broadley SA, Jorgensen L, Cheek A, et al. Early investigation and treatment of obstructive sleep apnea after stroke. J Clin Neurosci. 2007;14(4):328–33.
34. Noradina AT, Hamidon BB, Roslan H, et al. Risk factors for developing sleep-disordered breathing in patients with recent ischaemic stroke. Singap Med J. 2006;47(5):392–9.
35. Misiolek M, Marek B, Namyslowski G, et al. Sleep apnea syndrome and snoring in patients with hypothyroidism with relation to overweight. J Physiol Pharmacol. 2007;58(Suppl 1):77–85.

36. Resta O, Pannacciulli N, Di Gioia G, et al. High prevalence of previously unknown subclinical hypothyroid in obese patients referred to a sleep clinic for sleep disordered breathing. Nutr Metab Cardiovasc Dis. 2004;14(5):248–53.
37. Rajagopal KR, Abbrecht PH, Derderian SS, et al. Obstructive sleep apnea in hypothyroidism. Ann Intern Med. 1984;101(4):491–4.
38. Chasens ER, Umlauf MG, Weaver TE. Sleepiness, physical activity, and functional outcomes in veterans with type 2 diabetes. Appl Nurs Res. 2009;22(3):176–82.
39. Saaresranta T, Irjala K, Aittokallio T, et al. Sleep quality, daytime sleepiness and fasting insulin levels in women with chronic obstructive pulmonary disease. Respir Med. 2005;99(7):856–63.
40. Darbishire L, Risdale L, Seed PT. Distinguishing patients with chronic fatigue from those with chronic fatigue syndrome: a diagnostic study in UK primary care. Br J Gen Pract. 2003;53(491):441–5.
41. Zimmerman M, McGlinchey JB, Posternak MA, et al. Differences between minimally depressed patients who do and do not consider themselves to be in remission. J Clin Psychiatry. 2005;66(9):1134–8.
42. Posternak MA, Zimmerman M. Symptoms of atypical depression. Psychiatry Res. 2001;104(2):175–81.
43. Mitchell PB, Wilhelm K, Parker G, et al. The clinical features of bipolar depression: a comparison with matched major depressive disorder patients. J Clin Psychiatry. 2001;62(3):212–6.
44. Nofzinger EA, Thase ME, Reynolds CF, et al. Hypersomnia in bipolar depression: a comparison with narcolepsy using the multiple sleep latency test. Am J Psychiatry. 1991;148(9):1177–81.
45. Parker G, Malhi G, Hadzi-Pavlovic D, et al. Sleeping in? The impact of age and depressive sub-type on hypersomnia. J Affect Disord. 2006;90(1):73–6.
46. Kroenke K, Spitzer RL, Williams JB. The PHQ-9: validity of a brief depression severity measure. J Gen Intern Med. 2001;16(9):606–13.
47. Spitzer RL, Kroenke K, Williams JB, Lowe B. A brief measure for assessing generalized anxiety disorder: the GAD-7. Arch Intern Med. 2006;166(10):1092–7.
48. Kozlowska K, Nunn KP, Rose D, et al. Conversion disorder in Australian pediatric practice. J Am Acad Child Adolesc Psychiatry. 2007;46(1):68–75.
49. Hicks JA, Shapiro CM. Pseudo-narcolepsy: case report. J Psychiatry Neurosci. 1999;24(4):348–50.
50. Feldman MD, Russell JL. Factitious cyclic hypersomnia: a new variant of factitious disorder. South Med J. 1991;84(3):379–81.
51. Thorpy MJ, Wagner D, Spielman AJ, et al. Polysomnographic documentation of narcolepsy. Arch Neurol. 1983;40:126–7.
52. Friedman M, Tanyori H, La Rosa M, et al. Clinical predictors of obstructive sleep apnea. Laryngoscope. 1999;109(12):1901–7.
53. Gonzalez H, Minville V, Delanoue K, et al. The importance of increased neck circumference to intubation difficulties in obese patients. Anesth Analg. 2008;106(4):1132–6.
54. Taibah K, Ahmed M, Baessa E, et al. An unusual cause of obstructive sleep apnea presenting during pregnancy. J Laryngol Otol. 1998;112(12):1189–91.
55. Lin WN, Lee LA, Wang CC, et al. Obstructive sleep apnea syndrome in an adolescent girl with hypertrophic lingual thyroid. Pediatr Pulmonol. 2009;44(1):93–5.
56. Barnes TW, Olsen KD, Morgenthaler TI. Obstructive lingual thyroid causing sleep apnea: a case report and review of the literature. Sleep Med. 2004;5(6):605–7.
57. Lane TJ, Matthews DA, Manu P. The low yield of physical examinations and laboratory investigations of patients with chronic fatigue. Am J Med Sci. 1990;299:313–8.
58. Fukuda K, Straus SE, Hickie I, et al. The chronic fatigue syndrome: a comprehensive approach to its definition and study. International Chronic Fatigue Syndrome Study Group. Ann Intern Med. 1994;121(12):953–9.
59. McCarty DE. Resolution of hypersomnia following identification and treatment of vitamin D deficiency. J Clin Sleep Med. 2010;6(6):605–8.

60. Knutsen KV, Brekke M, Gjelstad S, et al. Vitamin D status in patients with musculoskeletal pain, fatigue and headache; a cross sectional descriptive study in a multi-ethnic general practice in Norway. Scand J Prim Health Care. 2010;28(3):166–71.

61. Kryger MH, Otake K, Foerster J. Low body stores of iron and restless legs syndrome: a correctable cause of insomnia in adolescents and teenagers. Sleep Med. 2002;3(2):127–32.

62. Kellinghaus C, Lüders HO. Frontal lobe epilepsy. Epileptic Disord. 2004;6(4):223–39.

63. Jeffree RL, Besser M. Colloid cyst of the third ventricle: a clinical review of 39 cases. J Clin Neurosci. 2001;8(4):328–31.

64. Riccitelli G, Rocca MA, Forn C, et al. Voxelwise assessment of the regional distribution of damage in the brains of patients with multiple sclerosis and fatigue. AJNR Am J Neuroradiol. 2011;32(5):874–9.

65. Pellicano C, Gallo A, Li X, et al. Relationship of cortical atrophy to fatigue in patients with multiple sclerosis. Arch Neurol. 2010;67(4):447–53.

66. de Lange FP, Koers A, Kalkman JS, et al. Increase in prefrontal cortical volume following cognitive behavioural therapy in patients with chronic fatigue syndrome. Brain. 2008;131(Pt 8):2172–80.

67. Littner M, Hirshkowitz M, Kramer M, Kapen S, Anderson WM, Bailey D, Berry RB, Davila D, Johnson S, Kushida C, Loube DI, Wise M. Woodson BT practice parameters for using polysomnography to evaluate insomnia: an update. Sleep. 2003;26(6):754–60.

68. Carskadon MA, Dement WC, Mitler MM, et al. Guidelines for the multiple sleep latency test (MSLT): a standard measure of sleepiness. Sleep. 1986;9(4):519–24.

69. Arand D, Bonnet M, Hurwitz T, et al. Standards of Practice Committee of the American Academy of Sleep Medicine. The clinical use of the MSLT and MWT. Sleep. 2005;28(1):123–44.

70. Levine B, Roehrs T, Zorick F, et al. Daytime sleepiness in young adults. Sleep. 1988;11(1):39–46.

71. Johns MW. Sensitivity and specificity of the multiple latency test (MSLT), the maintenance of wakefulness test and the Epworth sleepiness scale: failure of the MSLT as a gold standard. J Sleep Res. 2000;9(1):5–11.

72. Bliwise DL, Carskadon MA, Seidel WF, et al. MSLT-defined sleepiness and neuropsychological test performance do not correlate in the elderly. Neurobiol Aging. 1991;12(5):463–8.

73. Richardson GS, Carskadon MA, Flagg W, et al. Excessive daytime sleepiness in man: multiple sleep latency measurement in narcoleptic and control subjects. Electroencephalogr Clin Neurophysiol. 1978;45(5):621–7.

74. Hartse KM, Zorick F, Sicklesteel J, et al. Nap recordings in the diagnosis of daytime somnolence. Sleep Res. 1979;8:190.

75. Van den Hoed J, Kraemer H, Guilleminault C, et al. Disorders of excessive daytime somnolence: polygraphic and clinical data for 100 patients. Sleep. 1981;4(1):23–37.

76. Aldrich MS, Chervin RD, Malow BA. Value of the multiple sleep latency test (MSLT) for the diagnosis of narcolepsy. Sleep. 1997;20(8):620–9.

77. Mitler MM, Gujavarty KS, Browman CP. Maintenance of wakefulness test: a polysomnographic technique for evaluating treatment efficacy in patients with excessive somnolence. Electroencephalogr Clin Neurophysiol. 1982;53(6):658–61.

78. Doghramji K, Mitler MM, Sangal RB, et al. A normative study of the maintenance of wakefulness test (MWT). Electroencephalogr Clin Neurophysiol. 1997;103(5):554–62.

79. Littner MR, Kushida C, Wise M, et al. Standards of Practice Committee of the American Academy of Sleep Medicine. Practice parameters for clinical use of the multiple sleep latency test and the maintenance of wakefulness test. Sleep. 2005;28(1):113–21.

80. Stoohs RA, Philip P, Andries D, et al. Reaction time performance in upper airway resistance syndrome versus obstructive sleep apnea syndrome. Sleep Med. 2009;10(9):1000–4.

81. Lamond N, Jay SM, Dorrian J, et al. The sensitivity of a palm-based psychomotor vigilance task to sleep loss. Behav Res Methods. 2008;40(1):347–52.

82. Bombardier CH, Buchwald D. Chronic fatigue, chronic fatigue syndrome, and fibromyalgia. Disability and health-care use. Med Care. 1996;34:924.

83. Roehrs T, Roth T. Sleep, sleepiness, sleep disorders and alcohol use and abuse. Sleep Med Rev. 2001;5(4):287–97.
84. Manea L, Gilbody S, McMillan D. Optimal cut-off score for diagnosing depression with the Patient Health Questionnaire (PHQ-9): a meta-analysis. CMAJ. 2011;184(3):E191–6.
85. Swinson RP. The GAD-7 scale was accurate for diagnosing generalized anxiety disorder. Evid Based Med. 2006;11(6):184.
86. Lowe B, Decker O, Muller S, et al. Validation and standardization of the Generalized Anxiety Disorder Screener (GAD-7) in the general population. Med Care. 2008;46(3):266–74.

Chapter 8
Assessment of Medication and Recreational Drugs Associated with Fatigue

Amir Sharafkhaneh, Mary Rose, and Max Hirshkowitz

Introduction

Fatigue is a prevalent condition that increases the risk of errors, contributes to accidents, and impairs quality of life. Causes of fatigue include various medications and recreational agents. With the ever-increasing list of medications approved for managing chronic medical conditions, it can be difficult to ascertain the role of the agents in provoking or exacerbating fatigue. This is especially true when the medical condition for which the agent is prescribed is itself associated with fatigue. A detailed history is a crucial process for establishing the causal relationship between a psychoactive substance and fatigue. The temporal relationship between initiation and/or administration of a medicine and the onset of fatigue represents the most important clue. Sometimes, removal of the presumed agent and close follow-up of a patient is needed to ascertain such a role. With that in mind, there are certain groups of agents that may cause fatigue. In this chapter, we review pharmacological and recreational agents associated with fatigue.

A. Sharafkhaneh, MD, PhD (⊠)
Department of Medicine, Baylor College of Medicine, Houston, TX, USA

Medical Care Line, Michael E. DeBakey VA Medical Center, Houston, TX, USA
e-mail: amirs@bcm.edu

M. Hirshkowitz, PhD
Division of Public Mental Health and Population Sciences, School of Medicine, Stanford University, Stanford, CA, USA

Department of Medicine, Baylor College of Medicine, Houston, TX, USA

M. Rose, PsyD
Department of Medicine, Pulmonary, Critical Care and Sleep Section, Baylor College of Medicine and The Michael E. DeBakey Veterans Administration Hospital, Houston, TX, USA

© Springer Science+Business Media, LLC, part of Springer Nature 2018
A. Sharafkhaneh, M. Hirshkowitz (eds.), *Fatigue Management*,
https://doi.org/10.1007/978-1-4939-8607-1_8

Medications and Fatigue

Cardiac Medication

Cardiac conditions are major causes of fatigue. The armamentarium of medications for treatment of cardiac diseases has been expanding tremendously in the last few decades. Large-scale randomized trials scientifically demonstrate that many of these agents improve longevity, physical functioning, and quality of life. However, some of these agents may be associated with increased fatigue.

Beta blockers are widely used in management of various chronic cardiovascular disorders. Various studies reported fatigue as a frequent side effect and a main reason of beta-blocker discontinuation [1]. As high as 56% of patients with heart failure who were started on a beta blocker reported fatigue. In this group fatigue was the most common cause of discontinuing the medication [2]. Propranolol apparently has a higher rate of causing fatigue [1]. In contrast, meta-analysis of randomized trials of beta blockers in heart failure patients showed a very small increase or no increase in fatigue caused by the medication [3, 4]. The fatigue with beta blocker usually is seen shortly after the start of medication. Beta blockers can impair microvascular function by reducing resting capillary blood flow in skeletal muscles and thus promote fatigue [5, 6]. This effect has not been seen in a newer beta blocker (nebivolol) [7].

Results from various studies show that most of the patient can tolerate when switched to another beta blocker [1, 2]. Thus, in assessing the potential causal effect of fatigue in patients on beta blocker, history of illness and the symptom can help to establish any temporal relationship between the start or worsening of fatigue and initiation of the medication.

In contrast to beta blockers, fatigue due to other antihypertensive medications is less frequently reported [8]. In general, reported rate of fatigue due to these agents is less than 10% [9, 10]. The agents include ACE, angiotensin receptor blockers (ARB), and calcium channel blockers. Thus, these agents are not at top of the list for medication-induced fatigue.

Diuretics are frequently prescribed for management of hypertension, heart failure, and fluid overload. Diuretics can induce fatigue by creating electrolyte imbalance specially when combined with beta blockers [11].

Respiratory Medication

Chronic respiratory conditions like chronic obstructive pulmonary disease, asthma, pulmonary fibrosis, and pulmonary hypertension are associated with fatigue. Treatment of the conditions with proper pharmacotherapy and pulmonary rehabilitation can alleviate the fatigue and improve quality of life. Long-acting anticholinergics and long-acting beta agonists are first-line therapy for patients with

COPD. Systematic review of multiple studies did not show more report of fatigue compared to placebo [12]. In addition, other recommended therapies including inhaled corticosteroid, PDE4 inhibitor, and theophylline have not been reported to exacerbate fatigue.

Neurological and Psychiatric Medication

Neuropsychiatric disorders and injuries are major causes of lost years of healthy life as measured by disability-adjusted life years (DALYs) [13]. Pharmaceuticals designed to modify both disease progression and symptom management often have substantial side effects.

Iatrogenic causes of fatigue are common in many medications used to manage neurological and psychiatric conditions. In some cases, treatments can be substituted for less sedating products once the unintended side effects are identified. However, for some conditions, we have yet to develop pharmacological treatments which will not negatively impact vigilance and/or wakefulness or which are capable of targeting only the specific pathways desired for disease management. Though a comprehensive list of sedating medication for neurological and psychiatric conditions is beyond the scope of this chapter, mediating factors and strategies for optimizing management of sedation and fatigue provoking medications which may impede treatment will be reviewed. Terms such as fatigue, drowsiness, and sedation are often used interchangeably in the literature. The pathways of the brain affected during these experiences are similar, though fatigue and drowsiness may be differentiated here with drowsiness being a condition in which the individual desires to sleep or has difficulty maintaining wakefulness.

Mood stabilizers, antidepressants, and anxiolytics have been well established to have fatiguing side effects and routinely require additional pharmacotherapy to treat fatigue symptomatically using wake-promoting agents. In patients for whom adherence is already challenging, medications provoking fatigue create a substantial barrier, and some patients feel this adverse effect may outweigh the benefits they provide. Management of disorders such as schizophrenia and bipolar depression is a prime example. Both disorders are managed largely by medications whose side effect profiles commonly include sedation and/or fatigue. There are currently nine first-line atypical antipsychotic medications, five of which are associated with the adverse event of sedation [14].

Miller reports that adherence is poor in about 40% of those with schizophrenia [15]. Several studies have indicated that among those with first-episode psychosis (FEP), medication discontinuation is extremely common. McEvoy found in a large-scale study of 400 FEP patients that drowsiness was the most common adverse event for olanzapine, quetiapine, and risperidone [16]. Patients with schizophrenia have multiple vulnerabilities for treatment adherence difficulty. Judgment is often impaired in recognizing the negative consequences of being untreated, or that there is a disease process present at all. Additionally, schizophrenics may have paranoid ideation that prescribed medication is intended to control or do harm to them. The sedating effect of many antipsychotics affects not only physical fatigue and sedation but may impair mental alertness and active cognitive and emotional engagement. Phan points out that no single technique has been proven most effective in improving adherence, recommending continual reassessment and strategies directed toward the patient (and caregiver) and implemented throughout the course of the patient's illness [17].

Despite the negative impact of sedation on adherence in schizophrenia, sedation has been considered a more important contributor to adherence problems in bipolar depression than in schizophrenia [18]. The most commonly used pharmacologic therapies for bipolar depression include mood stabilizers, antidepressants, and atypical antipsychotics. The sedating side effects of these medications have been well established as problematic for adherence [19]. Adherence consequent to sedation is likely problematic in those with bipolar mood disorder consequent to the fact that the euthymic, and often euphoric and inflated, features of the condition itself, when hypomanic, are a substantial contributor to poor adherence. Relinquishing these symptoms has been a notoriously problematic adherence issue for those with bipolar depression, making a plan for rapid management of side effects essential.

Neurological conditions are extremely variable in their scope of severity and impact. Some of the most common neurological conditions whose conditions, as well as treatments may be associated with sedation, include Alzheimer's, Parkinson's, epilepsy, headaches, and neuropathic pain. Pain conditions such as headache and neuropathic pain are treated symptomatically and do not require disease-modifying treatments which require a prolonged absorption time. Thus, medications which may cause sedation can be strategically taken in the evening to diminish interference with daytime activities.

For neuropathic pain, there are several treatment options. First-line treatment options include tricyclic antidepressants (TCAs), gabapentin, pregabalin, and serotonin noradrenaline reuptake inhibitors (SNRIs) [20]. TCAs and SNRIs take some time to reach peak levels, and thus patients may experience side effects without much perceived benefit for 6–8 weeks, challenging adherence further. Amitriptyline and doxepin generally cause the most sedation of the currently available TCAs, consequent to their anticholinergic effects, which is why it is often used in patients with insomnia complaints [21]; thus, if sedation is a significant barrier to care, the clinician has multiple other options for treatment which are likely to have fewer sedating side effects. Gabapentin and pregabalin are associated with the side effect of significant sleepiness and daytime fatigue, which is the reason they are often dosed preferentially in the evening.

Alzheimer's and Parkinson's are more common in the elderly. Sedation may cause multiple problems for these patients, including higher risk for falls. As their progression is not deterred by the currently available treatments, it is important that those symptoms affecting overall quality of life be weighed with the individual patient. For these conditions, sedation that limits the patient from participating in daily activities and/or key life events is unlikely to be accepted, even if better management of cognitive functioning and/or of a movement disorder is the trade-off.

Common Alzheimer's medications to improve cognition include donepezil, rivastigmine, memantine, and galantamine. Of these, donepezil is the only listed as having sedation as a common side effect [22]. Parkinson's is most typically treated with levodopa for which sedation is a common side effect. Sedation side effects may increase the risk of falls in patients who are likely already experiencing balance and coordination difficulty.

There are numerous anti-epileptic medications currently on the market. Many of these are associated with sedation. Medication adherence is problematic in those with epilepsy, with a substantial discrepancy between what physicians prescribe and what patients report taking [23]. In one study, tiredness and sleepiness were among the most common adverse effects [24].

For all neuropsychiatric conditions which may require adjunct treatment to mitigate sedation side effects, the treating physician should develop a preemptive plan to manage possible problems with fatigue. At the time that an initial treatment plan is decided upon, possible side effects should be reviewed with the patient. A plan for a quick response to provide pharmacologic options for fatigue should be in place at the time that the potentially sedating treatment medication is started. The physician is also advised to assess the likelihood that sedation will obstruct adherence, so that the consequences of poor adherence, as well as alternative treatment options, may be reviewed. The likelihood that sedation may be temporary with some treatments and likely to subside over time may also provide some added boost to a patient's ability to bear through the initial challenge of adjustment.

Sedating side effects may result in difficulty with ADL, work, socialization, and overall quality of life. Additionally, circadian rhythm disorders may develop if side effects include daytime naps or if the wake-promoting agents given to manage the sedating medications result in difficulty initiating sleep.

Several agents are used to counteract sedating treatments. Many of these are used off-label, as very few are approved for disease-specific wake and vigilance promotion. The most commonly prescribed of these include methylphenidate, modafinil, armodafinil, dextroamphetamine, and lisdexamfetamine. In this group, only modafinil and armodafinil are not considered cardiotoxic. Regardless of the disease for which stimulants are used to counteract sedation, drowsiness, and/or fatigue, risks and limitations of the stimulant, such as sleeplessness, agitation, and restless legs syndrome, should be reviewed, as the physician may not have the chance to review these side effects directly with the patient before calling in the stimulant. As many of these medications are off-label for the above conditions, the prescribing physician should be prepared to submit the required paperwork needed for appeals.

In addition to pharmacologic management, behavioral strategies for managing fatigue and daytime sleepiness and careful attention to possible comorbid sleep disorders, such as obstructive sleep apnea, which may be either the primary cause of the reported "side effect" or magnifying the fatigue complaint, should be reviewed. Given that many patients may have comorbid cardiac disease, contraindicated medications, or overall negative side effects to the stimulant itself should be reviewed. Behavioral strategies such as exercise, adequate sleep time, weight loss, and diet should be reviewed as viable options to facilitate management of side effects of fatigue, particularly that lack of sleep, fatigue, and poor diet are well known to magnify and to even provoke relapse in several of the above-mentioned conditions, most notably bipolar mood disorder and epilepsy.

Though significant side effects such as fatigue and sedation are problematic to adherence, if the patient considers the benefits to be substantial, they are likely to forge through these side effects. However, it is the task of the physician to work with the patient to determine if the patient needs to tolerate these side effects or if there are safe tolerable countermeasures available.

Recreational Agents and Fatigue

Since time immemorial humans have used psychoactive substances recreationally. The effects range from producing mild euphoria to creating a mental state mimicking psychosis. Substances can be taken orally in liquid or solid form, inhaled, or injected. Such substance may be part of religious rituals. Others are used medicinally. However, the majority of use occurs in a social context. The pleasant sensation, anxiety reduction, and disinhibition lead to repeated use. Some agents produce a compulsive desire to readminister and are considered "psychologically" addicting. By contrast, some substances create physical addiction associated with severe abstinence syndromes when discontinued.

With respect to legality, recreational substances fall into several categories:

1. Some substances are legal but can require a minimum age limit for use (e.g., alcoholic beverages). Nonetheless, public intoxication can lead to arrest.
2. Some substances are legal in specific localities but illegal elsewhere (e.g., marijuana).
3. Some substances are legal with prescription but illegal when used by an individual for whom the medication is not prescribed (e.g., hydrocodone).
4. Some substances are always illegal and are available only through the black market (e.g., heroin).

The dictionary[1] definition for drug abuse is "excessive use of a drug (such as alcohol, narcotics, or cocaine); use of a drug without medical justification." We might add to that the illegal use of a drug or substance. Acquiring illegal drugs puts the user in contact with a criminal element of society. This contact escalates the danger to the user both during the "buy" because the seller can pose a threat of violence and the police pose a threat of arrest and incarceration. Other dangers exist as well, including the drugs being variable in potency, tainted, or being other than what they are purported to be (e.g., fentanyl, which is 50–100 times more potent than morphine).

---

[1] Merriam-Webster Online

Alcohol

Alcohol is the most widely used, legal recreational drug. A product of fermentation and/or distillation, it is widely available. It may take the form of beer, wine, mead, brandy, distilled spirits, or whiskey and ranges in potency form under 10% to more than 50% by volume. In enough quantity within a specified time period, it intoxicates the user and can produce effects ranging from mild euphoria to impaired coordination to loss of judgment to total inability to function. In high enough doses, it can cause death.

Other effects include drowsiness, loss of concentration, slowing of simple reaction times, and memory impairment. A typical alcoholic beverage takes between 30 and 120 min to be fully absorbed into the bloodstream and is metabolized by a healthy individual at about one quarter ounce per hour. These pharmacodynamics vary depending on an individual's weight, sex, metabolic rate, the presence or absence of concurrent food intake, and the overall composition of the beverage consumed (e.g., the beverage's concentration and sugar content). The individual's activity level, kidney function, and liver function also alter metabolic rates. Nonetheless, a 150 pound individual drinking one alcoholic beverage per hour adds approximately 0.01% with each drink over time. An individual who imbibes to a 0.10% alcohol level will have detectable alcohol levels for about 8 h. Because intoxicated individuals operating a motor vehicle or other dangerous equipment are putting themselves and others in danger, legal limits have been established. However, legal limits vary depending on the locality. Additionally, some employers set specific limits for their workers and may mandate pre-employment or random testing in the interests of safety.

Testing can employ several methodologies, including urine tests, blood tests, and breathalyzer tests. Urine tests can detect alcohol if it has been ingested. Some urine tests can detect if alcohol was ingested for up to 80 h. Urine tests are binary (positive or negative) but do not indicate intoxication level. Blood tests provide a quantitative index of blood alcohol content (BAC); consequently, they can detect if an individual is acutely intoxicated (and/or a chronic alcoholic). The legal system has established a per se rule for interpreting BAC, and if the level exceeds the local jurisdictional limit, it is considered a surrogate for establishing intoxication. Breathalyzer tests measure ethyl alcohol in an exhaled breath. Breathalyzers determine alcohol level using gas chromatography and can be used to estimate the amount of alcohol recently consumed.

Marijuana

Marihuana is a widely used psychoactive drug derived from *Cannabis sativa* and/or *Cannabis indica*. Although it is used worldwide as a recreational drug, it was outlawed in more than two dozen states in the USA between 1916 and 1931. Finally, in 1937, federal legislation was passed banning its production, distribution, and use. Anti-marijuana propaganda at the time claimed marijuana intoxication incited violent crimes and madness and produced a "lust for blood." State-based decriminalization began in the late 1990s, and marijuana products are now legal in some states for medical and recreational use. However, as of this writing, it is still illegal according to federal law.

Tetrahydrocannabinol (THC) is the primary psychoactive compound found in cannabis. However, there are more than a hundred other cannabinoids, the most important of which is cannabidiol (CBD). Marijuana and marijuana extracts can be smoked, vaped, or made into edible forms. When smoked or vaped, psychoactive effects begin within a few minutes; when eaten the effects may begin 30–60 min after ingestion. These effects include heightened sensations, distortions of time perception, mood changes, impaired coordination, impaired memory, and cognitive difficulties. In high doses, hallucinations, delusional thinking, and temporary psychosis may occur. Most individuals who regularly use marijuana experience euphoria. By contrast, some people experience anxiety, paranoia, and panic. Although not considered addicting, marijuana withdrawal symptoms include insomnia, irritability, anxiety, altered appetite, and craving for the drug.

Urine tests for THC may remain positive for 30 days after a single use and for 12 weeks for a chronic user who has discontinued use. Blood tests will detect a single use for 6–24 h after a single intoxication and for up to a week for a regular user. These tests may be helpful to determine general usage of the recreational drug but not specific for determining intoxication or impairment. Saliva tests are becoming popular as part of post-accident investigations because they are sensitive to use within the past 24 h.

With respect to fatigue management, for some individuals, THC and CBD produce sleepiness. In fact, insomnia is one of the touted medical uses of the drug.

Opioids and Other Narcotics

Opioids and other narcotics are widely used in pain management; however, their use recreationally has become epidemic. Opioids produce euphoria and are physiologically addicting. These drugs are unquestionably a powerful part of the medical arsenal for pain reduction, but as tolerance develops, effectiveness declines, dose escalation is common, dependence increases, and addiction can follow. Experts estimate 2 million, or more, individuals in the USA are dependent on opioids. Some are abusing prescription drugs, while others are obtaining them illegally. The most common pharmaceutically prescribed opioids are morphine, oxycodone, and hydrocodone. Illicit opioids include heroin and fentanyl. 2014 statistics estimate nationwide hydrocodone distribution at 7.8 billion and oxycodone at 4.9 billion pills.

The overall effects of opioids include sedation, nausea, vomiting, dizziness, constipation, and respiratory depression. Opioids also can provoke sleep-related breathing disorders. When "high" on opioids, the user typically has compromised cognitive function, diminished dexterity, and impaired judgment. Withdrawal is associated with fatigue, anxiety, irritability, muscle pain, abdominal cramping, nausea, and diarrhea. The pressure of the abstinence syndrome and the craving for drug can likewise adversely alter thought, coordination, and judgment.

Testing for opioids is complex and can be performed on saliva, urine, blood, and/ or hair. The different opioids have different amounts of time they are detectable. Clinical testing laboratories perform a wide spectrum of tests for opioids and other illicit drugs as part of orderable screening panels.

Tranquilizers

Tranquilizers, particularly the benzodiazepines, are commonly used medially to treat anxiety; however, they became a popular recreational drug in the 1960s. They are still used recreationally, often in conjunction with "uppers" to modulate the stimulant effects. Referred to on the street as "trancs" or "downers," these drugs include alprazolam (Xanax), diazepam (Valium), lorazepam (Ativan), and clonazepam (Klonopin), just to name a few. Effects include excessive sedation, disorientation, dizziness, unconsciousness, impaired dexterity, slowing of reflexes, confusion, and fatigue. They also can provoke dry mouth, headaches, nausea, and vomiting. With chronic uses they will produce tolerance, dependence, and addiction with possible tremors and convulsions during withdrawal. Drug abuse panels available from clinical testing laboratories can detect usage. Sedation and fatigue are prominent effects of these drugs.

Uppers

"Uppers" are drugs that produce alertness by stimulating the central nervous system. The stimulant effect largely comes from acutely increased availability of the catecholamine neurotransmitters (dopamine and norepinephrine). These drugs include amphetamines, methylphenidate (Ritalin), MDMA (3,4-methylenedioxyme thamphetamine – known by the street name ecstasy), ephedrine, and cocaine. These drugs are widely abused both recreationally and to allow the individual to remain awake for long durations and reduce time spent sleeping. College students studying for exams, long-distance driving, and all-night work sessions are some of the applications. Some of the drugs in this class are used by the military to improve alertness and fend off fatigue in combat situations. "Youth" culture makes use of these drugs as part of all-night dance parties (raves). These drugs, in contrast to caffeine (which also increases alertness), also induce tremendous euphoria in some individuals. Abusers are therefore most often chronically sleep deprived and will continue using until they can no longer maintain the pace (referred to as "crash"). The inability to remain awake can occur without warning and thus represents great danger if it happens while driving or operating dangerous equipment. During the "crash" period, extreme sleepiness and fatigue is continually present. Standard drug testing can detect prior use of "uppers" in saliva (for 24–72 h), urine (for 2–5 days), and hair (for 90 days). Use of uppers has many adverse effects on health that are a function of the particular drug, dosages, and duration of chronic use (which is beyond the scope of this chapter).

Hallucinogens

About a half century ago, hallucinogenic drugs became part of popular culture. Their use profoundly influenced art and music. There are a great many different psychoactive substances used recreationally that can induce hallucinations. They vary in mechanism of action, psychokinetics, and psychodynamics. The most notorious, perhaps, was lysergic acid diethylamide (LSD). As the term suggests, the common feature of these substances is after ingestion an individual may see, hear, or feel things appear very real but do not exist. The user may also experience rapid mood swings. Other drugs and substances fall within this category: phencyclidine (PCP), dimethyltryptamine (DMT), ketamine, psilocybin mushrooms, ayahuasca, datura, and peyote (mescaline). Newer "designer drugs" with hallucinogenic properties have been developed to circumvent legal prohibitions and to circumvent detection by testing assays. Hallucinogens do not produce fatigue but render most individuals unable to function in the workplace or able to safely operate machinery. As an aftereffect of the hallucinogenic experience (or "trip"), the individual may be lethargic, sleepy, and fatigued.

Acknowledgment This work is supported by the Department of Veterans Affairs Research and Development Care Line.

References

1. Helfand M, Peterson K, Christensen V, Dana T, Thakurta S. Drug class review: beta adrenergic blockers: final report update. Drug Class Reviews. 2009.
2. Butler J, Khadim G, Belue R, Chomsky D, Dittus RS, Griffin M, Wilson JR. Tolerability to beta-blocker therapy among heart failure patients in clinical practice. J Card Fail. 2003;9:203–9.
3. Ko DT, Hebert PR, Coffey CS, Curtis JP, Foody JM, Sedrakyan A, Krumholz HM. Adverse effects of beta-blocker therapy for patients with heart failure: a quantitative overview of randomized trials. Arch Intern Med. 2004;164:1389–94.
4. Ko DT, Hebert PR, Coffey CS, Sedrakyan A, Curtis JP, Krumholz HM. Beta-blocker therapy and symptoms of depression, fatigue, and sexual dysfunction. JAMA. 2002;288:351–7.
5. Pechan J, Mikulecky M, Srbecky M. Acute haemodynamic effect of metoprolol in essential hypertension. Cor Vasa. 1988;30:51–9.
6. Pechan J, Ondrejicka M, Janotka M, Kellerova E. The effect of guanethidine and propranolol on capillary blood flow in subcutaneous tissue and muscle in essential hypertension. Cardiology. 1974;59:172–83.
7. Velasco A, Solow EB, Price AL, Wang Z, Arbique D, Arbique G, Adams-Huet B, Schwedhelm E, Lindner JR, Vongpatanasin W. Differential effects of nebivolol vs metoprolol on microvascular function in hypertensive humans. Am J Physiol Heart Circ Physiol. 2016;311:H118.
8. Dahlof B, Sever PS, Poulter NR, Wedel H, Beevers DG, Caulfield M, Collins R, Kjeldsen SE, Kristinsson A, McInnes GT, et al. Prevention of cardiovascular events with an antihypertensive regimen of amlodipine adding perindopril as required versus atenolol adding bendroflumethiazide as required, in the Anglo-Scandinavian Cardiac Outcomes Trial-Blood Pressure Lowering Arm (ASCOT-BPLA): a multicentre randomised controlled trial. Lancet. 2005;366:895–906.

9. Julius S, Kjeldsen SE, Weber M, Brunner HR, Ekman S, Hansson L, Hua T, Laragh J, McInnes GT, Mitchell L, et al. Outcomes in hypertensive patients at high cardiovascular risk treated with regimens based on valsartan or amlodipine: the VALUE randomised trial. Lancet. 2004;363:2022–31.
10. Guay DR. Trandolapril: a newer angiotensin-converting enzyme inhibitor. Clin Ther. 2003;25:713–75.
11. Sica DA, Carter B, Cushman W, Hamm L. Thiazide and loop diuretics. J Clin Hypertens. 2011;13:639–43.
12. Ni H, Soe Z, Moe S. Aclidinium bromide for stable chronic obstructive pulmonary disease. Cochrane Database Syst Rev. 2014:CD010509.
13. Murray CJ, Vos T, Lozano R, Naghavi M, Flaxman AD, Michaud C, Ezzati M, Shibuya K, Salomon JA, Abdalla S, et al. Disability-adjusted life years (DALYs) for 291 diseases and injuries in 21 regions, 1990-2010: a systematic analysis for the Global Burden of Disease Study 2010. Lancet. 2012;380:2197–223.
14. Citrome L, Eramo A, Francois C, Duffy R, Legacy SN, Offord SJ, Krasa HB, Johnston SS, Guiraud-Diawara A, Kamat SA, et al. Lack of tolerable treatment options for patients with schizophrenia. Neuropsychiatr Dis Treat. 2015;11:3095–104.
15. Miller BJ. A review of second-generation antipsychotic discontinuation in first-episode psychosis. J Psychiatr Pract. 2008;14:289–300.
16. McEvoy JP, Lieberman JA, Perkins DO, Hamer RM, Gu H, Lazarus A, Sweitzer D, Olexy C, Weiden P, Strakowski SD. Efficacy and tolerability of olanzapine, quetiapine, and risperidone in the treatment of early psychosis: a randomized, double-blind 52-week comparison. Am J Psychiatry. 2007;164:1050–60.
17. Phan SV. Medication adherence in patients with schizophrenia. Int J Psychiatry Med. 2016;51:211–9.
18. Velligan DI, Weiden PJ, Sajatovic M, Scott J, Carpenter D, Ross R, Docherty JP. The expert consensus guideline series: adherence problems in patients with serious and persistent mental illness. J Clin Psychiatry. 2009;70(Suppl 4):1–46.
19. Kemp DE. Managing the side effects associated with commonly used treatments for bipolar depression. J Affect Disord. 2014;169(Suppl 1):S34–44.
20. Brix FN, Hein SS, Staehelin JT. Management of painful neuropathies. Handb Clin Neurol. 2013;115:279–90.
21. Doerr JP, Spiegelhalder K, Petzold F, Feige B, Hirscher V, Kaufmann R, Riemann D, Voderholzer U. Impact of escitalopram on nocturnal sleep, day-time sleepiness and performance compared to amitriptyline: a randomized, double-blind, placebo-controlled study in healthy male subjects. Pharmacopsychiatry. 2010;43:166–73.
22. U.S. Department of Health and Human Services. Alzheimer's. 3 Oct 2016. Ref type: online source.
23. Mevaag M, Henning O, Baftiu A, Granas AG, Johannessen SI, Nakken KO, Johannessen LC. Discrepancies between physicians' prescriptions and patients' use of antiepileptic drugs. Acta Neurol Scand. 2016;135:80.
24. Kowski AB, Weissinger F, Gaus V, Fidzinski P, Losch F, Holtkamp M. Specific adverse effects of antiepileptic drugs—a true-to-life monotherapy study. Epilepsy Behav. 2016;54:150–7.

Chapter 9
Treating Sleep-Related Breathing Disorders

Christine H. Won, Vahid Mohsenin, and Meir Kryger

Introduction

Sleep-disordered breathing (SDB) includes obstructive sleep apnea, central sleep apnea, periodic breathing, upper airway resistance syndrome, and nocturnal hypoventilation. Central sleep apnea (CSA) and periodic breathing are breathing disorders associated with abnormal respiratory drive. They may occur in association with heart failure, liver or renal disease, neurologic conditions, and medications such as opiates. Nocturnal hypoventilation is characterized by persistent hypoxemia and hypercapnia during sleep and may occur due to neuromuscular disease, obesity hypoventilation syndrome, or obstructive lung disease. Upper airway resistance syndrome (UARS) describes frequent arousals related to snoring and partial upper airway obstruction. Many patients with UARS are affected with daytime sleepiness and fragmented sleep, but the clinical significance to cardiovascular or mental health has yet to be described. Finally, obstructive sleep apnea (OSA), by far the most common presenting form of SDB, is characterized by recurring upper airway collapse associated with arousals, oxygen desaturations, and increased sympathetic neural activity. OSA has been associated with significant cardiovascular and metabolic derangements, as well as impairments in mental health and job performance. As such, untreated OSA poses risk to public health and public safety. The mainstay treatment for SDB, particularly OSA, is positive airway pressure (PAP) therapy.

C. H. Won, MD, MS · M. Kryger, MD (✉)
Yale University School of Medicine, Section of Pulmonary,
Critical Care and Sleep Medicine, New Haven, CT, USA

Veterans Affairs Connecticut Health Care System, West Haven, CT, USA
e-mail: Christine.won@yale.edu; meir.kryger@yale.edu

V. Mohsenin, MD
Yale University School of Medicine, Section of Pulmonary and Critical Care Medicine,
New Haven, CT, USA
e-mail: vahid.mohsenin@yale.edu

© Springer Science+Business Media, LLC, part of Springer Nature 2018
A. Sharafkhaneh, M. Hirshkowitz (eds.), *Fatigue Management*,
https://doi.org/10.1007/978-1-4939-8607-1_9

This treatment is highly effective. Unfortunately, adherence rates are low on the order of 40%, leaving the majority of OSA patients untreated.

Poor PAP adherence has led to the development of alternative treatments specifically for OSA and UARS. Some patients are successfully treated with surgeries. An oral appliance or mandibular advancement device may be appropriate for select patients. Adjunctive therapies include weight loss and positional sleeping. Medications have been tried with little success and are not considered mainstay therapies for SDB. There continues to be emerging alternatives to PAP therapy, and the results of these innovations are yet to be fully appreciated.

Positive Airway Pressure Therapy

PAP therapy was originally described by Sullivan et al. in 1981 [1] and since remains the gold standard treatment for OSA [2]. PAP therapy for OSA involves generating a continuous pressure throughout the inspiratory and expiratory cycle via a mask covering the nose and/or mouth while the patient sleeps. PAP acts as a pneumatic splint for the upper airway, preventing its collapse during sleep. A second mechanism by which PAP may affect upper airway size is by increasing lung volume. The increased lung volume provides a downward traction on the trachea which is hypothesized to stretch upper airway structures and increase upper airway size. PAP has been shown to be safe and effective for long-term use and is associated with very little serious side effects.

The optimal PAP setting for OSA can be achieved during a titration study [3]. Several attempts have been made to develop prediction models for PAP settings. However, the level of pressure needed to eliminate OSA for any individual varies and cannot be reliably predicted based on OSA severity or patient demographic or anatomic features. Thus, the current preferred method is to perform an attended in-laboratory titration study. Newer technology has allowed for titrations to occur at home with auto-titrating PAP machines. The auto-titrating PAP machine is responsive to the patient's breathing and reacts by increasing pressures for reduced respiratory flow. Most studies indicate auto-titrating PAP machines are effective in achieving good control of OSA and useful for determining optimal PAP settings [4–6]. Moreover, newer machines are able to differentiate between obstructive and central sleep apneas and will respond appropriately [7]. While auto-titrating PAP is a modality for determining optimal PAP settings in the home setting, some patients prefer the modality as definitive PAP therapy since the machine varies the pressure on a needed basis and effectively lowers the mean pressure for the night.

The first approach to central sleep apnea and periodic breathing is to address the underlying medical issue whether it be cardiac, neurologic, or liver disease or related to sedative or narcotic use. If SDB cannot be managed by addressing the underlying conditions, then treatment may be warranted. Continuous PAP (CPAP) has historically been used to treat CSA and periodic breathing with good effect.

The American Academy of Sleep Medicine (AASM) recommends CPAP as the initial treatment for CSA due to heart failure [8]. Nocturnal oxygen is also recommended in this case. A more recent PAP modality, adaptive servo-ventilation (ASV), has been shown to be highly effective in treating CSA and periodic breathing [9] and is also recommended by AASM for these sleep-related breathing disorders [10]. ASV delivers a set pressure during expiration to eliminate obstructive sleep apnea. Pressure support during inspiration varies in addition to correct periodic breathing. A backup rate delivers mandatory breaths in the event of central sleep apnea.

The clinical significance and the impact of therapy on health outcomes of CSA and periodic breathing are not yet fully understood. In the CANPAP study [11], CPAP attenuated central sleep apnea, improved nocturnal oxygenation, increased the ejection fraction, lowered norepinephrine levels, and increased the distance walked in 6 min; however, it did not affect survival of heart failure patients with CSA. Despite not understanding the full implications of CSA or periodic breathing, clinicians readily treat these conditions since treatment is very effective and patients often derive symptomatic benefit.

Effect of PAP on Sleep Quality and Daytime Function

PAP effectively reduces the number of apneas and hypopneas through the night and improves subjective and objective sleepiness. Studies also demonstrate benefits in sleep quality and quality of life for both the patient and bed partner [12, 13]. Some studies show PAP treatment improves vitality, energy, and productivity [14–16], while others show no improvement in quality of life or cognitive function [17]. These findings may result from the fact that PAP itself may create sleep disturbances and affect overall sleep quality. In fact as many as 20% of treated OSA patients continue to suffer from daytime sleepiness. For those who benefit from PAP therapy, however, the effects can be dramatic and in many cases life-altering.

Study results on the effects of PAP on neurophysiologic function are inconsistent. There are a number of challenges in performing these studies, including controlling for the effect of learning on repeated testing and the difficulties of interpreting studies with longer periods of treatment. With these limitations in mind, several studies have found PAP improves overall cognitive function without improvement in any specific cognitive domain. Some studies show an improvement in Digit Vigilance-Time, information processing speed, vigilance, and sustained attention and alertness [18–20].

OSA poses a public health problem as it has been shown that untreated patients have an increased risk of motor vehicle accidents anywhere between 2.5- and 6-fold [21–23]. Furthermore, commercial drivers and heavy equipment operators often encompass the two greatest risk factors for OSA, those being male and overweight. It is imperative to screen these high-risk patients since PAP therapy has shown to significantly reduce the rate of motor vehicle accidents [24, 25].

Effect of PAP on Cardiovascular Disease

Large population studies have demonstrated an increased risk for hypertension in those with OSA. However, the role of PAP therapy in reversing these risks is less well demonstrated. Becker et al. found that effective treatment of sleep apnea with nasal CPAP for ≥9 weeks lowered both nocturnal and daytime systolic and diastolic BP by approximately 10 mm Hg [26]. Meanwhile, other investigations have shown smaller or no effect on daytime blood pressure [27–29]. These conflicting results likely reflect differences in PAP adherence, treatment interval, or sleep apnea severity. Despite inconclusive data regarding the effects of PAP on blood pressure, the AASM recommends PAP as adjunctive treatment for systemic hypertension in patients with sleep apnea [2].

Patients with OSA also have increases in pulmonary arterial pressure secondary to hypoxic vasoconstriction and sympathetic overdrive. Patients with OSA and concomitant lung diseases such as chronic obstructive pulmonary disease (known as overlap syndrome) or obesity hypoventilation syndrome may have severe daytime pulmonary hypertension. Studies show even short-term PAP therapy reduces daytime hypercapnia [30, 31] and pulmonary arterial pressures [32].

There is considerable literature regarding the benefits of PAP therapy on a number of markers of cardiovascular health including decreased sympathetic activity, decreased markers of inflammation, and improved endothelial function [33–37]. There is also growing evidence to suggest a beneficial effect on cardiovascular function and clinical outcomes in OSA patients. PAP therapy improves left ventricular ejection fraction and improves symptoms of left heart failure [38, 39]. PAP therapy also reduces the risk of atrial fibrillation recurrence after cardioversion [40]. Fatal and nonfatal cardiovascular events such as ischemic heart disease, heart failure, and arrhythmias are also reduced by PAP therapy [41–43]. Finally, several large observational studies have found a benefit of PAP treatment on mortality [42, 44]. These findings support the use of PAP for OSA regardless of whether symptoms are present.

Effect of PAP on Other Diseases

PAP has shown to improve many health problems posed by untreated OSA. For example, PAP therapy has been shown to improve insulin sensitivity and reduce hemoglobin A1c in certain individuals [45, 46]. Adherent PAP users are also more likely to lose weight. Sexual dysfunction is an important problem for patients with OSA, and PAP therapy may improve erectile dysfunction [47]. Patients with OSA also appear to have increased nocturnal natriuresis which improves with PAP treatment [48].

PAP Adherence

Long-term adherence to PAP has historically been very poor with reported rates of approximately 40% [17, 49, 50]. This has led to the emergence of various modes of pressure delivery such as bi-level PAP, auto-adjusting CPAP, and ASV. While none of the variants of PAP improve adherence in unselected patients [51, 52], individual patients may respond favorably to changes in pressure mode. In addition, more choices of mask interface are now available to improve comfort and leaks. However, despite the increase in PAP equipment options, lack of acceptance and inadequate adherence remain the major causes of treatment failure. An integrative approach to PAP treatment including education, objective adherence monitoring, early intervention for side effects, and telephone and clinic support is essential for optimizing adherence.

In general, factors found to predict PAP adherence are increased severity of sleep apnea or higher apnea-hypopnea index (AHI; the average number of apneas and hypopneas per hour of sleep), greater daytime sleepiness, and perceived symptomatic benefit. Some studies suggest that heated humidification can improve PAP adherence, especially in patients with nasal congestion or dryness [53, 54]. Factors that negatively influence adherence are lack of daytime sleepiness, lack of perceived benefit, side effects from PAP, previous uvulopalatopharyngoplasty, nasal obstruction, and claustrophobia [55–59]. Interestingly, studies have not found pressure level to be predictive of adherence.

A number of social-cognitive models have been applied to PAP treatment. In one model, the patient's perception of the relative costs (e.g., side effects, inconvenience) versus benefits (e.g., symptom improvement) determines adherence [55]. The perception of risk from untreated sleep apnea and expectations regarding treatment outcome and volition to engage in treatment behavior may also determine PAP adherence [60]. These models provide a structure for social-cognitive interventions.

Side Effects of PAP

Many patients struggle to use or stop using PAP because of side effects. Most common adverse effects are related to the air pressure of the machine (e.g., air leaks, difficulty exhaling) and to the fit of the mask (e.g., skin irritation, excessive pressure or pain, rash). Ocular, nasal, and oral dryness are also off-putting experiences for patients who use PAP. Claustrophobia, while not technically a side effect of CPAP, can interfere with a patient's ability to use therapy. Less common complaints include aerophagia and gastric distention, ear or sinus infections, or concerns about disturbing a bed partner's sleep. Some patients report facial changes with chronic PAP use [61].

There have been many attempts by the PAP industry to address these common complaints. For example, most machines have a ramp feature in which the machine starts off by delivering a low pressure which gradually increases over time into the therapeutic range. This allows the patient time to fall asleep comfortably. Another common feature of newer machines is an expiratory pressure-reducing system in which the machine drops the pressure by a specified amount during early exhalation. This feature aims to make exhalation more comfortable. Although recent studies have not shown this technology to impact PAP adherence in unselected PAP users [62–64], it remains a useful tool to address individual patient's complaints about pressure intolerance.

Close clinical follow-up with attention to mask fit and comfort is essential for improving individual PAP adherence [65]. Proper interfaces should produce minimal leak, feel comfortable without excessive pressure points, and be easy for the patient to put on and remove. There are numerous available PAP interfaces, and patients often have to be tried on several before finding one that best suits their needs.

Alternatives to PAP Therapy

Positive airway pressure therapy is the standard treatment for sleep-disordered breathing. It is highly effective in eliminating sleep-disordered breathing and improves health outcomes, cognition, and performance. Unfortunately, adherence to PAP remains problematic, and as a result alternative therapies need to be explored. A number of studies have compared PAP to oral appliances [66, 67], position therapy [68], or upper airway surgery [69]. While PAP most effectively and reliably reduces the AHI and sleepiness, patient satisfaction with PAP compared to other treatments likely depends on patient preference.

Surgery

Upper airway surgery is an important treatment option for patients with obstructive sleep apnea, particularly for those who have failed or cannot tolerate PAP. Surgery aims to reduce anatomical upper airway obstruction in the nose, oropharynx, and hypopharynx. Procedures addressing nasal obstruction include septoplasty, turbinectomy, and radiofrequency ablation of the turbinates. Surgical procedures to reduce soft palate redundancy include uvulopalatopharyngoplasty, uvulopalatal flap, and radiofrequency ablation of the soft palate with adenotonsillectomy. More significant, however, particularly in cases of severe OSA, is hypopharyngeal or retrolingual obstruction related to an enlarged tongue base or more commonly due to maxillomandibular deficiency. Surgeries in these cases are aimed at reducing the bulk of the tongue base or providing more space for the tongue in the oropharynx so as to limit posterior collapse during sleep. These procedures include genioglossal advancement, hyoid suspension, distraction osteogenesis, tongue radiofrequency ablation, maxillomandibular advancement hypoglossal nerve stimulation.

Surgery is considered appropriate on a case-by-case basis in those who fail PAP therapy and have anatomical targets. Successful surgery depends on proper patient selection, proper procedure selection, and an experienced surgeon. In general, surgery for OSA is less effective than PAP (with the exception of tracheotomy). Phase I or soft tissue surgeries (nasal, palate reduction, and tongue advancement or reduction surgeries) have a reported success rate of 50–60% for significantly improving OSA by greater than 50% in select patients, whereas phase II or bone surgery (maxillomandibular advancement) has a success rate of greater than 90% [70, 71]. It should be emphasized that most literature uses the definition of surgical success as achieving a greater than 50% reduction in AHI and/or an AHI of less than 20 events per hour. Although sleep apnea surgeries may not be curative, they will often achieve enough treatment effect to require significantly less therapeutic PAP, making tolerance and adherence more favorable [72, 73].

Although fortunately rare, life-threatening complications have been associated with sleep apnea surgery [74, 75]. Fatalities in the early postoperative period have been related to upper airway collapse or obstruction secondary to pharmacological sedation and surgical edema [76]. Nasal PAP use during the perioperative period has shown to protect patients from airway obstruction and hypoxemia and is highly encouraged, especially in cases of severe OSA [77, 78].

Nasal Reconstruction

The goal of nasal reconstructive surgery is to improve nasal airway blockage caused by bony, cartilaginous, or hypertrophied tissues to restore normal breathing as well as to optimize nasal CPAP use. A patent nasal airway is important for minimizing mouth breathing, because mouth breathing worsens upper airway obstruction by forcing the lower jaw to rotate downward and backward and pushing the tongue into the posterior pharyngeal space. Nasal reconstructive surgeries include septal and/or bony intranasal reconstruction, alar valve or alar rim reconstruction, and turbinectomy. Radiofrequency treatments for turbinate hypertrophy may also be done in the outpatient office setting. These procedures are generally low in risk and successful at achieving nasal patency. However, by themselves, they are not likely to make a significant impact on moderate or severe sleep-disordered breathing. Nonetheless, it remains an essential part of treating OSA as a means of improving nasal PAP tolerance and adherence.

Uvulopalatopharyngoplasty

The palatal and lateral pharyngeal tissues are highly compliant and collapsible during sleep in certain patients. Uvulopalatopharyngoplasty (UPPP) aims to enlarge the retropalatal airway by trimming and reorienting the posterior and anterior lateral pharyngeal pillars and by excising the uvula and posterior portion of the palate. This surgery is often performed in conjunction with adenotonsillectomy or combined with limited resection, advancement, or radiofrequency ablation of the tongue base to achieve maximal enlargement of the retropalatal and retrolingual airway [79–81]. UPPP has a reported success rate of approximately 40–50% for improving mild to moderate OSA, although surgical efficacy appears to decrease over time [82]. It is recommended that the procedure be performed by experienced surgeons, as it may be associated with significant complications, including velopharyngeal insufficiency, dysphagia, persistent dryness, and nasopharyngeal stenosis [83–85].

Maxillomandibular Osteotomy

The first reports of mandibular skeletal surgery for OSA were done by Kuo et al. [86] in 1979 and Bear et al. [87] in 1980. This surgery specifically addresses hypopharyngeal or base-of-tongue obstruction. The maxilla and mandible are advanced simultaneously by means of LeFort I maxillary and sagittal-split mandibular osteotomies to enlarge the retrolingual and retropalatal airway. Achieving such clearance, especially for long-term improvement, usually necessitates an advancement of 10–15 mm of the maxilla and mandible. This surgery is perhaps the most effective surgery for improving OSA when performed on appropriately selected patients. Studies report reduction in postoperative respiratory disturbance index (RDI, another marker of the severity of sleep disordered breathing) by at least 50%, with an average improvement of greater than 85%, in approximately 90% of patients [88–90].

In 80% of patients, temporary numbness of the cheek and chin area can occur and usually resolves within 6–12 months after surgery. Skeletal relapse resulting in malocclusion can also occur in up to 15% of patients, and therefore, coordinated treatment with an orthodontist may be necessary when indicated [88].

Hypoglossal Nerve Stimulation

This recently introduced treatment involves implanting a pacemaker-like module subcutaneously. This system is used to stimulate a branch of the hypoglossal nerve. This has been shown to be effective in highly selected patients whose severe sleep apnea has not been adequately treated, whose upper airway collapse is not concentric (by sleep endoscopy), and whose BMI is 32 or less [91].

Tracheotomy

Tracheotomy, because it bypasses the entire upper airway, is considered curative for OSA. However, despite being the most effective surgical treatment for OSA, patient acceptance is low due to the associated morbidity and social implications. Permanent tracheostomy as a long-term treatment of OSA remains an important option in morbidly obese patients with obesity hypoventilation syndrome or in patients with significant craniofacial anomaly for whom all other forms of nonsurgical and surgical treatments have failed.

Oral Appliances

Oral appliances are alternatives to PAP for treatment of obstructive sleep apnea. They offer the advantages of being portable, less bulky and intrusive, and more comfortable than PAP. Oral appliances comprise of mandibular advancement and tongue-retaining devices. Mandibular advancement splints generally attach to the dental arches and mechanically protrude the mandible and the soft tissue structures attached to it. Tongue-retaining devices use suction pressure to maintain the tongue in a protruded position during sleep. Both devices in effect increase upper airway dimension and reduce its collapsibility [92, 93]. Mandibular advancement splints require the patient to have sufficient teeth, whereas tongue-retaining devices can be used by edentulous patients. Most research studies have used mandibular advancement splints, as they represent the most common type of oral appliance.

Compared to PAP, oral appliances are less efficacious for improving the AHI or oxygen saturation [94], though improvements in subjective and objective measures of daytime sleepiness may be similar [66, 95, 96]. A complete response (reduction of the AHI to <5) can be expected in approximately 35–40% of patients with an oral appliance and a partial response (≥50% reduction in AHI but residual AHI >5) in 25% of patients. Treatment failure occurs in approximately 35–40% of patients [97, 98]. Although the efficacy of oral appliances may be inferior and less reliable than PAP therapy, the AASM supports their use for mild-to-moderate OSA or for patients with severe OSA who are unable to tolerate or refuse treatment with PAP.

Adherence to oral appliances is approximately 77% at 1 year [99]. A study using a novel intraoral monitoring device to assess objective adherence found that the average use of the oral appliance was 6.8 h per night, which is similar to self-reported adherence in other studies [100]. In contrast, only 46% of patients use CPAP for at least 4 h per night for >70% of nights [101].

The impact of an oral appliance on cardiovascular and other outcomes is limited to a few studies demonstrating only a modest reduction in blood pressure [95, 97]. Study results are conflicting regarding the impact of the oral appliance on neuropsychological functioning in OSA patients. Some studies show improvement in psychomotor speed; others found no difference or inferiority to PAP in several aspects of neuropsychological functioning [66, 102]. Improvements in objective measures of sleepiness using the maintenance of wakefulness test [103] and the multiple sleep latency test [97] have been demonstrated, but there are no published studies of the effect of oral appliance treatment on motor vehicle accident risk or workplace safety.

It is important to remember that individual patient factors as well as oral appliance type and design will affect treatment efficacy and outcome. Therefore oral appliances should be considered on a case-by-case basis. Some studies have found female gender, lower age, lower body mass index, smaller neck circumference, lower baseline AHI, and supine-dependent OSA to be predictive of successful oral appliance treatment outcomes [104–106]. Various cephalometric predictors of successful oral appliance treatment outcome have also been demonstrated such as shorter soft palate, larger retropalatal airway space, decreased distance between the hyoid and mandibular plane, narrower angle from the sella to the nasion to the supramentale point, and wider angle from the sella to the nasion to the subspinale point [107].

Mandibular advancement splints generate reciprocal forces on the teeth and jaw and can result in acute symptoms, as well as long-term dental and skeletal changes. Complaints associated with oral appliances are usually minor and self-limiting and include excessive salivation, mouth dryness, tooth pain, gum irritation, headaches, and temporomandibular joint discomfort. The frequencies of these adverse effects vary widely, ranging from 6 to 86% of patients [99]. The long-term adverse effects include changes in the occlusion and dental arch, increase in the lower facial height, increase in the mandibular plane angle, increase in the degree of mouth opening, and changes in the inclination of the incisors [108–110]. The duration of oral appliance use correlates with the extent of changes in the bite relationship and mandibular posture.

Weight Loss

Several risk factors such as age, male gender, menopause in women, and craniofacial abnormalities have been identified in the development of OSA, but undoubtedly, the strongest risk factor for OSA is obesity reflected by several markers including body mass index (BMI), neck circumference, and waist-to-hip ratio [111–114]. More than half of the prevalence of OSA is attributable to excess body weight. In fact, for each unit increase in BMI, the adjusted odds ratio for developing OSA is 1.14 (95% CI 1.10–1.19) [113]. However, the impact of BMI on OSA becomes much less significant after age 60, and weight changes have a lesser impact on the severity of OSA in the elderly. In subjects with no OSA or mild OSA at baseline (AHI <15), a 10% weight gain increases the odds of developing moderate (AHI ≥15) or worse OSA by sixfold. A 10% weight gain predicts an approximate 32% increase in the AHI. A 10% weight loss predicts a 26% decrease in the AHI [115]. In randomized controlled trials examining the effect of weight loss on OSA, average AHI appeared to be only modestly affected when comparing the weight loss group with the control group; however, the degree of improvement was associated with degree of weight loss, and there were greater OSA remissions (AHI <5) in the successful weight loss group [116, 117].

Bariatric surgery is an effective treatment for morbid obesity and has shown some benefit for treating sleep-disordered breathing. Studies have shown improvement in self-reported symptoms of snoring, witnessed apneas, and subjective daytime sleepiness in 70–80% of successful bariatric surgery patients. The effect was greatest in those with the most weight loss [118, 119]. The study showed more than 70% reduction in AHI associated with dramatic weight loss following bariatric surgery, though only 38% achieved remission or cure (AHI <5) [120]. It should be noted that the majority of patients remained obese despite incredible weight loss at the time of their repeat polysomnography. Interestingly, a prospective study found approximately half of the patients who had mild OSA following bariatric surgery developed severe OSA 7 years postoperatively despite no significant weight changes [121].

Taken together, the limited studies that assessed OSA pre- and postsurgical weight loss demonstrate a significant improvement in OSA severity and symptoms. However, a significant proportion of patients will continue to have moderate and in some cases severe OSA and should therefore be continued on PAP therapy.

Positional Therapy

The influence of body position on OSA is well recognized. Sleep-disordered breathing severity worsens in the supine posture, most likely due to an increase in upper airway collapsibility and to a posterior displacement of the tongue [122–124]. It is estimated that 50–60% of all OSA patients have positional obstructive sleep, depending how positional sleep apnea is defined.

Numerous positional therapy strategies have been employed to prevent OSA patients from sleeping in a supine position including head-positioning pillows and the "tennis ball technique" (a tennis ball or other obtrusive object fastened to the back with a belt or sewn into the patient's shirt). These tactics have shown to significantly decrease supine sleep time and to decrease AHI [125, 126]. Positional therapy however is clearly inferior to PAP therapy [127]. In addition, adherence is very poor. Objective and self-reported measurements show 74% adherence rates at 3 months, 38% after 6 months, and less than 6% at 2.5 years, with high variability between individuals and age groups [128–130]. Given these poor results, this type of therapy is considered second-line therapy for those who fail PAP or other conventional strategies.

Medications

Pharmacological alternatives to PAP are enticing and continue to be investigated though with limited progress. Drugs that have been tried for the treatment of OSA may be classified into three categories: (1) upper airway tone promoters, (2) respiratory stimulants, and (3) sleep-stage stabilizers. Serotonergic receptors may play a role in upper airway tone, which has led to the trial of many serotonin-modulating medications such as protriptyline [131–133], paroxetine [134], ondansetron [135], and buspirone [136]. Unfortunately, none of these medications have reliably shown to treat OSA. There is some evidence to suggest estrogen replacement in postmenopausal women may improve AHI by possibly improving airway tone [137]; however, this too is unreliable, and estrogen therapy is not indicated as standard treatment for OSA in postmenopausal women. Likewise, ventilatory stimulants such as progestogens [136], acetazolamide [133], and theophyllines [138, 139] have not been shown to be effective for the management of OSA. Tricyclic antidepressant drugs and clonidine [139] have been studied because of their known property for reducing rapid eye movement (REM) sleep and because sleep apnea is known to be worse during this stage of sleep. Unfortunately, they have failed to show significant improvement in OSA and are not considered standard therapy. Sodium oxybate, the standard treatment for cataplexy, induces stage N3 or delta sleep, a stage in which OSA seems particularly absent. The theoretical benefit of induced delta sleep in OSA management has yet to be studied.

There is currently insufficient evidence to recommend any systemic pharmacologic treatment for OSA. Currently the role of medications in OSA treatment is largely adjunctive to standard PAP therapy. For example, medications that reduce nasal congestion such as inhaled steroids may facilitate PAP use and improve PAP adherence. Similarly, early hypnotic use has shown to improve adherence to PAP therapy [140, 141]. Finally, wake-promoting medications are used in OSA patients to treat sleepiness refractory to PAP therapy. As many as 22% of patients who use PAP for more than 6 h per night experience persistent daytime sleepiness, and 52% have evidence of objective sleepiness on the multiple sleep latency test [142–144]. Modafinil, a newer generation non-amphetamine-based wake-promoting medication, has shown to improve functional outcomes in OSA patients with residual sleepiness despite regular PAP use [145].

Conclusion

The mainstay treatment for sleep-disordered breathing is positive airway pressure therapy. There is robust evidence to suggest PAP therapy improves cardiovascular, metabolic, psychiatric, and mental health outcomes. In addition, patients enjoy significant symptomatic benefit as well as improvement in neuropsychomotor function. Unfortunately, many patients also experience side effects, and as a result PAP tolerability and adherence are low. As a result, research is ongoing to determine means of improving PAP adherence, as well as to develop effective alternatives.

References

1. Sullivan CE, Issa FG, Berthon-Jones M, Eves L. Reversal of obstructive sleep apnoea by continuous positive airway pressure applied through the nares. Lancet. 1981;1(8225):862–5.
2. Kushida CA, Littner MR, Hirshkowitz M, et al. Practice parameters for the use of continuous and bilevel positive airway pressure devices to treat adult patients with sleep-related breathing disorders. Sleep. 2006;29(3):375–80.

3. Kushida CA, Chediak A, Berry RB, et al. Clinical guidelines for the manual titration of positive airway pressure in patients with obstructive sleep apnea. J Clin Sleep Med. 2008;4(2):157–71.
4. Ayas NT, Patel SR, Malhotra A, et al. Auto-titrating versus standard continuous positive airway pressure for the treatment of obstructive sleep apnea: results of a meta-analysis. Sleep. 2004;27(2):249–53.
5. Hukins C. Comparative study of autotitrating and fixed-pressure CPAP in the home: a randomized, single-blind crossover trial. Sleep. 2004;27(8):1512–7.
6. Berry RB, Parish JM, Hartse KM. The use of auto-titrating continuous positive airway pressure for treatment of adult obstructive sleep apnea. An American Academy of Sleep Medicine review. Sleep. 2002;25(2):148–73.
7. Farre R, Montserrat JM, Rigau J, Trepat X, Pinto P, Navajas D. Response of automatic continuous positive airway pressure devices to different sleep breathing patterns: a bench study. Am J Respir Crit Care Med. 2002;166(4):469–73.
8. Aurora RN, Chowdhuri S, Ramar K, et al. The treatment of central sleep apnea syndromes in adults: practice parameters with an evidence-based literature review and meta-analyses. Sleep. 2012;35(1):17–40.
9. Morgenthaler TI, Gay PC, Gordon N, Brown LK. Adaptive servoventilation versus noninvasive positive pressure ventilation for central, mixed, and complex sleep apnea syndromes. Sleep. 2007;30(4):468–75.
10. Randerath WJ, Nothofer G, Priegnitz C, et al. Long-term auto servo-ventilation or constant positive pressure in heart failure and co-existing central with obstructive sleep apnea. Chest. 2012;142:440–7.
11. Bradley TD, Logan AG, Kimoff RJ, et al. Continuous positive airway pressure for central sleep apnea and heart failure. N Engl J Med. 2005;353(19):2025–33.
12. Beninati W, Harris CD, Herold DL, Shepard JW Jr. The effect of snoring and obstructive sleep apnea on the sleep quality of bed partners. Mayo Clinic Proc. 1999;74(10):955–8.
13. Parish JM, Lyng PJ. Quality of life in bed partners of patients with obstructive sleep apnea or hypopnea after treatment with continuous positive airway pressure. Chest. 2003;124(3):942–7.
14. Jenkinson C, Davies RJ, Mullins R, Stradling JR. Comparison of therapeutic and subtherapeutic nasal continuous positive airway pressure for obstructive sleep apnoea: a randomised prospective parallel trial. Lancet. 1999;353(9170):2100–5.
15. Sin DD, Mayers I, Man GC, Ghahary A, Pawluk L. Can continuous positive airway pressure therapy improve the general health status of patients with obstructive sleep apnea?: a clinical effectiveness study. Chest. 2002;122(5):1679–85.
16. Monasterio C, Vidal S, Duran J, et al. Effectiveness of continuous positive airway pressure in mild sleep apnea-hypopnea syndrome. Am J Respir Crit Care Med. 2001;164(6):939–43.
17. Barbe F, Mayoralas LR, Duran J, et al. Treatment with continuous positive airway pressure is not effective in patients with sleep apnea but no daytime sleepiness. a randomized, controlled trial. Ann Intern Med. 2001;134(11):1015–23.
18. Bardwell WA, Ancoli-Israel S, Berry CC, Dimsdale JE. Neuropsychological effects of one-week continuous positive airway pressure treatment in patients with obstructive sleep apnea: a placebo-controlled study. Psychosom Med. 2001;63(4):579–84.
19. Henke KG, Grady JJ, Kuna ST. Effect of nasal continuous positive airway pressure on neuropsychological function in sleep apnea-hypopnea syndrome. A randomized, placebo-controlled trial. Am J Respir Crit Care Med. 2001;163(4):911–7.
20. Lim W, Bardwell WA, Loredo JS, et al. Neuropsychological effects of 2-week continuous positive airway pressure treatment and supplemental oxygen in patients with obstructive sleep apnea: a randomized placebo-controlled study. J Clin Sleep Med. 2007;3(4):380–6.
21. Tregear S, Reston J, Schoelles K, Phillips B. Continuous positive airway pressure reduces risk of motor vehicle crash among drivers with obstructive sleep apnea: systematic review and meta-analysis. Sleep. 2010;33(10):1373–80.
22. Teran-Santos J, Jimenez-Gomez A, Cordero-Guevara J. The association between sleep apnea and the risk of traffic accidents. Cooperative Group Burgos-Santander. N Engl J Med. 1999;340(11):847–51.

23. Sassani A, Findley LJ, Kryger M, Goldlust E, George C, Davidson TM. Reducing motor-vehicle collisions, costs, and fatalities by treating obstructive sleep apnea syndrome. Sleep. 2004;27(3):453–8.
24. George CF. Reduction in motor vehicle collisions following treatment of sleep apnoea with nasal CPAP. Thorax. 2001;56(7):508–12.
25. Findley L, Smith C, Hooper J, Dineen M, Suratt PM. Treatment with nasal CPAP decreases automobile accidents in patients with sleep apnea. Am J Respir Crit Care Med. 2000;161(3 Pt 1):857–9.
26. Becker HF, Jerrentrup A, Ploch T, et al. Effect of nasal continuous positive airway pressure treatment on blood pressure in patients with obstructive sleep apnea. Circulation. 2003;107(1):68–73.
27. Pepperell JC, Ramdassingh-Dow S, Crosthwaite N, et al. Ambulatory blood pressure after therapeutic and subtherapeutic nasal continuous positive airway pressure for obstructive sleep apnoea: a randomised parallel trial. Lancet. 2002;359(9302):204–10.
28. Faccenda JF, Mackay TW, Boon NA, Douglas NJ. Randomized placebo-controlled trial of continuous positive airway pressure on blood pressure in the sleep apnea-hypopnea syndrome. Am J Respir Crit Care Med. 2001;163(2):344–8.
29. Dimsdale JE, Loredo JS, Profant J. Effect of continuous positive airway pressure on blood pressure: a placebo trial. Hypertension. 2000;35(1 Pt 1):144–7.
30. Rapoport DM, Sorkin B, Garay SM, Goldring RM. Reversal of the "Pickwickian syndrome" by long-term use of nocturnal nasal-airway pressure. New Engl J Med. 1982;307(15):931–3.
31. Sullivan CE, Berthon-Jones M, Issa FG. Remission of severe obesity-hypoventilation syndrome after short-term treatment during sleep with nasal continuous positive airway pressure. Am Rev Respir Dis. 1983;128(1):177–81.
32. Sajkov D, Wang T, Saunders NA, Bune AJ, McEvoy RD. Continuous positive airway pressure treatment improves pulmonary hemodynamics in patients with obstructive sleep apnea. Am J Respir Crit Care Med. 2002;165(2):152–8.
33. Chin K, Ohi M, Kita H, et al. Effects of NCPAP therapy on fibrinogen levels in obstructive sleep apnea syndrome. Am J Respir Crit Care Med. 1996;153(6 Pt 1):1972–6.
34. Lavie L, Kraiczi H, Hefetz A, et al. Plasma vascular endothelial growth factor in sleep apnea syndrome: effects of nasal continuous positive air pressure treatment. Am J Respir Crit Care Med. 2002;165(12):1624–8.
35. Dyugovskaya L, Lavie P, Lavie L. Increased adhesion molecules expression and production of reactive oxygen species in leukocytes of sleep apnea patients. Am J Respir Crit Care Med. 2002;165(7):934–9.
36. Schulz R, Mahmoudi S, Hattar K, et al. Enhanced release of superoxide from polymorpho-nuclear neutrophils in obstructive sleep apnea. Impact of continuous positive airway pressure therapy. Am J Respir Crit Care Med. 2000;162(2 Pt 1):566–70.
37. Yokoe T, Minoguchi K, Matsuo H, et al. Elevated levels of C-reactive protein and interleukin-6 in patients with obstructive sleep apnea syndrome are decreased by nasal continuous positive airway pressure. Circulation. 2003;107(8):1129–34.
38. Malone S, Liu PP, Holloway R, Rutherford R, Xie A, Bradley TD. Obstructive sleep apnoea in patients with dilated cardiomyopathy: effects of continuous positive airway pressure. Lancet. 1991;338(8781):1480–4.
39. Kaneko Y, Floras JS, Usui K, et al. Cardiovascular effects of continuous positive airway pressure in patients with heart failure and obstructive sleep apnea. N Engl J Med. 2003;348(13):1233–41.
40. Kanagala R, Murali NS, Friedman PA, et al. Obstructive sleep apnea and the recurrence of atrial fibrillation. Circulation. 2003;107(20):2589–94.
41. Peker Y, Hedner J, Norum J, Kraiczi H, Carlson J. Increased incidence of cardiovascular disease in middle-aged men with obstructive sleep apnea: a 7-year follow-up. Am J Respir Crit Care Med. 2002;166(2):159–65.

42. Marin JM, Carrizo SJ, Vicente E, Agusti AG. Long-term cardiovascular outcomes in men with obstructive sleep apnoea-hypopnoea with or without treatment with continuous positive airway pressure: an observational study. Lancet. 2005;365(9464):1046–53.
43. Doherty LS, Kiely JL, Swan V, McNicholas WT. Long-term effects of nasal continuous positive airway pressure therapy on cardiovascular outcomes in sleep apnea syndrome. Chest. 2005;127(6):2076–84.
44. He J, Kryger MH, Zorick FJ, Conway W, Roth T. Mortality and apnea index in obstructive sleep apnea. Experience in 385 male patients. Chest. 1988;94(1):9–14.
45. Babu AR, Herdegen J, Fogelfeld L, Shott S, Mazzone T. Type 2 diabetes, glycemic control, and continuous positive airway pressure in obstructive sleep apnea. Arch Intern Med. 2005;165(4):447–52.
46. Harsch IA, Schahin SP, Radespiel-Troger M, et al. Continuous positive airway pressure treatment rapidly improves insulin sensitivity in patients with obstructive sleep apnea syndrome. Am J Respir Crit Care Med. 2004;169(2):156–62.
47. Goncalves MA, Guilleminault C, Ramos E, Palha A, Paiva T. Erectile dysfunction, obstructive sleep apnea syndrome and nasal CPAP treatment. Sleep Med. 2005;6(4):333–9.
48. Krieger J, Follenius M, Sforza E, Brandenberger G, Peter JD. Effects of treatment with nasal continuous positive airway pressure on atrial natriuretic peptide and arginine vasopressin release during sleep in patients with obstructive sleep apnoea. Clin Sci. 1991;80(5):443–9.
49. Pepin JL, Krieger J, Rodenstein D, et al. Effective compliance during the first 3 months of continuous positive airway pressure. A European prospective study of 121 patients. Am J Respir Crit Care Med. 1999;160(4):1124–9.
50. Sin DD, Mayers I, Man GC, Pawluk L. Long-term compliance rates to continuous positive airway pressure in obstructive sleep apnea: a population-based study. Chest. 2002;121(2):430–5.
51. Smith I, Lasserson TJ. Pressure modification for improving usage of continuous positive airway pressure machines in adults with obstructive sleep apnea. Cochrane Database Syst Rev. 2009;4:CD003531.
52. Kushida CA, Berry RB, Blau A, et al. Positive airway pressure initiation: a randomized controlled trial to assess the impact of therapy mode and titration process on efficacy, adherence, and outcomes. Sleep. 2011;34(8):1083–92.
53. Massie CA, Hart RW, Peralez K, Richards GN. Effects of humidification on nasal symptoms and compliance in sleep apnea patients using continuous positive airway pressure. Chest. 1999;116(2):403–8.
54. Neill AM, Wai HS, Bannan SP, Beasley CR, Weatherall M, Campbell AJ. Humidified nasal continuous positive airway pressure in obstructive sleep apnoea. Eur Respir J. 2003;22(2):258–62.
55. Engleman HM, Wild MR. Improving CPAP use by patients with the sleep apnoea/hypopnoea syndrome (SAHS). Sleep Med Rev. 2003;7(1):81–99.
56. Meslier N, Lebrun T, Grillier-Lanoir V, et al. A French survey of 3,225 patients treated with CPAP for obstructive sleep apnoea: benefits, tolerance, compliance and quality of life. Eur Respir J. 1998;12(1):185–92.
57. McArdle N, Devereux G, Heidarnejad H, Engleman HM, Mackay TW, Douglas NJ. Long-term use of CPAP therapy for sleep apnea/hypopnea syndrome. Am J Respir Crit Care Med. 1999;159(4 Pt 1):1108–14.
58. Meurice JC, Dore P, Paquereau J, et al. Predictive factors of long-term compliance with nasal continuous positive airway pressure treatment in sleep apnea syndrome. Chest. 1994;105(2):429–33.
59. Janson C, Noges E, Svedberg-Randt S, Lindberg E. What characterizes patients who are unable to tolerate continuous positive airway pressure (CPAP) treatment? Respir Med. 2000;94(2):145–9.
60. Weaver TE, Maislin G, Dinges DF, et al. Self-efficacy in sleep apnea: instrument development and patient perceptions of obstructive sleep apnea risk, treatment benefit, and volition to use continuous positive airway pressure. Sleep. 2003;26(6):727–32.

61. Tsuda H, Almeida FR, Tsuda T, Moritsuchi Y, Lowe AA. Craniofacial changes after 2 years of nasal continuous positive airway pressure use in patients with obstructive sleep apnea. Chest. 2010;138(4):870–4.
62. Bakker J, Campbell A, Neill A. Randomized controlled trial comparing flexible and continuous positive airway pressure delivery: effects on compliance, objective and subjective sleepiness and vigilance. Sleep. 2010;33(4):523–9.
63. Berry RB, Kryger MH, Massie CA. A novel nasal expiratory positive airway pressure (EPAP) device for the treatment of obstructive sleep apnea: a randomized controlled trial. Sleep. 2011;34(4):479–85.
64. Aloia MS, Stanchina M, Arnedt JT, Malhotra A, Millman RP. Treatment adherence and outcomes in flexible vs standard continuous positive airway pressure therapy. Chest. 2005;127(6):2085–93.
65. Ballard RD, Gay PC, Strollo PJ. Interventions to improve compliance in sleep apnea patients previously non-compliant with continuous positive airway pressure. J Clin Sleep Med. 2007;3(7):706–12.
66. Engleman HM, McDonald JP, Graham D, et al. Randomized crossover trial of two treatments for sleep apnea/hypopnea syndrome: continuous positive airway pressure and mandibular repositioning splint. Am J Respir Crit Care Med. 2002;166(6):855–9.
67. Ferguson KA, Ono T, Lowe AA, Keenan SP, Fleetham JA. A randomized crossover study of an oral appliance vs nasal-continuous positive airway pressure in the treatment of mild-moderate obstructive sleep apnea. Chest. 1996;109(5):1269–75.
68. Jokic R, Klimaszewski A, Sridhar G, Fitzpatrick MF. Continuous positive airway pressure requirement during the first month of treatment in patients with severe obstructive sleep apnea. Chest. 1998;114(4):1061–9.
69. Woodson BT, Steward DL, Weaver EM, Javaheri S. A randomized trial of temperature-controlled radiofrequency, continuous positive airway pressure, and placebo for obstructive sleep apnea syndrome. Otolaryngol Head Neck Surg. 2003;128(6):848–61.
70. Riley RW, Powell NB, Li KK, Troell RJ, Guilleminault C. Surgery and obstructive sleep apnea: long-term clinical outcomes. Otolaryngol Head Neck Surg. 2000;122(3):415–21.
71. Grote L, Hedner J, Grunstein R, Kraiczi H. Therapy with nCPAP: incomplete elimination of sleep related breathing disorder. Eur Respir J. 2000;16(5):921–7.
72. Zonato AI, Bittencourt LR, Martinho FL, Gregorio LC, Tufik S. Upper airway surgery: the effect on nasal continuous positive airway pressure titration on obstructive sleep apnea patients. Eur Arch Otorhinolaryngol. 2006;263(5):481–6.
73. Friedman M, Schalch P, Joseph NJ. Palatal stiffening after failed uvulopalatopharyngoplasty with the pillar implant system. Laryngoscope. 2006;116(11):1956–61.
74. Hogan PW, Argalious M. Total airway obstruction after maxillomandibular advancement surgery for obstructive sleep apnea. Anesth Analg. 2006;103(5):1267–9.
75. Kim JA, Lee JJ, Jung HH. Predictive factors of immediate postoperative complications after uvulopalatopharyngoplasty. Laryngoscope. 2005;115(10):1837–40.
76. Rennotte MT, Baele P, Aubert G, Rodenstein DO. Nasal continuous positive airway pressure in the perioperative management of patients with obstructive sleep apnea submitted to surgery. Chest. 1995;107(2):367–74.
77. Riley RW, Powell NB, Guilleminault C, Pelayo R, Troell RJ, Li KK. Obstructive sleep apnea surgery: risk management and complications. Otolaryngol Head Neck Surg. 1997;117(6):648–52.
78. Schechter MS, Section on Pediatric Pulmonology SoOSAS. Technical report: diagnosis and management of childhood obstructive sleep apnea syndrome. Pediatrics. 2002;109(4):e69.
79. Nelson LM. Combined temperature-controlled radiofrequency tongue reduction and UPPP in apnea surgery. Ear Nose Throat J. 2001;80(9):640–4.
80. Jacobowitz O. Palatal and tongue base surgery for surgical treatment of obstructive sleep apnea: a prospective study. Otolaryngol Head Neck Surg. 2006;135(2):258–64.
81. Walker-Engstrom ML, Tegelberg A, Wilhelmsson B, Ringqvist I. 4-year follow-up of treatment with dental appliance or uvulopalatopharyngoplasty in patients with obstructive sleep apnea: a randomized study. Chest. 2002;121(3):739–46.

82. Fairbanks DN. Uvulopalatopharyngoplasty complications and avoidance strategies. Otolaryngol Head Neck Surg. 1990;102(3):239–45.
83. Haavisto L, Suonpaa J. Complications of uvulopalatopharyngoplasty. Clin Otolaryngol Allied Sci. 1994;19(3):243–7.
84. Zohar Y, Finkelstein Y, Talmi YP, Bar-Ilan Y. Uvulopalatopharyngoplasty: evaluation of post-operative complications, sequelae, and results. Laryngoscope. 1991;101(7 Pt 1):775–9.
85. Li HY, Li KK, Chen NH, Wang PC. Modified uvulopalatopharyngoplasty: The extended uvulopalatal flap. Am J Otolaryngol. 2003;24(5):311–6.
86. Kuo PC, West RA, Bloomquist DS, McNeil RW. The effect of mandibular osteotomy in three patients with hypersomnia sleep apnea. Oral Surg Oral Med Oral Pathol. 1979;48(5):385–92.
87. Bear SE, Priest JH. Sleep apnea syndrome: correction with surgical advancement of the mandible. J Oral Surg. 1980;38(7):543–9.
88. Prinsell JR. Maxillomandibular advancement surgery in a site-specific treatment approach for obstructive sleep apnea in 50 consecutive patients. Chest. 1999;116(6):1519–29.
89. Waite PD, Wooten V, Lachner J, Guyette RF. Maxillomandibular advancement surgery in 23 patients with obstructive sleep apnea syndrome. J Oral Maxillofac Surg. 1989;47(12):1256–61. Discussion 1262.
90. Guilleminault C, Partinen M, Praud JP, Quera-Salva MA, Powell N, Riley R. Morphometric facial changes and obstructive sleep apnea in adolescents. J Pediatr. 1989;114(6).997–9.
91 Woodson BT, Strohl KP, Soose RJ, et. al. Upper Airway Stimulation for Obstructive Sleep Apnea: 5-Year Outcomes. Otolaryngol Head Neck Surg. 2018 Mar 1:194599818762383. doi: https://doi.org/10.1177/0194599818762383. [Epub ahead of print].
92. Ryan CF, Love LL, Peat D, Fleetham JA, Lowe AA. Mandibular advancement oral appliance therapy for obstructive sleep apnoea: effect on awake calibre of the velopharynx. Thorax. 1999;54(11):972–7.
93. Ng AT, Gotsopoulos H, Qian J, Cistulli PA. Effect of oral appliance therapy on upper airway collapsibility in obstructive sleep apnea. Am J Respir Crit Care Med. 2003;168(2):238–41.
94. Ahrens A, McGrath C, Hagg U. A systematic review of the efficacy of oral appliance design in the management of obstructive sleep apnoea. Eur J Orthod. 2011;33(3):318–24.
95. Barnes M, McEvoy RD, Banks S, et al. Efficacy of positive airway pressure and oral appliance in mild to moderate obstructive sleep apnea. Am J Respir Crit Care Med. 2004;170(6):656–64.
96. Tan YK, L'Estrange PR, Luo YM, et al. Mandibular advancement splints and continuous positive airway pressure in patients with obstructive sleep apnoea: a randomized cross-over trial. Eur J Orthod. 2002;24(3):239–49.
97. Gotsopoulos H, Chen C, Qian J, Cistulli PA. Oral appliance therapy improves symptoms in obstructive sleep apnea: a randomized, controlled trial. Am J Respir Crit Care Med. 2002;166(5):743–8.
98. Mehta A, Qian J, Petocz P, Darendeliler MA, Cistulli PA. A randomized, controlled study of a mandibular advancement splint for obstructive sleep apnea. Am J Respir Crit Care Med. 2001;163(6):1457–61.
99. Ferguson KA, Cartwright R, Rogers R, Schmidt-Nowara W. Oral appliances for snoring and obstructive sleep apnea: a review. Sleep. 2006;29(2):244–62.
100. Lowe AA, Sjoholm TT, Ryan CF, Fleetham JA, Ferguson KA, Remmers JE. Treatment, airway and compliance effects of a titratable oral appliance. Sleep. 2000;23(Suppl 4):S172–8.
101. Kribbs NB, Pack AI, Kline LR, et al. Objective measurement of patterns of nasal CPAP use by patients with obstructive sleep apnea. Am Rev Respir Dis. 1993;147(4):887–95.
102. Naismith S, Winter V, Gotsopoulos H, Hickie I, Cistulli P. Neurobehavioral functioning in obstructive sleep apnea: differential effects of sleep quality, hypoxemia and subjective sleepiness. J Clin Exp Neuropsychol. 2004;26(1):43–54.
103. Menn SJ, Loube DI, Morgan TD, Mitler MM, Berger JS, Erman MK. The mandibular repositioning device: role in the treatment of obstructive sleep apnea. Sleep. 1996;19(10):794–800.
104. Marklund M, Stenlund H, Franklin KA. Mandibular advancement devices in 630 men and women with obstructive sleep apnea and snoring: tolerability and predictors of treatment success. Chest. 2004;125(4):1270–8.

105. Ng AT, Qian J, Cistulli PA. Oropharyngeal collapse predicts treatment response with oral appliance therapy in obstructive sleep apnea. Sleep. 2006;29(5):666–71.
106. Liu Y, Lowe AA, Fleetham JA, Park YC. Cephalometric and physiologic predictors of the efficacy of an adjustable oral appliance for treating obstructive sleep apnea. Am J Orthod Dentofacial Orthop. 2001;120(6):639–47.
107. Mayer G, Hochban W, Meier-Ewert K. Differential therapeutic aspects in treatment of obstructive sleep apnea syndrome. Der Nervenarzt. 1995;66(4):293–8.
108. Pantin CC, Hillman DR, Tennant M. Dental side effects of an oral device to treat snoring and obstructive sleep apnea. Sleep. 1999;22(2):237–40.
109. Robertson CJ. Dental and skeletal changes associated with long-term mandibular advancement. Sleep. 2001;24(5):531–7.
110. Rose EC, Staats R, Virchow C Jr, Jonas IE. Occlusal and skeletal effects of an oral appliance in the treatment of obstructive sleep apnea. Chest. 2002;122(3):871–7.
111. Young T, Peppard PE, Gottlieb DJ. Epidemiology of obstructive sleep apnea: a population health perspective. Am J Respir Crit Care Med. 2002;165(9):1217–39.
112. Palmer LJ, Buxbaum SG, Larkin E, et al. A whole-genome scan for obstructive sleep apnea and obesity. Am J Hum Genet. 2003;72(2):340–50.
113. Tishler PV, Larkin EK, Schluchter MD, Redline S. Incidence of sleep-disordered breathing in an urban adult population: the relative importance of risk factors in the development of sleep-disordered breathing. JAMA. 2003;289(17):2230–7.
114. Young T, Palta M, Dempsey J, Skatrud J, Weber S, Badr S. The occurrence of sleep-disordered breathing among middle-aged adults. N Engl J Med. 1993;328(17):1230–5.
115. Peppard PE, Young T, Palta M, Dempsey J, Skatrud J. Longitudinal study of moderate weight change and sleep-disordered breathing. JAMA. 2000;284(23):3015–21.
116. Tuomilehto HP, Seppa JM, Partinen MM, et al. Lifestyle intervention with weight reduction: first-line treatment in mild obstructive sleep apnea. Am J Respir Crit Care Med. 2009;179(4):320–7.
117. Foster GD, Borradaile KE, Sanders MH, et al. A randomized study on the effect of weight loss on obstructive sleep apnea among obese patients with type 2 diabetes: the Sleep AHEAD study. Arch Intern Med. 2009;169(17):1619–26.
118. Grunstein RR, Stenlof K, Hedner JA, Peltonen M, Karason K, Sjostrom L. Two year reduction in sleep apnea symptoms and associated diabetes incidence after weight loss in severe obesity. Sleep. 2007;30(6):703–10.
119. Dixon JB, Schachter LM, O'Brien PE. Sleep disturbance and obesity: changes following surgically induced weight loss. Arch Intern Med. 2001;161(1):102–6.
120. Valencia-Flores M, Orea A, Herrera M, et al. Effect of bariatric surgery on obstructive sleep apnea and hypopnea syndrome, electrocardiogram, and pulmonary arterial pressure. Obes Surg. 2004;14(6):755–62.
121. Pillar G, Peled R, Lavie P. Recurrence of sleep apnea without concomitant weight increase 7.5 years after weight reduction surgery. Chest. 1994;106(6):1702–4.
122. Penzel T, Moller M, Becker HF, Knaack L, Peter JH. Effect of sleep position and sleep stage on the collapsibility of the upper airways in patients with sleep apnea. Sleep. 2001;24(1):90–5.
123. Teerapraipruk B, Chirakalwasan N, Simon R, et al. Clinical and polysomnographic data of positional sleep apnea and its predictors. Sleep Breath. 2012;16:1167–72.
124. van Kesteren ER, van Maanen JP, Hilgevoord AA, Laman DM, de Vries N. Quantitative effects of trunk and head position on the apnea hypopnea index in obstructive sleep apnea. Sleep. 2011;34(8):1075–81.
125. Van Maanen JP, Richard W, Van Kesteren ER, et al. Evaluation of a new simple treatment for positional sleep apnoea patients. J Sleep Res. 2012;21:322–9.
126. Svatikova A, Chervin RD, Wing JJ, Sanchez BN, Migda EM, Brown DL. Positional therapy in ischemic stroke patients with obstructive sleep apnea. Sleep Med. 2011;12(3):262–6.

127. Permut I, Diaz-Abad M, Chatila W, et al. Comparison of positional therapy to CPAP in patients with positional obstructive sleep apnea. J Clin Sleep Med. 2010;6(3):238–43.
128. Heinzer RC, Pellaton C, Rey V, et al. Positional therapy for obstructive sleep apnea: an objective measurement of patients' usage and efficacy at home. Sleep Med. 2012;13:425–8.
129. Bignold JJ, Deans-Costi G, Goldsworthy MR, et al. Poor long-term patient compliance with the tennis ball technique for treating positional obstructive sleep apnea. J Clin Sleep Med. 2009;5(5):428–30.
130. Oksenberg A, Silverberg D, Offenbach D, Arons E. Positional therapy for obstructive sleep apnea patients: a 6-month follow-up study. Laryngoscope. 2006;116(11):1995–2000.
131. Brownell LG, West P, Sweatman P, Acres JC, Kryger MH. Protriptyline in obstructive sleep apnea: a double-blind trial. N Engl J Med. 1982;307(17):1037–42.
132. Stepanski EJ, Conway WA, Young DK, Zorick FJ, Wittig RM, Roth T. A double-blind trial of protriptyline in the treatment of sleep apnea syndrome. Henry Ford Hosp Med J. 1988;36(1):5–8.
133. Whyte KF, Gould GA, Airlie MA, Shapiro CM, Douglas NJ. Role of protriptyline and acetazolamide in the sleep apnea/hypopnea syndrome. Sleep. 1988;11(5):463–72.
134. Kraiczi H, Hedner J, Dahlof P, Ejnell H, Carlson J. Effect of serotonin uptake inhibition on breathing during sleep and daytime symptoms in obstructive sleep apnea. Sleep. 1999;22(1):61–7.
135. Stradling J, Smith D, Radulovacki M, Carley D. Effect of ondansetron on moderate obstructive sleep apnoea, a single night, placebo-controlled trial. J Sleep Res. 2003;12(2):169–70.
136. Mendelson WB, Maczaj M, Holt J. Buspirone administration to sleep apnea patients. J Clin Psychopharmacol. 1991;11(1):71–2.
137. Polo-Kantola P, Rauhala E, Helenius H, Erkkola R, Irjala K, Polo O. Breathing during sleep in menopause: a randomized, controlled, crossover trial with estrogen therapy. Obstet Gynecol. 2003;102(1):68–75.
138. Mulloy E, McNicholas WT. Theophylline in obstructive sleep apnea. A double-blind evaluation. Chest. 1992;101(3):753–7.
139. Hein H, Behnke G, Jorres RA, Magnussen H. The therapeutic effect of theophylline in mild obstructive sleep Apnea/Hypopnea syndrome: results of repeated measurements with portable recording devices at home. Eur J Med Res. 2000;5(9):391–9.
140. Lettieri CJ, Shah AA, Holley AB, et al. Effects of a short course of eszopiclone on continuous positive airway pressure adherence: a randomized trial. Ann Intern Med. 2009;151(10):696–702.
141. Lettieri CJ, Collen JF, Eliasson AH, Quast TM. Sedative use during continuous positive airway pressure titration improves subsequent compliance: a randomized, double-blind, placebo-controlled trial. Chest. 2009;136(5):1263–8.
142. Weaver TE, Maislin G, Dinges DF, et al. Relationship between hours of CPAP use and achieving normal levels of sleepiness and daily functioning. Sleep. 2007;30(6):711–9.
143. Black J. Sleepiness and residual sleepiness in adults with obstructive sleep apnea. Respir Physiol Neurobiol. 2003;136(2–3):211–20.
144. Santamaria J, Iranzo A, Ma Montserrat J, de Pablo J. Persistent sleepiness in CPAP treated obstructive sleep apnea patients: evaluation and treatment. Sleep Med Rev. 2007;11(3):195–207.
145. Weaver TE, Chasens ER, Arora S. Modafinil improves functional outcomes in patients with residual excessive sleepiness associated with CPAP treatment. J Clin Sleep Med. 2009;5(6):499–505.

Chapter 10
Treating Narcolepsy and Idiopathic Hypersomnia

Tony J. Masri, Vikas Jain, and Christian Guilleminault

Introduction

According to the 2005 International Classification of Sleep Disorders (ICSD-2), narcolepsy and idiopathic hypersomnia are considered hypersomnias of central origin [1]. In this chapter we will review the treatment of these two conditions. The pathophysiology of idiopathic hypersomnia remains unclear. Large systematic studies are lacking due to the rare prevalence of idiopathic hypersomnia. Treatment is mostly focused on excessive daytime sleepiness (EDS). We will discuss presently available and emerging treatment options for narcolepsy. Symptomatic treatment options for narcolepsy are used for EDS in patients with idiopathic hypersomnia.

Diagnosis and Clinical Features of Narcolepsy

Narcolepsy as a distinct syndrome was first characterized by Gelineau in 1880. Excessive daytime sleepiness, sleep paralysis, hypnagogic hallucinations, and cataplexy known as "the clinical tetrad" were reported by Yoss, Daly, and Vogel in the late 1950s [2, 3]. Our understanding of narcolepsy was greatly enhanced by the discovery of cataplexy in knockout mice and the hypocretin mutation in narcoleptic Doberman pinschers. It is important to note that cataplexy is the only feature of the tetrad that is unique to narcolepsy. The presence of a history of excessive daytime

T. J. Masri, MD · V. Jain, MD, FAASM, CCSH · C. Guilleminault, MD, D Bio (✉)
Stanford University Division of Sleep Medicine, Redwood City, CA, USA
e-mail: cguil@stanford.edu

© Springer Science+Business Media, LLC, part of Springer Nature 2018
A. Sharafkhaneh, M. Hirshkowitz (eds.), *Fatigue Management*,
https://doi.org/10.1007/978-1-4939-8607-1_10

sleepiness as well as a positive multiple sleep latency test (MSLT) defined as mean sleep latency less than 8 min with two or more sleep-onset REM periods (SOREMP) is essential for the diagnosis of narcolepsy. The most specific genetic marker for narcolepsy is HLA DQB1*0602. It is found in 95% of patients with narcolepsy with cataplexy [4, 5]. However, HLA DQB1*0602 can be positive in as many as 18–35% of the general population as shown by Mignot's group [4]. Research at Stanford and elsewhere has identified hypocretin as a major sleep-modulating neurotransmitter [6]. In order to confirm the diagnosis of narcolepsy, CSF levels of hypocretin can be measured, and using the Stanford University technique, CSF hypocretin-1 levels below 110 ng/L have a positive predictive value of 94% for narcolepsy with cataplexy [7, 8]. The prevalence of narcolepsy is estimated to be around 0.04%.

Diagnosis and Clinical Features of Idiopathic Hypersomnia

Bedrich Roth was the first to describe idiopathic hypersomnia characterized by excessive daytime sleepiness, prolonged sleep, and somnolence. It was defined by the absence of sleep attacks, cataplexy, sleep paralysis, and hallucinations [9]. The 2005 International Classification of Sleep Disorders (ICSD-2) recognizes two types of idiopathic hypersomnia marked by either long sleep or short sleep (see Table 10.1). Idiopathic hypersomnia with long sleep is the classical form of hypersomnia characterized by excessive daytime sleepiness with unwanted and unrefreshing naps usually once or twice a day along with prolonged nocturnal sleep (more than 10 h) with difficulty waking up in the mornings or from naps. It has been hypothesized that in some cases there is an abnormal homeostatic functioning of sleep [10]. Patients do not independently wake up and require repeated prompting from others and often remain somnolent after waking up. They also commonly suffer from what is best described as "sleep drunkenness." Nocturnal polysomnography (PSG) would have to exclude any other causes of excessive daytime sleepiness.

By definition idiopathic hypersomnia is a diagnosis of exclusion. The differential diagnosis includes narcolepsy with cataplexy, narcolepsy without cataplexy, sleep-related breathing disorders, restless leg syndrome, behaviorally induced insufficient sleep syndrome, chronic sleep insufficiency, long sleepers, chronic fatigue syndrome, and hypersomnia induced by a psychiatric or medical condition. When upper airway resistance syndrome is suspected, esophageal pressure monitoring (Pes) should be included in the sleep study. Otherwise the PSG could be falsely negative.

There are no large epidemiologic studies of idiopathic hypersomnia. Prevalence data is extrapolated from clinical experience at large sleep centers. It is estimated that the ratio of idiopathic hypersomnia to narcolepsy is at 10.3–16.2%. This suggests that the prevalence of idiopathic hypersomnia is between 2 and 8 per 100,000 [11, 12]. Our knowledge of the pathophysiological mechanism of idiopathic

Table 10.1 Criteria for the diagnosis of idiopathic hypersomnia based on the 2005 International Classification of Sleep Disorders (ICSD-2)

	IH with long sleep	IH without long sleep
A.	The patient has a complaint of excessive daytime sleepiness occurring almost daily for at least 3 months	The patient has a complaint of excessive daytime sleepiness occurring almost daily for at least 3 months
B.	The patient has prolonged nocturnal sleep time (more than 10 h) documented by interview, actigraphy, or sleep logs. Waking up in the morning or at the end of naps is almost always laborious	The patient has normal nocturnal sleep (greater than 6 h but less than 10 h), documented by interviews, actigraphy, or sleep logs
C.	Nocturnal polysomnography has excluded other causes of daytime sleepiness	Nocturnal polysomnography has excluded other causes of daytime sleepiness
D.	The polysomnogram demonstrates a short sleep latency and a major sleep period that is prolonged to more than 10 h in duration	Polysomnography demonstrates a major sleep period that is normal in duration (greater than 6 h but less than 10 h)
E.	If an MSLT is performed following overnight polysomnography, a mean sleep latency of less than 8 min is found and fewer than two SOREMPs are recorded. Mean sleep latency in IH with long sleep time has been shown to be 6.2 ± 3.0 min	An MSLT following overnight polysomnography demonstrates a mean sleep latency of less than 8 min and fewer than two SOREMPs. Mean sleep latency in IH has been shown to be 6.2 ± 3.0 min
F.	The hypersomnia is not better explained by another sleep disorder, medical or neurological disorder, mental disorder, medication use, or substance use disorder	The hypersomnia is not better explained by another sleep disorder, medical or neurological disorder, mental disorder, medication use, or substance use disorder

hypersomnia is limited, in part due to the lack of natural animal models. Therefore, it is very difficult to come up with targeted therapeutic agents. A recent study found that patients with narcolepsy and idiopathic hypersomnia had low levels of histamine in the cerebrospinal fluid (CSF) compared to normal levels in patients with obstructive sleep apnea [13]. We might then conclude that there is a common contributing pathology to hypersomnias of central origin. Of the currently available pharmacological treatments, amphetamines, methylphenidate, and modafinil are the most closely studied therapies for idiopathic hypersomnia. We will discuss these agents along with all available treatment options in the following sections dedicated to the treatment of the two conditions.

Behavioral Treatment Options

Counseling patients on the importance of practicing good sleep hygiene and keeping a regular sleep/wake schedule should be an integral part of therapy. Short naps lasting for only 15–20 min a few times a day can be very refreshing for patients with narcolepsy. Large carbohydrate-rich meals should be avoided because of their sedating effects. In patients with idiopathic hypersomnia, increasing sleep time during week-end as been shown to be un-helpful [10]. There is some anecdotal evidence that restricting total sleep time may be beneficial in some patients with idiopathic hypersomnia. Patients with narcolepsy and idiopathic hypersomnia are often frustrated due to the difficulty involved in their diagnosis. Many patients typically go undiagnosed for 10–15 years following the onset of their initial symptoms. Support groups such as the National Sleep Foundation and the Narcolepsy Network are very helpful.

Pharmacological Treatment

Sodium Oxybate

Sodium oxybate is the sodium salt of gamma-hydroxybutyrate acid (GHB). GHB is naturally found in the central nervous system with the highest concentration in the hypothalamus and basal ganglia. GHB in its physiologic form acts as a neurotransmitter affecting other monoamines such as serotonin and dopamine. Sodium oxybate is the only medication that affords clinicians the ability to treat EDS, cataplexy, and disturbed nocturnal sleep with a single agent.

The exact mechanism of GHB is unclear; however, it is thought that it acts on gamma-aminobutyric acid (GABA)$_B$ receptors. High-affinity and low-affinity binding sites have been identified [14]. There is strong consensus that the clinical benefits of GHB are mediated through its action as an agonist at GABA$_B$ receptors. These clinical benefits have been studied over the past 40 years. Sodium oxybate has been FDA approved since 2002 for the treatment of cataplexy and EDS in patients with narcolepsy. It also has been used off-label for the treatment of insomnia and fibromyalgia among others. Broughton and Mamelak were the first to demonstrate improvement in sleep quality, frequency of sleep attacks, and cataplexy. They also noticed an increase in slow-wave sleep with GHB [15–17]. In a double-blind crossover study of 20 patients with narcolepsy for a period of 4 weeks, Scrima et al. [18] demonstrated both decreased cataplexy when compared to placebo and decreased subjective arousals from sleep. PSG and daytime multiple sleep latency test (MSLT) analysis also revealed an increase in slow-wave sleep. They documented a significant increase in wakefulness on MSLT when compared to placebo. In another placebo-controlled, double-blind crossover study of 24 patients, Lammers et al. [19] demonstrated a reduction of hypnogogic hallucinations, daytime sleep attacks, the severity of subjective daytime sleepiness, awakenings out of REM sleep, and percentage of wakefulness during REM sleep. In addition, they noted some decrease of cataplexy attacks, but it was not statistically significant. As previously seen in other studies, there has been a clear trend toward an increase in slow-wave sleep. Larger studies by the US Xyrem multicenter study group looking at the administration of sodium oxybate over a longer period of time have replicated similar results [20]. Upon discontinuation of treatment, patients who were administered GHB did not have evidence of rebound cataplexy, and there were no adverse events or any features of acute withdrawals noted when compared to placebo [21]. When it comes to the effects of GHB on nocturnal awakenings, increase in slow-wave sleep, and improved concentration, researchers observed a clear dose-dependent effect. The higher doses were 7.5 g and 9 g [22]. Of note, the therapeutic effects of GHB are not simultaneous; if the effects on cataplexy and sleep are seen quickly after administration of the therapeutic dose, the effect of daytime sleepiness takes 2–3 months to be observed. This strongly suggests that the effect is not primary but that GHB induces other changes that progressively lead to an alerting action. It has been suggested – but never proven – that an interaction between GHB and dopamine secretion is behind the progressive development of the alerting effect. Such delayed alerting response means that initially sleepy patients should be treated with another drug until GHB is effective.

Side Effects of Sodium Oxybate

The most common side effects include nausea, headache, dizziness, and enuresis. To a lesser extent, viral infections, pain, and weight loss have been noted. In our experience, it would be best to begin with a low dose and titrate upward slowly as nausea and enuresis typically resolve within the first few weeks.

Administration of Sodium Oxybate

Sodium oxybate is typically divided into two nocturnal doses separated by 2.5–4 h. The first dose is given at bedtime and should be at least 2 h after the last meal to allow for optimal absorption. An appropriate starting dose can be 2–2.5 g, twice nightly. This dose can be titrated upward to a maximum of 9 g based on nocturnal total sleep, sleep paralysis, and cataplexy. The half-life of sodium oxybate is between 90 and 120 min. Given the immediate onset of somnolence, patients should be instructed to lie down and remain in bed immediately after ingestion. The effective dose begins at 6 g. Generally the effects of GHB are noticed within the first few days of administration; however it may take 2–3 months to achieve a full response. There has also been a demonstrated sustained improvement of cataplexy for over 12 months while maintaining efficacy on daytime sleepiness. Multiple studies have not revealed a negative effect on respiratory parameters [20, 23–28]. In patients with concomitant sleep apnea, the recommended optimal treatment should include treatment with nasal continuous positive airway pressure (CPAP). We do not recommend the use of sodium oxybate in pregnant patients. In patients with hepatic failure, the dose should be reduced. Also given the high sodium load, sodium oxybate should be given with caution in patients with congestive heart failure. GHB has been previously used as a party drug with the potential to produce disinhibition, euphoric state, and amnesia when abused. However, clinically monitored dosing is relatively safe and has low risk for dependence [29]. Patients should be instructed to avoid alcohol when using GHB. Also, if the first nocturnal dose was missed, patients should not double up on the second dose. Until present, there have not been any studies using GHB for the treatment of idiopathic hypersomnia, and therefore we do not recommend its use for the treatment of excessive daytime sleepiness in this population. GHB has been used in children as young as 6 years of age; usually the starting dose is lower than in adults, and the total dosage is around 6 g till teenage with decent body weight.

Treatment of Excessive Daytime Sleepiness with Stimulants (Table 10.2)

Modafinil

Modafinil is the recommended first-line treatment for EDS. The exact mechanism of action by which modafinil promotes wakefulness is unclear. Modafinil is not chemically related to other stimulants such as amphetamines and methylphenidate. There is strong evidence that modafinil has effects on the presynaptic dopaminergic mechanisms [30, 31]. Based on in vivo microdialysis studies, modafinil has been shown to increase extracellular levels of dopamine in the brain [32–34]. It has also been suggested that modafinil has a stimulating action on histaminergic neurons involved in alertness.

In a double-blind placebo-controlled comparison trial of modafinil, sodium oxybate, or the combination for the treatment of EDS in 270 adult patients with narcolepsy, effectiveness was demonstrated with both medications with an additive benefit when used together [35]. As both modafinil and GHB are metabolized through the liver, when administrated together, we recommend regular hepatic function testing.

Anderson et al., through a retrospective study, looked at 54 patients who started on modafinil of which 39% remained on this drug alone: 24 patients had a drop of more than 4 points on their Epworth Sleepiness Scale (ESS), 8 were switched to amphetamines, and 7 had no reported benefit [36]. In a similar study

Table 10.2 Recommended pharmacologic dosages for the treatment of excessive daytime sleepiness

Medication	Starting dose	Maximum dose
Modafinil	100 mg/day	400 mg/day
Armodafinil	50 mg/day	250 mg/day
Sodium oxybate (GHB)	5 g/day divided into 2 doses	9 g/day
Methylphenidate	10 mg/day	60 mg/day
Atomoxetine	10 mg/day	25 mg/day
Dextroamphetamine	5 mg/day	60 mg/day
Methamphetamine	20 mg/day	25 mg/day

by Ali et al., 25 out of 50 patients remained on modafinil, 18 had complete symptomatic relief, while 4 had a partial response [37]. In a recent study on modafinil in patients with idiopathic hypersomnia and narcolepsy, Lavault et al. demonstrated a similar benefit [38].

Within 2 h of administration, modafinil reaches its peak bioavailability. The administration half-life ranges between 10 and 17 h and reaches its steady state within 2–4 days. European studies suggest twice-daily administration in the morning and around noon. We recommend starting with a low dose of 100 mg daily and titrating upward to 400 mg per day as needed. This dosage can be divided into a morning and afternoon dose for those patients with persistent afternoon sleepiness. Modafinil can induce cytochrome p450 hepatic enzymes; therefore, plasma levels of other medications such as phenytoin, propranolol, warfarin, tricyclic antidepressants, and oral contraceptives can be altered. Women of childbearing age who are prescribed with modafinil should be advised to use an alternative form of contraception. The effectiveness of steroid contraceptives can remain reduced for up to 1 month after discontinuation. Modafinil has a low potential for abuse due to the lack of addictive quality, and tolerance has not been demonstrated. The most common side effects include headache and to a lesser extent nervousness, dry mouth, and nausea. Modafinil may increase blood pressure, and therefore careful monitoring is crucial in patients with hypertension or heart disease. There have also been two reported cases of Stevens-Johnson syndrome with the use of modafinil. Modafinil is considered by the FDA to be a pregnancy category B drug. The European Regulatory Agency has discontinued recommendation of usage of modafinil in OSA patients treated with nasal CPAP due to cardiovascular concern. There is no clear evidence that modafinil has such side effects in narcolepsy patients [39].

Armodafinil

The FDA approved armodafinil in 2007 for the treatment of excessive daytime sleepiness. Armodafinil is a longer-lasting R-enantiomer of racemic modafinil. The effective half-life is approximately 15 h with a similar mean maximum plasma concentration as modafinil. However, plasma concentrations were found to be higher in patients during wakefulness later in the day when compared to modafinil. This is particularly beneficial for patients suffering from idiopathic hypersomnia with persistent afternoon excessive daytime sleepiness. The side effect profile is similar to modafinil. Bioavailability is not usually affected by food intake; however, absorption can be delayed up to 2–4 h if taken with food.

One hundred ninety-six patients with narcolepsy were studied in a multicenter randomized double-blind placebo-controlled trial and were found to have a significant improvement in excessive daytime sleepiness throughout the day [40–42]. There are no studies providing head-to-head comparisons of modafinil to armodafinil.

Amphetamines

Amphetamines and derivatives are potent central nervous system stimulants. At low doses these stimulants increase the release of dopamine, norepinephrine, and serotonin; and at higher doses they can inhibit the reuptake of amines by dopamine transporters [43]. Amphetamine through its D-isomer is more selective for dopamine transmission. Methamphetamine is more lipophilic than D-amphetamine and as a result has a more rapid onset of action. The elimination half-life of amphetamines varies between 10 and 30 h. Ali and associates looked at seven patients who received dextroamphetamine. None of them had a complete or partial response to the drug. Five patients received methamphetamine, and three patients had a complete response. Amphetamines can improve the performance of simple motor and cognitive tasks. They can also enhance endurance, coordination, as well as mental and physical alertness. The highest benefit is noted in monotonous situations [44]. The lowest effective dose should be prescribed. These medications should be administered in the morning, lunchtime, and in the afternoon, but no later than 3 pm. The most common side effects of amphetamines include irritability, mood changes, headache, hyperactivity, and weight loss. These side effects are more prominent at the higher than recommended dose by the American Academy of Sleep Medicine. At such high doses, side effects can include psychosis and paranoia, and patients might require psychiatric hospitalization. There is little evidence of abuse or addiction in patients with narcolepsy [35]. However, the same cannot be reported with patients with idiopathic hypersomnia due to a lack of data. Dextroamphetamine is classified by the FDA as pregnancy category B, and methamphetamine is FDA pregnancy category C. Amphetamines may induce a rebound hypersomnia that has been related to its mechanism of action: amphetamine inhibits reuptake and depletes presynaptic vesicles of the involved neurotransmitters. At one point, therapeutic action will clearly decline which may necessitate the drug being given more often or increasing the dosage without truly addictive behavior.

Based on our clinical experience, methylphenidate is superior to amphetamines. Our patients derive a similar benefit with methylphenidate as they do from modafinil. In a study by Ali et al., 61 patients received methylphenidate, and 40 reported a complete response and 14 had a partial response [37]. Methylphenidate has a shorter elimination half-life that allows for it to be given in 2–3 doses throughout the day. Slow-release form may be helpful if subjects do not want to have multiple intakes. We do not recommend higher than 60 mg per day of either methylphenidate or amphetamines. Overall methylphenidate has a better therapeutic index with a more limited reduction of appetite and less increase in blood pressure when compared to amphetamines [45]. As with amphetamines, the abuse potential with methylphenidate is low in patients with narcolepsy. The FDA classifies methylphenidate as pregnancy category C. Of note, none of the currently available stimulants have been systematically studied in parallel with a placebo control or in comparison with each other in patients with narcolepsy.

Other Drugs

Atomoxetine, a specific noradrenergic reuptake inhibitor, has shown some benefit in improving daytime sleepiness in children. However it is not as effective as modafinil or sodium oxybate in older teenagers and adults [40, 46]. Atomoxetine can also help with cataplexy.

Selegiline is an irreversible monoamine oxidase B inhibitor. Through its active metabolites, L-amphetamine and L-methamphetamine, it provides improvement of excessive daytime sleepiness with a dose of 20 mg per day to a maximum of 40 mg per day [40, 46]. There is a risk of hypertensive emergencies; therefore, a diet low in tyramine is recommended. This potentially serious adverse effect makes this drug far less appealing.

Treatment of Cataplexy (Table 10.3)

Cataplexy is the result of REM-associated muscle atonia inappropriately occurring during periods of wakefulness in narcolepsy patients. Muscarinic, cholinergic, and noradrenergic systems at various receptor levels in addition to glycinergic and glutaminergic receptors are involved in the inhibitory pathway affecting lower motor neuron control. We discuss medications that target these receptors and help alleviate cataplexy.

Monoamine Inhibitors and Other Antidepressants

The first medications used to treat cataplexy included imipramine, clomipramine, and protriptyline [29, 47, 48]. These medications are all tricyclic antidepressants which inhibit serotonin, norepinephrine, and dopamine reuptake and block

Table 10.3 Recommended pharmacologic dosages for the treatment auxiliary effects such as cataplexy

Medication[a]	Starting dose (mg/day)	Maximum dose (mg/day)
Venlafaxine	75	300
Fluoxetine	20	60
Viloxazine	50	200
Protriptyline	2.5	20
Imipramine	25	200
Clomipramine	25	200
Desipramine	25	200

[a]Note for Table 10.3: The use of the antidepressant medications listed is not approved by the US Food and Drug Administration (FDA) for the treatment of cataplexy. The only medication specifically approved by the FDA for cataplexy is sodium oxybate (see Table 10.3 for dosage)

cholinergic, histaminergic, and adrenergic transmission. There is a significant anticholinergic side effect profile. As a result, patients commonly suffer from dry mouth, sweating, tachycardia, constipation, and sexual side. They are by no means the first line of treatment for cataplexy. Some clinicians use low doses of clomipramine as a treatment option for cataplexy [49, 50]. The abrupt discontinuation of tricyclic antidepressants can worsen cataplexy and might lead in some cases to status cataplecticus [51].

Selective serotonin reuptake inhibitors (SSRI) such as fluoxetine have been studied in the treatment of cataplexy [52]. We recommend starting fluoxetine at 20 mg in the morning, to be slowly increased at first to 60 mg and if needed up to 80 mg a day divided into twice-daily dosing. In addition, fluvoxamine at doses varying from 25 to 200 mg per day has had some benefits. These drugs, particularly fluoxetine, mostly act through their active metabolites such as norfluoxetine, a noradrenaline reuptake blocker. Typical side effects with these medications include nausea, some sexual difficulties, and central nervous system excitation. However, they are far better tolerated than older tricyclic antidepressants. SSRIs are FDA pregnancy category C. A slow withdrawal should be used in order to avoid rebound cataplexy which typically occurs 3–4 days after withdrawal and peaks near the tenth day following discontinuation.

Venlafaxine, a newer antidepressant, which acts as an inhibitor of serotonin and noradrenergic reuptake and to a lesser extent an inhibitor of dopamine reuptake, is commonly used. Similar to other newer antidepressants, it has beneficial effects on cataplexy, hypnogogic/hypnopompic hallucinations, and sleep paralysis. We typically begin with a dose of 75 mg and slowly titrate up to a dose of 150 mg a day. When faced with a decision of whether to use venlafaxine or sodium oxybate for the treatment of cataplexy, there are several practical considerations. Sodium oxybate has a more significant effect on daytime sleepiness, but it will take several weeks before such effect is noted. However, venlafaxine is more affordable and is readily available.

Emerging Treatments

Based on new discoveries of the pathophysiology of narcolepsy, new treatment modalities are being studied. The two major areas of focus are excessive daytime sleepiness and cataplexy. These treatment categories include hypocretin-based treatments, gene therapy, cell transplantation, immunotherapy, thyrotrophin (TRH) agonists and analogs, and histamine (H3 receptor) antagonists.

Hypocretin-Based Therapy

In the future, replacing hypocretin will become the gold standard for treatment of narcolepsy [53]. Low and undetectable levels of hypocretin are reported in 95% of patients with narcolepsy and cataplexy [8, 54]. As a result, restoring the function of the hypocretin neurons would alleviate cataplexy and improve excessive daytime sleepiness. Hypocretin supplementation is now being investigated with some promising results. In a study by John et al., canines who underwent systemic administration of hypocretin experienced an increase in wake times and activity levels, along with reduced sleep fragmentation. In addition, cataplexy was reduced in a dose-dependent fashion [55]. This is only one example of several animal studies that has shown promising results. The major challenge of these therapies is the delivery of hypocretin across the blood-brain barrier. Alternative methods of delivery have also shown some promise in animal studies. These include intracerebroventricular hypocretin replacement, hypocretin stem cell transplantation, and intranasal hypocretin administration. In particular, intranasal delivery of hypocretin can bypass the blood-brain barrier with the benefits of a short onset of action and limited peripheral side effects [56]. A study conducted by Hanson et al. showed intranasal delivery of hypocretin in awake mice led to significant drug delivery in the spinal cord and brain. The highest concentration of hypocretin was found to be in the hypothalamus and trigeminal nerve [56]. A recent short study by Baier et al. showed that when administered before bedtime intranasally, there was an effect on REM sleep and decrease in the number of transition wake-REM sleep [57]. Another alternative to provide delivery of hypocretin would be peptide analogs that could traverse the blood-brain barrier. The challenge would be to find peptide analogs with the appropriate combination and high selective activation to keep peripheral side effects at a minimum. Diurnal fluctuations in hypocretin secretions have been observed. As a result, any therapy would require time-controlled administration to account for circadian variations [58]. Hypocretin agonists might actually be effective in patients suffering from excessive daytime sleepiness in the absence of narcolepsy.

Gene Therapy

Stimulating the production of hypocretin through gene therapy would theoretically address the hypocretin deficiency seen in narcolepsy. A study by Mieda et al. revealed that deficiency or the absence of hypocretin does not always result in permanent loss of function. The study suggests hypocretin gene therapy with viral vectors as a potential treatment option [59]. There is also evidence looking at molecular genetics of narcolepsy that suggests targeting monoaminergic genes and immune-related genes. A genetic panel would then provide the treating physician a predictive value to predetermine the responsiveness to specific combination of therapies.

Cell Transplantation

It is estimated that normal humans have about 70,000 hypocretin neurons. An estimated loss of 85–95% of these neurons occurs before symptoms are produced in patients with narcolepsy. As a result, a minimum of 10% of hypocretin-producing cells would be necessary to obtain a therapeutic effect [8, 60]. Transplanting hypocretin-producing cells as seen in similar studies with dopaminergic neurons in Parkinson's patients could be a treatment option [61]. Limitations to this approach include cost-effectiveness, graft reactions, and the available supply of hypocretin neurons [62].

Immunotherapy

An autoimmune process is hypothesized to be responsible for the mechanism by which hypocretin neurons are destroyed. Some investigations with immuno-therapy such as intravenous immunoglobulin (IVIG) have been explored in animal models and in humans. Combination therapy of methylprednisolone, azathioprine, and methotrexate applied at birth to canines with narcolepsy resulted in an initial delay of onset of symptoms and reduction of cataplexy by as much as 90% [63]. Canines treated at a later stage in life had a lesser response. Based on small case reports in humans, treatment with prednisone and plasma-pheresis alone has not yet shown long-term clinical benefit [64, 65]. However, treatment with IVIG especially within 1–2 months from the onset of symptoms has been shown to have long-lasting benefits on cataplexy and EDS in small case series [66, 67]. However, immunosuppressive agents are not always effective. Their therapeutic potential may be directly related to the timing of the administration. If hypocretin deficiency is due to the reversible destruction of hypocretin-producing cells rather than an irreversible destruction of these neurons, immunotherapy may continue to work in abating the symptoms beyond the initial phase.

Thyrotropin-Releasing Agents

Thyrotropin-releasing hormone (TRH) is a tripeptide hormone found throughout the central nervous system. It stimulates the release of thyroid-stimulating hormone and prolactin. Nishino and associates studied the effectiveness of three TRH analogs in the treatment of excessive daytime sleepiness and narcolepsy in canines [68]. Two out of the three compounds had benefits on excessive daytime sleepiness, while all three had a significant impact on the frequency of cataplexy. The most potent compound, CG-3703, had an anticataplectic potency equal to similar doses of desipramine and clomipramine. Its effective dose in producing wakefulness was similar to a comparable dose of d-amphetamine. With further research, TRH agonists may be applied in the treatment of humans with narcolepsy.

Histamine₃ Receptor Antagonists

Histamine plays a key role in the regulation of the sleep-wake cycle. Histaminergic neurons projecting from the tuberomammillary nucleus in the hypothalamus constitute the only source of histamine in the central nervous system. During wakefulness histaminergic activity is at its peak, while its decline produces sleepiness. Nishino and associates reported a decrease of histamine in the CSF of patients suffering from narcolepsy and idiopathic hypersomnia [69]. As a result, histamine is a crucial treatment target for excessive daytime sleepiness in patients with idiopathic hypersomnia. H_3R is a subtype of histamine receptors. Research on H_3R antagonists has shown that it can activate histaminergic neurons and increase the levels of histamine while producing wakefulness [70]. In addition, H_3R is involved in the regulation of other neurotransmitters such as serotonin, dopamine, and norepinephrine. Out of the ten largest pharmaceutical companies, eight are involved in research looking at histamine H_3R [71]. New drugs with high selectivity for this receptor are being developed. The first of such medications is tiprolisant or BF2.649 which has passed clinical phase 2 trials for the treatment of excessive daytime sleepiness in patients suffering from narcolepsy [70]. A small single-blinded study with 22 subjects receiving tiprolisant after taking placebo for 1 week had a reduced Epworth sleepiness score by 5.9 points compared to 1.0 in placebo [72]. The main challenges in the development of these drugs involve in addition to the delivery process of long-term effects and circadian variations of histamine.

Conclusion

As in similarly rare disorders, large randomized, double-blind placebo-controlled trials evaluating the pathophysiology and treatment of narcolepsy and idiopathic hypersomnia are greatly limited. However, breakthroughs in basic neurobiology and neurogenetics, such as the ones we have outlined, will continue to enhance our understanding and offer new insights. This long journey of great discoveries has paved the way for more effective treatment modalities.

References

1. American Academy of Sleep Medicine. International classification of sleep disorders. Diagnostic and coding manual. 2nd ed. Westchester: American Academy of Sleep Medicine; 2005.
2. Westphal C. Eigenthümliche mit Einschläfen verbundene Anfälle. Arch Psychiatr. 1677;7:631–5.
3. Fisher F. Epileptoide schlafzustände. Arch Psychiatr. 1878;8:200–3.

4. Mignot E, Hayduk R, Black J, et al. HLA-DQB1*0602 is associated with narcolepsy in 509 narcoleptic patients. Sleep. 1997;20:1012–20.

5. Zeman A, Britton T, Douglas N, et al. Narcolepsy and excessive daytime sleepiness. BMJ. 2004;329:724–8.

6. Lin L, Faraco R, Li R, et al. The sleep disorder canine narcolepsy is caused by a mutation in the hypocretin (orexin) receptor 2 gene. Cell. 1999;98:365–76.

7. Dauviliers Y, Arnulf I, Mignot E. Narcolepsy with cataplexy. Lancet. 2007;369:499–511.

8. Mignot E, Lammers GJ, Ripley B, et al. The role of cerebrospinal fluid hypocretin measurement in the diagnosis of narcolepsy and other hypersomnias. Arch Neurol. 2002;59:1553–62.

9. Roth B. In: Roth B, editor. Narkolepsie und hypersomnie. Berlin: VEB Verlag; 1962.

10. Bassetti C, Pelayo R, Guilleminault C. Idiopathic hypersomnia. In: Kryger MH, Roth T, Dement WC, editors. Principle and practice of sleep medicine. 4th ed; 2005. p. 791–800.

11. Bassetti C, Aldrich MS. Idiopathic hypersomnia. A series of 42 patients. Brain. 1997;120(Pt 8):1423–35.

12. Billiard M, Dauvilliers Y. Idiopathic hypersomnia. Sleep Med Rev. 2001;5(5):351–60.

13. Kanbayashi T, Kodama T, Kondo H, et al. CSF histamine contents in narcolepsy, idiopathic hypersomnia and obstructive sleep apnea syndrome. Sleep. 2009;32(2):175–80.

14. Snead OC 3rd, Liu CC. Gamma-hydroxybutyric acid binding sites in rat and human brain synaptosomal membranes. Biochem Pharmacol. 1984;33:2587–90.

15. Mamelak M, Escriu JM, Stokan O. The effects of gamma hydroxybutyrate on sleep. Biol Psychiatry. 1977;12:273–88.

16. Broughton R, Mamelak M. The treatment of narcolepsy-cataplexy with nocturnal gamma-hydroxybutyrate. Can J Neurol Sci. 1979;6:1–6.

17. Broughton R, Mamelak M. Effects of nocturnal gamma hydroxybutyrate on sleep/waking patterns in narcolepsy-cataplexy. Can J Neurol Sci. 1980;7:23–31.

18. Scrima L, Hartman PG, Johnson FH Jr, Hiller FC. Efficacy of gamma-hydroxybutyrate versus placebo in treating narcolepsy cataplexy: double-blind subjective measures. Biol Psychiatry. 1989;26:331–43.

19. Lammers GJ, Arends J, Declerck AC, et al. Gamma hydroxybutyrate and narcolepsy: a double-blind placebo-controlled study. Sleep. 1993;16:216–20.

20. A randomized, double blind, placebo-controlled multicenter trial comparing the effects of three doses of orally administered sodium oxybate with placebo for the treatment of narcolepsy. Sleep. 2002;25: 42–9.

21. U.S. Xyrem Multicenter Study Group. Sodium oxybate demonstrates long-term efficacy for the treatment of cataplexy in patients with narcolepsy. Sleep Med. 2004;5:119–23.

22. Mamelak M, Black J, Montplaisir J, Ristanovic R. A pilot study on the effects of sodium oxybate on sleep architecture and daytime alertness in narcolepsy. Sleep. 2004;27:1327–34.

23. Borgen LA, Okerholm RA, Lai A, et al. The pharmacokinetics of sodium oxybate oral solution following acute and chronic administration to narcoleptic patients. J Clin Pharmacol. 2004;44:253–7.

24. Scharf MB. Assessment of sodium oxybate for the long-term treatment of narcolepsy. Sleep. 2001;23(Abstract Suppl):A234.

25. Hornfeltdt C, Pertile T. Lack of withdrawal symptoms following abrupt cessation of therapeutically administered sodium oxybate. Sleep. 2001;24(Abstract Suppl):A236.

26. Black J, Ristanovic R, Mamelak M, et al. Dose response effects of sodium oxybate on polysomnographic (PSG) measures in narcolepsy patients; preliminary findings. Sleep. 2001;24(Abstract Suppl):A321.

27. Ristanovic RA, Black J, Mamelak M, et al. Effect of increasing doses of sodium oxybate on nocturnal respiratory disturbances. Sleep. 2002;25(Abstract Suppl):A473–4.

28. Black J, Ristanovic RA, Mamelak M, et al. Effect of increasing doses of sodium oxybate on nocturnal oxygen saturation: preliminary findings. Sleep. 2002;25(Abstract Suppl):A474–5.

29. Hishikawa Y, Ida H, Nakai K, et al. Treatment of narcolepsy with imipramine (tofranil) and desmethylimipramine (pertofran). J Neurol Sci. 1965;3:453–61.

30. Nishino S, Mao J, Sampathkumaran R, et al. Increased dopaminergic transmission mediates the wake-promoting effects of CNS stimulants. Sleep Res Online. 1998;1(1):49–61.
31. Minzenberg MJ, Carter CS. Modafinil: a review of neurochemical actiosn and effects on cognition. Neuropsychopharmacology. 2008;33(7):1477–502.
32. De Saint-Hilaire Z, Orosco M, Rouch C, et al. Variations in extra-cellular monoamines in the prefrontal cortex and median hypothalamus after modafinil administration: a microdialysis study in rats. Neuroreport. 2001;12(16):3533–7.
33. Wisor JP, Nishino S, Sora I, et al. Dopaminergic role in stimulant-induced wakefulness. J Neurosci. 2001;21(5):1787–94.
34. Murillo-Rodriguez E, Haro R, Palomero-Rivero M, et al. Modafinil enhances extracellular levels of dopamine in the nucleus accumbens and increases wakefulness in rats. Behav Brain Res. 2007;176(2):353–7.
35. Parkes JD, Dahlitz M. Amphetamine prescription. Sleep. 1993;16(3):201–3.
36. Anderson KN, Pilsworth S, Sharpless LD, et al. Idiopathic hypersomnia: a study of 77 cases. Sleep. 2007;30(10):1274–81.
37. Ali M, Auger RR, Slocumb NL, et al. Idiopathic hypersomnia: clinical features and response to treatment. J Clin Sleep Med. 2009;5(6):562–8.
38. Lavault S, Dauvilliers Y, Drouot X, et al. Benefit and risk of modafinil in idiopathic hypersomnia vs. narcolepsy with cataplexy. Sleep Med. 2011;12(6):550–6.
39. Hedner J, Zou D. Pharmacological management of sleep disordered breathing. In: McNicholas WT, Bonsignore MR, editors. Sleep apnoea, vol. 50. Sheffield: European Respiratory Society; 2010. p. 321–39.
40. Billiard M. Narcolepsy: current treatment options and future approaches. Neuropsychiatr Dis Treat. 2008;4:557–66.
41. Lankford DA. Armodafinil: a new treatment for excessive sleepiness. Expert Opin Investig Drugs. 2008;17:565–73.
42. Harsh JR, Hayduk R, Rosenberg R, et al. The efficacy and safety of armodafinil as treatment for adults with excessive sleepiness associated with narcolepsy. Curr Med Res Opin. 2006;22:761–74.
43. Seiden LS, Sabol KE, Ricaurte GA. Amphetamine: effects on catecholamine systems and behavior. Annu Rev Pharmacol Toxicol. 1993;33:639–77.
44. Mitler M, Erman M, Hajdukovic R. The treatment of excessive somnolence with stimulant drugs. Sleep. 1993;16:203–6.
45. Guilleminault C, Carskadon MA, Dement WC. On the treatment of rapid eye movement narcolepsy. Arch Neurol. 1974;30(1):90–3.
46. Roth T. Narcolepsy: treatment issues. J Clin Psychiatry. 2007;68(Suppl. 13):16–9.
47. Akimoto H, Honda Y, Takahashi Y. Pharmacotherapy in narcolepsy. Dis Nerv Syst. 1960;21:1–3.
48. Schmidt HS, Clark RW, Hyman PR. Protriptyline: an effective agent in the treatment of the narcolepsy-cataplexy syndrome and hypersomnia. Am J Psychiatry. 1977;134:183–5.
49. Billiard M, Bassetti C, Dauvilliers Y, EFNS Task Force, et al. EFNS guidelines on management of narcolepsy. Eur J Neurol. 2006;13(10):1035–48.
50. Parkes D. Introduction to the mechanism of action of different treatments of narcolepsy. Sleep. 1994;17:S93–6.
51. Lammers GJ. In: Barkoukis T, Matheson J, Ferber R, Doghramji K, editors. Therapy in sleep medicine. 1st ed. Philadelphia: Elsevier; 2011. p. 293.
52. Langdon N, Bandak S, Shindler J, et al. Fluoxetine in the treatment of cataplexy. Sleep. 1986;9:371–2.
53. Mignot E, Nishino S. Emerging therapies in narcolepsy-cataplexy. Sleep. 2005;28(6):754–63.
54. Nishino S, ripley B, Overeem S, et al. Hypocretin (orexin) deficiency in human narcolepsy. Lancet. 2000;355:39–40.
55. John J, Wu MF, Siegel JM. Systemic administration of hypocretin-1 reduces cataplexy and normalizes sleep and waking durations in narcoleptic dogs. Sleep Res Online. 2000;3:23–8.

56. Hanson LR, Martinez PM, Taheri M, et al. Intranasal administration of hypocretin 1 (orexin A) bypasses the blood-brain barrier and target the brain: a new strategy for the treatment of narcolepsy. Drug Deliv Technol. 2004;4:1–10.
57. Baier PC, Hallschmid M, Seeck-Hirschner M, et al. Sleep Med. 2011;12(10):941–6.
58. Zeitzer JM, Buckmaster CL, parker KJ, et al. Circadian and homeostatic regulation of hypocretin in a primate model: implications for the consolidation of wakefulness. J Neurosci. 2003;23:3555–60.
59. Mieda M, Willie JT, Hara J, et al. Orexin peptides prevent cataplexy and improve wakefulness in an orexin neuron-ablated model of narcolepsy in mice. Proc Natl Acad Sci U S A. 2004;101:4649–54.
60. Thannickal TC, Moore RY, Nienhuis R, et al. Reduced number of hypocretin neurons in human narcolepsy. Neuron. 2000;27:469–74.
61. Thorpy M. Therapeutic advances in narcolepsy. Sleep Med. 2007;8:427–40.
62. Arias-Carrion O, MurilloRodriguez E, Xu M, et al. Transplantation of hypocretin neurons into the pontine reticular formation: preliminary results. Sleep. 2004;27:1465–70.
63. Boehmer LN, Wu MF, John J, et al. Treatment with immunosuppressive and anti-inflammatory agents delays onset of canine genetic narcolepsy and reduces symptom severity. Exp Neurol. 2004;188:292–9.
64. Hect M, Lin L, Kushida CA, et al. Report of a case of immunosuppression with prednisone in an 8-year-old boy with an acute onset of hypocretin-deficiency narcolepsy. Sleep. 2003;26:809–10.
65. Chen W, black J, Call P, et al. Late-onset narcolepsy presenting as rapidly progressing muscle weakness: response to plasmapheresis. Ann Neurol. 2005;58:489–90.
66. Dauvilliers Y, Carlander B, rivier F, et al. Successful management of cataplexy with intravenous immunoglobulins at narcolepsy onset. Ann Neurol. 2004;56:905–8.
67. Zuberi SM, Mignot E, Ling L, et al. Variable response to intravenous immunoglobulin therapy in childhood narcolepsy. J Sleep Res. 2004;13(Suppl 1):828.
68. Nishino S, Arrigoni J, Shelton J, et al. Effects of thyrotropin-releasing hormone and its analogs on daytime sleepiness and cataplexy in canine narcolepsy. J Neurosci. 1997;17:6401–8.
69. Nishino S, Sakurai E, Nevsimalova S, et al. Decreased CSF histamine in narcolepsy with and without low CSF hypocretin-1 in comparison to healthy controls. Sleep. 2009;32:175–80.
70. Lin JS, Sakai K, Vanni-Mercier G, et al. Involvement of histaminergic neurons in arousal mechanisms demonstrated with H3-receptor ligands in the cat. Brain Res. 1990;523:325–30.
71. Wijtmans M, Leurs R, de Esch I. Histamine H3 receptor ligands break ground in a remarkable plethora of therapeutic areas. Expert Opin Investig Drugs. 2007;16:967–85.
72. Lin JS, Dauvilliers Y, Arnulf I, et al. An inverse agonist of the histamine H(3) receptor improves wakefulness in narcolepsy: studies in orexin−/− mice and patients. Neurobiol Dis. 2008;30:74–83.

Chapter 11
Assessment of Sleep Duration, Sleep Habits, Napping, and Circadian Rhythms in the Patient Complaining of Fatigue

John Herman

Introduction

When a patient complains of job-related fatigue or chronic fatigue, a critical component of his or her evaluation is to determine if the fatigue is secondary to the patient's sleep schedule, or to a sleep disorder, or to a circadian rhythm disorder. This chapter provides the reader with a description of how that evaluation should proceed and what tests, studies, and procedures to employ.

First, this chapter describes how to determine if the patient is obtaining adequate sleep or is chronically sleep deprived. Secondly, it describes how to determine if a sleep disorder is present. Finally, it explains how to determine if a circadian rhythm disorder is the cause of chronic fatigue. For each of these, the chapter will discuss scales, diaries, sleep logs, and actigraphy for ruling in or out a diagnosis with a reasonable degree of certainty.

Assessment of Sleep Duration

On average, adults spend about 7.5 h in bed to obtain slightly under 7 h of sleep. Throughout the life span, sleep latency increases as does the amount of awake after sleep onset, but time in bed remains constant [1]. Also deep sleep decreases. There is a corresponding increase in light sleep [1]. Overall, sleep quality decreases, with aging. However, this does not relate to increased fatigue in older compared to younger adults. The incidence of insomnia increases with age, especially in women, but the frequency of daytime impairment does not [2]. Such data indicates that fatigue does not increase with age despite poorer sleep quality.

J. Herman, PhD, FAASM
UT Southwestern Medical Center, Dallas, TX, USA

© Springer Science+Business Media, LLC, part of Springer Nature 2018
A. Sharafkhaneh, M. Hirshkowitz (eds.), *Fatigue Management*,
https://doi.org/10.1007/978-1-4939-8607-1_11

Research has shown a U-shaped curve with a nadir in mortality for those who sleep approximately 7 h and increased mortality of 15% in those who sleep more than 9 h and in those who sleep less than 4.5 h [3]. This study examined medical records of 1.1 million adults, age 30–102 years, over a 6-year period.

Knowing that the average number of hours of sleep required by an adult is 7 h has little to do with an individual's sleep requirement. Kripke et al.'s interval of 4.5–9 h, in the above publication, provides a wide window that includes the number of hours of sleep required by most individuals. If an individual requires more or less than those amounts, it is reasonable to look for a mental or medical cause, such as sleep apnea, chronic pain, an anxiety disorder, or bipolar disorder.

I know several extremely productive, successful, and healthy adults who sleep less than 4.5 h. I know other adults who sleep more than 9 h. None of them have any complaints regarding sleep, alertness, or fatigue. The clinician should not assume that idiosyncratic total sleep time is problematic, especially if the individual has no complaints. Total sleep time may resemble a two-tailed normal curve, with outliers three or more standard deviations from the mean, which is to be expected.

The Sleep Disorder Evaluation of an Individual with Fatigue

During the interview for assessment of fatigue, the clinician should establish the patient's normal bedtime and time of awakening. The clinician should also inquire about the number of times the patient awakens and how long he or she is awake on average. The clinician is then able to estimate total sleep time. The clinician should inquire about how difficult it is for the patient to awaken for work, how groggy the patient is, and how long the grogginess continues before the patient experiences normal wakefulness.

If the individual with fatigue has difficulty awakening, followed by a period of grogginess lasting over 1 h, it is important that time in bed is adequate. If the individual sleeps late on weekends, waking two or more hours later than workdays, and experiences less grogginess on weekends, then inadequate time in bed could be contributing to fatigue. Also, if the patient has an undiagnosed sleep disorder, it could lead to unrefreshing sleep, work impairment, and the complaint of fatigue.

Estimating Sleep Duration

We may estimate sleep duration from an interview, a questionnaire, having the patient maintain a sleep diary or complete a sleep log. A published and generally accepted questionnaire regarding sleep duration is the Sleep Timing Questionnaire (STQ) [4]. Please also visit the American Thoracic Society's website (http://www. thoracic.org/members/assemblies/assemblies/srn/questionaires/stq.php).

The Prevalence of Short Sleep Duration and Sleep Disorders

In 2009, the Centers for Disease Control and Prevention administered the Behavioral Risk Factor Surveillance System (BRFSS) survey that included a core question regarding perceived insufficient rest or sleep. It included four questions on sleep behavior. Data from the 2009 BRFSS sleep module assessed the prevalence of unhealthy/sleep behaviors by selected sociodemographic factors and geographic variations in 12 states [5].

This survey determined that, among 74,571 adult respondents, 35.3% reported having <7 h of sleep on average during a 24 h period, 48.0% reported snoring, 37.9% reported unintentionally falling asleep during the day at least 1 day in the preceding 30 days, and 4.7% reported nodding off or falling asleep while driving in the preceding 30 days. In all probability, what is referred to as less than 7 h of sleep is actually less than 7 h in bed. Subtracting normal sleep latency and wake after sleep onset yields less than 6.5 h of sleep. It is relevant to this chapter that 37.9% of the sample of adults fell asleep at least once unintentionally in the preceding 30 days, 4.7% while driving. This insufficient sleep that resulted in excessive daytime sleepiness could easily be perceived as chronic fatigue.

Also note that 48% of the sample reported snoring, some of whom could have obstructive sleep apnea, a condition that leads to excessive daytime sleepiness. Some with OSA might view their symptoms as chronic fatigue. Other sleep disorders not included could increase the number of individuals with poor sleep quality.

Sleep Quality

Sleep quality can be assessed via questionnaire using the Sleep Quality Scale (SQS) [6]. A 28-item scale has been validated in individuals age 18–59. The SCS evaluates daytime symptoms, restoration after sleep, problems initiating and maintaining sleep, difficulty awakening, and sleep satisfaction. Please also visit http://link.springer.com/chapter/10.1007/978-1-4419-9893-4_85#page-1.

Long Work Hours and Fatigue

In 2008 the National Sleep Foundation conducted a phone survey called Sleep in America in which they questioned 1000 Americans who work 30 or more hours per week about employment, work performance, and sleep [7]. They found that long work hours are associated with shorter sleep times and shorter sleep times are associated with more work impairments. Thirty-seven percent of respondents were classified as at-risk for any sleep disorder. These individuals had more negative work outcomes as compared with those not at-risk for a sleep disorder. The inability to work to normal capacity was a significant problem for individuals with insomnia symptoms, obstructive sleep apnea, and restless legs syndrome as compared with respondents without sleep disorders. These results suggest that long work hours may contribute to chronic sleep loss, which may in turn result in work impairment. An untreated sleep disorder is a form of insufficient sleep that may lead to fatigue.

The clinician should advise the patient with work-related fatigue and inadequate time in bed how much time in bed is required for an adult to obtain adequate sleep. If the clinician suspects a sleep disorder, the clinician should address the problem or refer the patient to a sleep disorder specialist. The sleep specialist will perform a sleep disorder-orientated evaluation to determine an initial diagnosis and perform indicated testing to confirm the diagnosis. In many diagnoses, such as insomnia, a circadian rhythm disorder, or restless legs syndrome, a sleep study is not indicated, but in some disorders, such as OSA, a sleep study is required.

Chronic Insomnia and Fatigue

The above section focused on the patient with inadequate sleep as a cause of job-related fatigue. This section examines chronic insomnia as a cause of fatigue. Individuals with insomnia may have trouble with sleep onset, sleep maintenance, or early morning awakenings or some combination of the three. Sleep-onset insomnia is defined as requiring more than 30 min to initiate sleep. Sleep-maintenance insomnia refers to excessive wake after sleep onset. Most individuals with either of these disorders remain in bed excessively. Unlike the too-little-time-in-bed group, these individuals may experience anxiety related to sleep. Some have been found to be chronically over aroused, as indicated by increased waking brain waves during sleep (alpha and beta), failure to suppress cortisol secretion during sleep, and increased brain metabolism during sleep as measured by positron-emission tomography [8].

The presence of insomnia is established by interview, diary, sleep log, or questionnaire. There are several well-accepted questionnaires for establishing the presence of insomnia and its severity. One such scale is the Insomnia Severity Index (ISI) [9]. The ISI is a brief scale for rating the presence and severity of insomnia. It consists of seven items each using a Likert-type scale. It evaluates sleep quality, severity of insomnia symptoms, sleep satisfaction, the degree to which insomnia interferes with functioning, how noticeable the respondent's symptoms are to others, and the level of distress secondary to insomnia. A copy of the ISI is included in the reference to it or may be downloaded from the Department of Veterans Affairs (https://www.myhealth.va.gov/mhv-portal-web/insomnia-severity-index).

The clinician should ask about common sleep disorders including insomnia, obstructive sleep apnea, and restless legs syndrome, each of which is associated with work impairment and fatigue.

Individuals with chronic insomnia frequently complain of fatigue and are diagnosed with chronic fatigue syndrome. Insomnia is best treated by cognitive behavioral therapy of insomnia (CBT-I). Studies have demonstrated that individuals with chronic insomnia and hyperarousal respond well to CBT-I [10]. One of these studies found dramatic improvements in sleep latency, sleep efficiency, and quality of morning awakenings. Any psychologist trained in CBT can easily follow the readily available instructions for CBT-I.

An alternative is a hypnotic agent such as a benzodiazepine or a benzodiazepine receptor agonist. This may be prescribed by the patient's PCP, or the patient may be referred to a sleep medicine specialist for further evaluation and treatment.

There are many available questionnaires that enhance a clinician's ability to evaluate and diagnose a sleep disorder. The most widely accepted instrument for assessing daytime sleepiness and its severity is the Epworth Sleepiness Scale [11] (http://epworthsleepinessscale.com/).

The Pittsburgh Sleep Quality Index (PSQI) is a widely recognized scale for assessing the quality of sleep [12]. The PSQI was developed to evaluate sleep quality in individuals with psychiatric symptoms. Its 19 items are in 7 domains: subjective sleep quality, sleep latency, sleep duration, sleep efficiency, sleep disturbances, use of sleep medication, and daytime impairment. Please also visit the following website: (http://www.opapc.com/uploads/documents/PSQI.pdf).

Fatigue severity, especially as it is related to sleep disorders, is frequently evaluated with the Fatigue Severity Scale (FSS) of sleep disorders [13]. It is a nine-item instrument that assesses fatigue as a symptom of various chronic conditions including medical disorders. The FSS evaluates the effect of fatigue on motivation, physical activity, work, family, and social activities. The FSS establishes how easily an individual is fatigued and how severely fatigue impacts the individual's life.

Evaluating Sleep-Related Breathing Disorders

One scale frequently used to assess the risk of OSA is the Berlin Questionnaire [14]. The questionnaire identifies individuals with a high risk of sleep apnea. Questions target three domains of sleep apnea symptoms: snoring, daytime sleepiness, and obesity or hypertension. It is without copyright and may easily be obtained online.

Another widely used questionnaire for assessing the risk of OSA is the STOP-Bang Questionnaire [15]. It consists of four yes/no and four fill-in-the-blank questions based upon the mnemonic "STOP-Bang": S is for snore, T for tired, O for observed stop breathing, P for high blood pressure, B for BMI, A for age, N for neck circumference, and G for gender. It is well validated in older adults only [16]. Validation studies claim that the STOP-Bang scale has a sensitivity and specificity of greater than 90% in patients with moderate to severe OSA. It is readily available online (http://www.stopbang.ca/).

If a bed partner is available to serve as an informant, a questionnaire frequently employed to assess sleep disorders in general is the Mayo Clinic Sleep Questionnaire, which is completed by the patient's bed partner [17]. This questionnaire is available at the Mayo Clinic's website (http://www.mayoclinic.org/documents/msq-copyrightfinal-pdf/doc-20079462).

The Varied Presentations of OSA

Most sleep disorders present to the care provider as excessive daytime sleepiness, fatigue, or insomnia. For example, OSA can prevent the initiation of sleep with partial airway blockage causing repeated awakenings while an individual is attempting to initiate sleep. This is perceived as sleep-onset insomnia. OSA can also appear to be sleep-maintenance insomnia caused by awakenings to breathe. A third way that OSA may be perceived is that patient presents with complaints of daytime sleepiness, fatigue, or loss of energy.

If there is no bed partner, obstructive sleep apnea may be occult. It is frequently associated with an upper or lower jaw posterior placement encroaching on the pharyngeal airway. Droopy eyelids, crowded teeth, a receding chin, retrognathia, "buck teeth," a large tongue, occlusion of a nare, broken nose, a crowded airway (Mallampati Class II or III), tonsillar hypertrophy, a large neck (typically 17 in. or greater), central obesity, and edema of the extremities are all risk factors for OSA [18]. Hypertension, especially hypertension that is not responsive to treatment, is associated with OSA.

Napping

Napping is almost universal in infants, and most children do not nap by age 7 [19]. Napping is common in the elderly and is associated with excessive daytime sleepiness and an increased risk of mortality [20]. In adults with long work hours, such as medical interns and trans-Atlantic airline pilots, napping has been shown to alleviate fatigue [21]. In an adult population, napping and fatigue are associated with poorer mental or physical health status [22]. An evaluation of a patient with fatigue should always include questions about napping frequency and duration.

It is important to assess if the patient feels refreshed or continues to be sleepy or fatigued after a nap. Refreshing naps are more likely to be associated with normal buildup of sleep pressure that is alleviated by a nap, frequently in individuals with inadequate sleep at night. So called "power naps" have been shown to alleviate daytime sleepiness and are frequently used by busy individuals with crowded schedules. Non-refreshing naps are more likely to be associated with fatigue, a psychiatric disorder, a sleep disorder, or a physical disorder.

Circadian Rhythms and Fatigue

Circadian rhythms are the biological rhythms of virtually every behavioral and metabolic variable in human existence, sleep being one of them. As part of our circadian rhythms, there is a consistent relationship between our temperature peak and the onset of melatonin secretion, which precedes sleep by about 2 h.

Under normal conditions, our circadian drive for alertness increases rapidly after the hour of awakening and remains high throughout our normal waking hours, with the exception of a brief postprandial dip after lunch hour. Circadian alertness then drops rapidly at the time of desired sleep. Circadian alertness is critical for the normal perception of vigor and vitality.

Unlike the consistent association between temperature peak and melatonin onset seen in normals, some individuals with chronic fatigue lack this association [24]. Normal individuals have a predictable albeit somewhat enigmatic peak and troth in circadian alertness: they rate themselves as most alert about 2 h before the normal onset of sleep and least alert at the time of morning awakening. In other words, after the homeostatic drive for sleep has been building throughout the day, circadian alertness overrides sleepiness, and after the homeostatic drive for sleep has been satiated at the time of morning awakening, the absence of circadian alertness overrides the satiation of the drive to sleep.

The failure for circadian alertness to be present at normal working hours may be experienced as fatigue. Additionally, many individuals with delayed sleep phase disorder show chronic fatigue. One study of 90 consecutive adults with delayed sleep phase disorder found 64% to be depressed with fatigue and psychomotor retardation [16].

In normal individuals, the concordance between nocturnal sleep and the synchronous rise and fall in circadian alertness is the bedrock of the sleep and wake system. Shift work or "social jet lag" is a discordance between an individual's phase of his or her circadian rhythm (see below) and the required time of work, school, or social activities. The effects of shift work or social jet lag are similar to travel across multiple time zones.

Measurement of Circadian Rhythms

The timing of sleep and napping may be estimated subjectively by clinical interview with the patient, the patient's bed partner, or by the scales described above. Wrist actigraphy for 1–2 weeks is widely accepted as an objective technique for measuring sleep and wakefulness, including a position statement by the American Academy of Sleep Medicine [24]. A patient may wear one of several widely accepted actigraphy devices on the dominant wrist for 1–2 weeks, collecting data about wrist movement every 30 s. Sometimes light wavelength and intensity are simultaneously collected. The data is downloaded to a computer. Software installed on the computer enables it to create 24 h graphs for each of the day the device is activated. Due to the relative absence of wrist movement during sleep, several software products are available that display the timing and duration of sleep as the actigraph shows little or no movement during sleep. One available product is manufactured by Philips Electronics [25].

Chronotype

Each of us possesses a chronotype, or an interval during our wake period when we experience greatest alertness. Following a normal night of sleep, the majority of individuals experience alertness throughout most of the waking period including an interval in the morning, afternoon, or evening when the individual feels most alert. This is the normal chronotype.

Some have difficulty waking, become alert during midday or in the evening, and have a tendency to stay awake later than he or she wishes. Such individuals tend to sleep late weekends or holidays. This is an evening chronotype. Others wake up early, have their largest appetite and greatest productivity early in the day, and are ready to retire at a relatively early hour. This is the morning chronotype.

Circadian Rhythm Disorders

When morningness or eveningness becomes so severe as to interfere with social, school, or professional activities, it becomes a circadian rhythm disorder, advanced sleep phase disorder, or delayed sleep phase disorder, respectively [26]. A commonly used instrument for assessing circadian phase is the Morningness-Eveningness Questionnaire [27]. This is a 19-item instrument that assesses individual differences in morning vs evening preference. Scale items establish preferred sleep and wake times and optimal time for accomplishing physically or mentally demanding tasks. A copy can be found in the above reference, and the questionnaire is readily available online.

Another scale developed to establish morningness-eveningness preference is the Munich Chronotype Questionnaire (MCTQ) [28]. This 19-item instrument examines actual hours of bedtime and wake time on weekdays and weekends, energy levels at various times of day, sleep latency, and time of day of sunlight exposure. The respondent selects one of the seven chronotypes that best matches his or her preference for engaging in activities, from extremely early to extremely late. Please also visit https://www.thewep.org/documentations/mctq.

Measuring the Phase of Circadian Rhythms by Dim Light Melatonin Onset (DLMO)

DLMO has become a widely accepted biomarker for measuring the beginning of the dark phase of the circadian rhythm. DLMO is associated with sleep onset in diurnal species and wake onset in nocturnal species. Measuring the phase of the individual's circadian rhythm is most typically accomplished by having the patient complete a log for 2 weeks that includes time in bed, time of sleep onset, and time of awakening. The time of DLMO correlates with the time of sleep onset, the time of body temperature minimum, and the wake-up time [28]. DLMO establishes the phase of an individual's circadian rhythm. If DLMO is early, for example, before 8:00 pm, the individual is phase advanced. If DLMO is late, for example, after midnight, the individual is phase delayed. Melatonin secretion begins approximately 2 h before sleep onset [29].

To measure DLMO, a patient who has completed the log described above begins to swab his or her cheek to collect salivary melatonin in cotton 3 h before his or her habitual time of sleep onset and continues to do so every 20 min until falling asleep. The patient must remain in extremely dim light (less than 5 lux), as light suppresses melatonin secretion. The patient places the saliva-containing cotton in a labeled test tube which is refrigerated.

Conclusions

A clinician evaluating an individual complaining of fatigue inquires about time in bed, sleep time, sleep disorders, and circadian rhythm disorders. Problems with any of the above items could be the root of the complaint of fatigue. Taking a good history is the basis for diagnosing many possible causes of fatigue.

This chapter describes a number of easily obtainable clinical scales that are related to these issues. The clinician should consider asking the patient to complete some of these scales before the clinical interview, allowing the clinician to review them an hone in on suspected causes of fatigue rapidly. Well-validated scales are underutilized by clinicians in general. They are time-saving instruments. They enable the clinician to identify problem areas before the patient arrives.

Diaries and logs of sleep habits provide soft data that buttresses the patient's description of his or her habits. Many patients are extremely vague when asked to answer the simplest questions about bedtime or sleep-onset time. The diary or log helps the patient and the clinician to more accurately assess the patient's complaint. Data that are more objective are required in some cases, such as actigraphy or the measurement of DLMO.

If the clinician uses the above interview techniques, diaries, logs, and instrumentation to rule in or out a sleep or circadian rhythm disorder and documents that the patient has adequate time in bed, then and only then does the patient's complaint of fatigue crystallize as an independent entity not secondary to a sleep or circadian rhythm issue.

References

1. Ohayon M, Carskadon MA, Guilleminault C, et al. Meta-analysis of quantitative sleep parameters from childhood to old age in healthy individuals: developing normative sleep values across the human lifespan. Sleep. 2004;27(7):1255–73.
2. Maurice M, Ohayon MM. Epidemiology of insomnia: what we know and what we still need to learn. Sleep Med Rev. 2002;6(2):97–111.

3. Kripke DF, Lawrence Garfinkel L, Wingard DI, et al. Mortality associated with sleep duration and insomnia. Arch Gen Psychiatry. 2002;59(2):131–6.

4. Monk TH, Buysse DJ, Kennedy KS, et al. Measuring sleep habits without using a diary: the sleep timing questionnaire. Sleep. 2003;26(2):208–12.

5. http://www.cdc.gov/features/dssleep/ read on 10 Jan 2013.

6. Yi H, Shin K, Shin C. Development of the sleep quality scale. J Sleep Res. 2006;15(3):309–16.

7. Swanson LM, Arendt JT, Rosekind MR, et al. J Sleep Res. 2011;20:487–94.

8. Riemann D, Kloepfer C, Berger M. Functional and structural brain alterations in insomnia: implications for pathophysiology. Eur J Neurosci. 2009;29(9):1754–60.

9. Bastien CH, Vallieres A, Morin CM. Validation of the insomnia severity index as an outcome measure for insomnia research. Sleep Med. 2001;2:297–307.

10. Gałuszko-Węgielnik M, Jakuszkowiak-Wojten K, Wiglusz MS, et al. The efficacy of cognitive-behavioural therapy (CBT) as related to sleep quality and hyperarousal level in the treatment of primary insomnia. Psychiatr Danub. 2012;24(Suppl 1):S51–5.

11. Johns MW. A new method for measuring daytime sleepiness: the Epworth sleepiness scale. Sleep. 1991;14(6):540–5.

12. Buysse DJ, Reynolds CF 3rd, Monk TH, et al. The Pittsburgh Sleep Quality Index: a new instrument for psychiatric practice and research. Psychiatry Res. 1989;28(2):193–213.

13. Lichstein KL, Means MK, Noe SL, et al. Fatigue and sleep disorders. Behav Res Ther. 1997;35(8):733–40.

14. Netzer NC, Stoohs RA, Netzer CM, Clark K, Strohl KP. Using the Berlin Questionnaire to identify patients at risk for the sleep apnea syndrome. Ann Intern Med. 1999;131(7):485–91.

15. Cheng F, Yegneswran B, Islam S, et al. STOP questionnaire—a tool to screen patients for obstructive sleep apnea. Anesthesiology. 2008;108(5):812–21.

16. Farney RJ, Walker BS, Rarney RM, et al. The STOP-Bang equivalent model and prediction of severity of obstructive sleep apnea: relation to polysomnographic measurements of the apnea/hypopnea index. J Clin Sleep Med. 2011;7(5):459–65.

17. http://www.mayoclinic.org/pdfs/MSQ-copyrightfinal.pdf read on 11 Jan 2013.

18. Kryger MH. Atlas of clinical sleep medicine. Philadelphia: Saunders/Elsevier; 2010. p. 149–66.

19. Weissbluth M. Naps in children: 6 months-7 years. Sleep. 1995;18(2):82–7.

20. Hays JC, Blazer DG, Foley DJ. Risk of napping: excessive daytime sleepiness and mortality in an older community population. J Am Geriatr Soc. 1996;44(6):693–8.

21. Arora V, Dunphy C, Chang VY, et al. The effects of on-duty napping on intern sleep time and fatigue. Ann Intern Med. 2006;144(11):792–8.

22. Briones B, Adams N, Strauss M, et al. Relationship between sleepiness and general health status. Sleep. 1996;19(7):583–8.

23. Williams G, Pirmohamed J, Minors D, et al. Dissociation of body-temperature and melatonin secretion circadian rhythms in patients with chronic fatigue syndrome. Clin Physiol. 1996;16(4):327–37.

24. Ancoli-Israel S, Cole R, Alessi C, et al. The role of actigraphy in the study of sleep and circadian rhythms. American Academy of Sleep Medicine Review Paper. Sleep. 2003;26(3):342–92.

25. Philips Home Health Care Solutions, Shevlin Corporate Park, Building C, 920 SW Emkay Ave, Suite 100, Bend, Oregon 97702.

26. American Academy of Sleep Medicine. International classification of sleep disorders: diagnostic and coding manual. 2nd ed. Westchester: American Academy of Sleep Medicine; 2005. p. 118–23.

27. Horne JA, Ostberg O. A self-assessment questionnaire to determine morningness-eveningness in human circadian rhythms. Int J Chronobiol. 1976;4:97–110.

28. Zavada A, Gordijn MC, Beersma DG, et al. Comparison of the Munich Chronotype Questionnaire with the Horne-Östberg's morningness-eveningness score. Chronobiol Int. 2005;22(2):267–78.

29. Crowley SJ, Acebo C, Fallone G, et al. Estimating dim light melatonin onset (DLMO) phase in adolescents using summer or school-year sleep/wake schedules. Sleep. 2006;29(12):1632–41.

Chapter 12
Treating Fatigue in Patients with Chronic Heart and Lung Disease

Shahram Moghtader, Faisal Kanbar-Agha, and Amir Sharafkhaneh

Introduction

Fatigue is prevalent in chronic cardiorespiratory conditions. Fatigue is a symptom complex that affects the quality of life markedly. It correlates strongly with other measures of quality of life and depression. Change in muscle structure and function, deteriorated nutritional status, sleep deprivation, hypoxia (awake, exertional and nocturnal), adverse effects of medications, and comorbid conditions are among many pathophysiologic mechanisms that may promote fatigue in these patients. Comprehensive assessment of all the promoting causes is required for better understanding and management of fatigue in these patients. In the following sections, we will briefly review fatigue in cardiac and respiratory conditions and discuss the effect of disease-specific therapy on fatigue.

S. Moghtader, MD
Section of Pulmonary and Critical Care and Sleep Medicine, Baylor College of Medicine, Houston, TX, USA

Sleep Disorders and Research Center, Michael E. DeBakey VA Medical Center, Houston, TX, USA

F. Kanbar-Agha, MD
Sleep Disorders and Research Center, Michael E. DeBakey VA Medical Center, Houston, TX, USA

A. Sharafkhaneh, MD, PhD (✉)
Department of Medicine, Baylor College of Medicine, Houston, TX, USA

Medical Care Line, Michael E. DeBakey VA Medical Center, Houston, TX, USA
e-mail: amirs@bcm.edu

© Springer Science+Business Media, LLC, part of Springer Nature 2018
A. Sharafkhaneh, M. Hirshkowitz (eds.), *Fatigue Management*,
https://doi.org/10.1007/978-1-4939-8607-1_12

Cardiac Diseases and Fatigue

Heart failure remains the most common cause of hospitalization and morbidity-mortality in the elderly population [1]. Its associated symptoms of dyspnea, lower extremity edema, and fatigue often prove debilitating to those affected. While these symptoms may cause functional limitations, they also significantly impact patients' psychological and social welfare. Fatigue, as a frequent manifestation of heart failure, remains particularly hard to characterize, given its subjectivity and unquantifiable nature. It is important, however, to effectively evaluate fatigue as a symptom as it has important and independent long-term prognostic implications [2]. It manifests physically, cognitively, and emotionally and is therefore necessary for physicians to identify [1]. The importance of defining, recognizing, and targeting fatigue given its impact on prognosis in cardiac disease was shown in an analysis of the 3029 patients randomized in the Carvedilol or Metoprolol European Trial (COMET) [2].

In a univariate analysis, fatigue was significantly related to reduced survival ($p < 0.001$) and the development of worsening heart failure. In a multivariate Cox regression analysis including the 16 baseline covariates (including demographics, New York Heart severity classification, baseline comorbid conditions, and baseline cardiovascular medications), fatigue still proved to be a significant predictor for worsening heart failure (RR 1.09 per unit; 95% CI 1.02–1.17; p 0.02). Multivariate regression analysis showed that fatigue offered an increased relative risk of 11% for mortality ($p = 0.009$), 26% for all-cause hospitalization ($p < 0.0001$), and 28% for worsening heart failure ($p < 0.0001$). This data shows the importance of fatigue as a symptom given that its severity predicts an increased risk of death and morbidity.

Research regarding the etiology of fatigue in cardiac disease has focused on vasoconstriction and endothelial dysfunction leading to impaired muscular blood flow [3]. Even with adequate blood flow, muscles can become fatigued if they have primary structural or functional abnormalities. Multiple etiologies of fatigue in heart failure have been postulated, including reduced cardiac output, reduced oxygen delivery, impaired muscle blood flow, and abnormal skeletal muscle [4].

There are many symptoms which have been reported in association with fatigue. The main symptom associated with fatigue is dyspnea. Dyspnea is also associated with sleep disorders and depression. A study comparing fatigue and other variables between those with heart failure and those without showed associations between fatigue, anxiety, and depression and that the three partially explained dyspnea variability in the heart failure patients [5]. Another factor correlated with fatigue in research was the body mass index—when higher than or equal to 25, fatigue was more intense [6].

Insomnia is also very prevalent in patients with heart failure. One review found that sleep-disordered breathing (SDB) and insomnia were the most common causes of sleep disturbances in CHF. Insomnia occurred in 33% of all patients with CHF. The more frequently reported symptoms were inability to sleep in the supine position (51%), restless sleep (44%), trouble falling asleep (40%), and early awakening (39%). There was no correlation between these sleep complaints and the severity of their CHF or clinical status. Using the Epworth Sleepiness Scale (ESS), approximately 20% of participants in the Cardiovascular Health Study (total of 4578 elderly participants) were identified as being usually sleepy in the daytime.

Management of Fatigue in Heart Failure

The last decade or two has seen significant progress in various management strategies that resulted in improved longevity and quality of life in patients with advanced heart disease. Among those, multiple pharmacotherapeutic agents are now part of the standard regimen for management of heart failure. In addition, cardiac rehabilitation takes a very important place in management of dyspnea and fatigue in patients with advanced heart disease.

Pharmacotherapeutic Interventions

Pharmacotherapeutic management of heart failure improves various outcomes including mortality, quality of life, and fatigue. Beta-blockers are proven medication in the management of heart failure. However, they are mentioned as the important reasons for fatigue that results in discontinuation of beta-blocker. It is not clear if beta-blockers will improve fatigue in patients with heart failure [7]. In contrast to beta-blockers, angiotensin-converting enzyme inhibitors and angiotensin receptor blockers may improve fatigue in patients with heart failure [8, 9]. Diuretics are main among important medications used for management of heart failure-related fluid overload. Reigel et al. in an observational study of 280 patients with heart failure identified lack of taking diuretics as a predictor of fatigue [10]. The mechanism(s) that diuretics may improve fatigue is not clear.

Various new medications are tested in patients with heart failure. Among those, levosimendan treatment, a calcium sensitizer, enhanced both objective echocardiographic estimations and the subjective quality of life questionnaires. Minnesota Living with Heart Failure Questionnaire and Left Ventricular Dysfunction 36 demonstrate a significant improvement in quality of life in heart failure patients following a 6-month time of month-to-month intermittent administration of levosimendan. The Specific Activity Questionnaire demonstrated a little change, since it depicts more strenuous action, a circumstance uncommon for these patients, who are severely symptom limited [11].

In a randomized trial, the addition of tolvaptan, a vasopressin antagonist, to standard therapy for acute heart failure syndromes, improves physician-assessed signs and symptoms like fatigue during hospitalization without serious adverse short- or long-term effects [12].

Agents as part of alternative medicine has been assessed in management of heart failure. In a randomized double-blinded placebo control study, Kumar et al.

evaluated effects of combination of ubiquinol and carnitine in various outcomes in patients with systolic heart failure. Patients in active arm of the study had significant improvement in fatigue, dyspnea, palpitation, and 6 min walk test [13]. In another study of natural agents, exercise tolerance was essentially expanded by Hawthorn extract. The pressure-heart rate product, an index of cardiac oxygen consumption, also showed a beneficial decrease with Hawthorn treatment. Symptoms such as shortness of breath and fatigue enhanced altogether with Hawthorn treatment compared to placebo [14]. Treatment of symptomatic, iron-deficient heart failure patients with ferric carboxymaltose over a 1-year time frame resulted in sustainable improvement in functional capacity, fatigue, and quality of life and may be associated with risk reduction of hospitalization for worsening heart failure [15].

Non-pharmacologic Intervention

Cardiac rehabilitation including exercise programs has been around for several decades. The program not only includes exercise but also nutritional counseling, psychological counseling, and self-management education. A recent meta-analysis of the studies conducted from 1945 to 2005 by Puetz et al. showed a consistent improvement in energy and fatigue in cardiac patients who receive supervised exercise programs [16].

Various components of a comprehensive cardiac rehabilitation program may reduce fatigue. A pilot study randomized heart failure subjects to aerobic and resistance exercise three times a week versus no exercise. The intervention group altogether had less fatigue (Piper Fatigue Scale) compared to the control group [17].

Education of patients with chronic medical conditions plays an important part in long-term management of the patients. In an education intervention study, Albert et al. compared standard education (SE) during discharge from a heart failure admission to standard education and video education (SE + VE) on various clinical outcomes. In the follow-up phone evaluation, the individuals randomized to SE + VE had significantly less fatigue with exertion compared to the standard education group [18].

In a randomized trial, Colin-Ramirez et al. assessed impact of salt- and water-limited eating routine on symptoms, leg edema, and fatigue. The salt-limited group demonstrated significant reduction in fatigue and edema in 6 months [19].

Treatment of Associated Comorbid Conditions

Sleep disorders including insomnia and sleep-disordered breathing is frequently seen in patients with chronic cardiac conditions. Management of sleep disorders may impact patients' quality of life and fatigue. In patients with sleep-disordered breathing, continuous positive airway pressure (CPAP) therapy decreases fatigue, maintenance insomnia, depressive symptoms, and sensitivity to pain [20].

Depression is prevalent in patients with chronic medical condition including heart failure. In a meta-analysis of several studies, 20% of patients with heart failure had depression, and this estimate increased twofolds in patients with more severe heart failure. Presence of depression is linked to worse clinical outcomes in these patients [21, 22]. Treatment of depression in patients with heart failure, using medications or cognitive behavioral therapy or other modalities, may help in reducing fatigue [23, 24].

Respiratory Disorders and Fatigue

Like in cardiac diseases, patients with chronic obstructive pulmonary disease (COPD), interstitial lung disease (ILD), and other chronic respiratory conditions often present with fatigue as one of the main symptoms. Chronic obstructive pulmonary disease (COPD) is the most studied among chronic respiratory conditions. In patients with COPD, fatigue is a common complaint. When evaluating a COPD patient on a daily basis, fatigue presents in 68–80% of patients [25–28]. Similar to COPD, fatigue is also commonly reported in ILD. Assessment for the presence of fatigue is an integral part of the assessment of quality of life in lung diseases [18]. Fatigue out of proportion to lung function impairment may be considered a reason against lung transplant [29, 30]. Fatigue is also reported in other chronic respiratory conditions including cystic fibrosis and asthma [31–33].

The exact pathophysiology of fatigue in COPD and ILD is not clear. Fatigue may result from the disease processes, adverse effects of medications used, and comorbid conditions. In chronic respiratory conditions, fatigue manifests as muscle weakness, poor exercise tolerance, and decrease in overall function. Like other chronic medical conditions, respiratory conditions may result in a catabolic state, muscle breakdown, and muscle atrophy that may manifest as fatigue [34, 35]. Further, overlap between chronic respiratory conditions including COPD and sleep-related breathing disorders and insomnia can cause or intensify fatigue [36, 37].

In addition to the disease processes, use of various medications can promote fatigue. A classic example is chronic corticosteroid use in COPD for treatment of acute exacerbations or in some rare occasions as a maintenance therapy. It is well known that steroids cause muscle fatigue and osteoporosis [38, 39]. Some of respiratory inhalational medications can cause insomnia that may further promote fatigue [37].

Various studies reported high prevalence of chronic fatigue in patients with COPD (39–58%) [40–42]. In a survey comparing COPD patients with general population, Theander et al. reported higher odds on frequency, duration, and severity of fatigue in patients with COPD [43]. Further, 51% of COPD patients reported fatigue as the worst or one of the worst symptoms [43]. Using Fatigue

Impact Scale (FIS) scores, patients with COPD reported higher scores in cognitive, physical, and psychological domains indicating significant effect of fatigue of the above domain [41].

Baltzan et al. studied exercise capacity in COPD patients with and without high fatigue scores. The high fatigue score group had lower exercise capacity, worse quality of life, and higher depressive symptoms and was less engaged in moderate-intensity activities [42]. In a large study of 3000 patients with and without COPD, high fatigue score (using Functional Assessment of Chronic Illness Therapy-Fatigue questionnaire) correlated with high depressive symptoms [44, 45]. Baghai-Ravary et al. studied 107 COPD patients and 30 age-matched controls. The study showed that the increase in fatigue was associated with reduced time spent outdoors, depression, and exacerbation frequency [46]. Further, fatigue increased during exacerbation episodes, and this change was related to increased depression [46].

Pathophysiology of fatigue in COPD is multifactorial. The work of breathing increases in COPD resulting in increased resting metabolic demand up to twice the normal level [25, 26]. Also the increased work of breathing is further complicated with altered nutrition leading in to muscle wasting and fatigue. Further, patients with advanced COPD may not be able to maintain adequate dietary intake (quantity and quality nutrition) due to decreased appetite and physical and/or financial limitations. This in turn results in cachexia and leads to weakness of the diaphragm and accessory muscles of ventilation and creates a vicious cycle. Data indicates higher mortality in COPD patients with lower body mass index [47].

In addition to COPD-related pathophysiological disturbances, presence of comorbid conditions particularly sleep deprivation may promote fatigue in patient with COPD. Studies report high prevalence of insomnia in COPD patients [37, 48–50]. The increased insomnia stems from COPD-related nocturnal symptoms and medication-related side effects that may disturb sleep [37]. In addition to insomnia, presence of sleep-disordered breathing with COPD may increase fatigue [36, 37, 51].

Management of Fatigue in COPD

It is generally accepted that the treatment of the underlying disorders is necessary for the management of patients with fatigue. In the case of patients with COPD, fatigue can be related to the underlying lung disease as well as other accompanying condition such as anxiety; depression; malnutrition; deconditioning; coexisting sleep problems such as insomnia and sleep-disordered breathing; coexisting heart disease such as coronary artery disease and congestive heart failure; coexisting endocrine problems such as diabetes and thyroid disease as the more common ones; coexisting chronic kidney and liver diseases; medication effects such as those used for the treatment of hypertension, insomnia, anxiety, and pain; chronic infections such as hepatitis C or atypical mycobacterial disease; occult malignancy; chronic anemia; rheumatic diseases; and allergies to name a few [52].

In this section we will primarily discuss fatigue management in COPD from a pulmonary perspective and briefly discuss other more common fatigue management considerations pertaining to patients with COPD such as depression, sleep-disordered breathing, and insomnia.

Both pharmacologic and non-pharmacologic interventions are important in the management of fatigue in COPD. The Global Initiative for Chronic Obstructive Lung Disease (GOLD) is the approach mostly used in the USA to guide therapies. Pharmacologic therapies are generally added in a stepwise fashion unless the patient presents with severe disease at which point multiple therapies are concurrently started to control the symptoms. Non-pharmacologic interventions include oxygen therapy, pulmonary rehabilitation, vaccinations, smoking cessations, and reduction of other risk factors [53].

Pharmacologic Therapies

The fundamentals of pharmacologic therapies include bronchodilators (beta agonists and anticholinergics) given alone or in combination with inhaled steroids depending upon severity of disease, risk of exacerbations, disease impact, and response to therapy [53].

These treatments are generally administered via inhalation in the forms of metered dose inhalers, dry powder inhaler, and soft mist inhaler, and some are given via nebulization. For maintenance therapies, long-acting agents are mostly recommended. Oral bronchodilators such as theophylline and albuterol have more systemic side effects and interactions with other medications and are less often used unless the patient is refractory to the inhalational therapies.

Long-acting bronchodilators are the mainstay of therapies in patients with COPD. These include beta agonists, anticholinergics, and less commonly used theophylline. They have consistently shown to improve dyspnea, cough, and sputum production which likely indirectly improve fatigue in these patients [54]. In addition to long-acting bronchodilators, inhaled corticosteroids are approved for use in patients with COPD [55].

In summary, although inhaled and oral bronchodilator therapy in the management of COPD has not been specifically studied in the management of fatigue, the improvement in dyspnea, quality of life, and exercise capacity with these agents may conceivably improve fatigue.

Oxygen Therapy

Many patients with stable severe COPD (especially GOLD stage IV) have chronic hypoxemia and benefit from O_2 therapy that has been shown to improve survival and quality of life in hypoxemic patients [56].

Pulmonary Rehabilitation in COPD

Optimal bronchodilation by long-acting bronchodilators is the first step in the treatment of patients with COPD. However, greater treatment effects (e.g., improvements in exercise performance, symptoms, and health-related quality of life including fatigue) are often achieved with the addition of pulmonary rehabilitation [57]. Comprehensive pulmonary rehabilitation programs aim at tackling the systemic consequences of COPD as well as the behavioral and educational deficiencies observed in many patients. Pulmonary rehabilitation is defined by the American Thoracic Society and the European Respiratory Society as a comprehensive intervention based on a thorough patient assessment followed by patient-tailored therapies that include, but are not limited to, exercise training, education, and behavioral modification designed to improve the physical and psychological condition of people with chronic respiratory disease and to promote the long-term adherence to health-enhancing behaviors [58].

Other important therapeutic modalities that are stressed in many rehabilitation programs include smoking cessation, oxygen therapy, nutritional support, and respiratory muscle training and adequate rest.

In general, patients with advanced COPD tend to limit their exercise due to dyspnea, and this leads to more musculoskeletal deconditioning. The goal of pulmonary rehabilitation in these patients is to break this cycle. Benefits of pulmonary rehabilitation include reduced dyspnea, improved health-related quality of life, decreased health-care utilization and fewer days of hospitalization [59]. Several studies have demonstrated improved quality of life following both inpatient and outpatient pulmonary rehab programs [60].

In addition to disease-specific management, attention to and treatment of comorbid conditions like depression, insomnia, and sleep apnea may improve quality of life and fatigue.

Conclusion

Fatigue is prevalent in patients with cardiac or respiratory conditions. Fatigue can stem from many causes including primary disease itself, medications, and comorbid conditions. Disease targeted therapy is the first line that can improve fatigue. In addition, enrollment of patients in rehabilitation program may, to some degree, reverse physical and psychological effects of the disease. In addition, close attention to secondary comorbid conditions particularly sleep problems and depression is warranted.

Acknowledgment This work is supported by the Department of Veterans Affairs Research and Development Care Line.

References

1. Fini A, de Almeida Lopes Monteiro da Cruz D. Characteristics of fatigue in heart failure patients: a literature review. Rev Lat Am Enfermagem. 2009;17:557–65.
2. Ekman I, Cleland JG, Swedberg K, Charlesworth A, Metra M, Poole-Wilson PA. Symptoms in patients with heart failure are prognostic predictors: insights from COMET. J Card Fail. 2005;11:288–92.
3. Drexler H, Coats AJ. Explaining fatigue in congestive heart failure. Annu Rev Med. 1996;47:241–56.
4. Sharafkhaneh A, Melendez J, Akhtar F, Lan C. Fatigue in cardiorespiratory conditions. In: Hirshkowtiz M, Sharafkhaneh A, editors. Fatigue Elsevier; 2013. p. 221–8.
5. Redeker NS. Somatic symptoms explain differences in psychological distress in heart failure patients vs a comparison group. Prog Cardiovasc Nurs. 2006;21:182–9.
6. Tiesinga LJ, Dassen TW, Halfens RJ. DUFS and DEFS: development, reliability and validity of the Dutch fatigue scale and the Dutch exertion fatigue scale. Int J Nurs Stud. 1998;35:115–23.
7. Aurich-Barrera B, Wilton LV, Shakir SA. Use and risk management of carvedilol for the treatment of heart failure in the community in England: results from a modified prescription-event monitoring study. Drug Saf. 2009;32:43–54.
8. Cohn JN, Tognoni G. A randomized trial of the angiotensin-receptor blocker valsartan in chronic heart failure. N Engl J Med. 2001;345:1667–75.
9. Beller B, Bulle T, Bourge RC, Colfer H, Fowles RE, Giles TD, Grover J, Whipple JP, Fisher MB, Jessup M, et al. Lisinopril versus placebo in the treatment of heart failure: the Lisinopril heart failure study group. J Clin Pharmacol. 1995;35:673–80.
10. Riegel B, Ratcliffe SJ, Sayers SL, Potashnik S, Buck HG, Jurkovitz C, Fontana S, Weaver TE, Weintraub WS, Goldberg LR. Determinants of excessive daytime sleepiness and fatigue in adults with heart failure. Clin Nurs Res. 2012;21:271–93.
11. Papadopoulou EF, Mavrogeni SI, Dritsas A, Cokkinos DV. Assessment of quality of life using three activity questionnaires in heart failure patients after monthly, intermittent administration of levosimendan during a six-month period. Hellenic J Cardiol. 2009;50:269–74.
12. Pang PS, Gheorghiade M, Dihu J, Swedberg K, Khan S, Maggioni AP, Grinfeld L, Zannad F, Burnett JC Jr, Ouyang J, et al. Effects of tolvaptan on physician-assessed symptoms and signs in patients hospitalized with acute heart failure syndromes: analysis from the efficacy of vasopressin antagonism in heart failure outcome study with tolvaptan (EVEREST) trials. Am Heart J. 2011;161:1067–72.
13. Kumar A, Singh RB, Saxena M, Niaz MA, Josh SR, Chattopadhyay P, Mechirova V, Pella D, Fedacko J. Effect of carni Q-gel (ubiquinol and carnitine) on cytokines in patients with heart failure in the Tishcon study. Acta Cardiol. 2007;62:349–54.
14. Pittler MH, Guo R, Ernst E. Hawthorn extract for treating chronic heart failure. Cochrane Database Syst Rev. 2008;1:CD005312.
15. Ponikowski P, van Veldhuisen DJ, Comin-Colet J, Ertl G, Komajda M, Mareev V, McDonagh T, Parkhomenko A, Tavazzi L, Levesque V, et al. Beneficial effects of long-term intravenous iron therapy with ferric carboxymaltose in patients with symptomatic heart failure and iron deficiency dagger. Eur Heart J. 2015;36:657–68.
16. Puetz TW, Beasman KM, O'Connor PJ. The effect of cardiac rehabilitation exercise programs on feelings of energy and fatigue: a meta-analysis of research from 1945 to 2005. Eur J Cardiovasc Prev Rehabil. 2006;13:886–93.
17. Pozehl B, Duncan K, Hertzog M. The effects of exercise training on fatigue and dyspnea in heart failure. Eur J Cardiovasc Nurs. 2008;7:127–32.
18. Albert NM, Buchsbaum R, Li J. Randomized study of the effect of video education on heart failure healthcare utilization, symptoms, and self-care behaviors. Patient Educ Couns. 2007;69:129–39.

19. Colin RE, Castillo ML, Orea TA, Rebollar GV, Narvaez DR, Asensio LE. Effects of a nutritional intervention on body composition, clinical status, and quality of life in patients with heart failure. Nutrition. 2004;20:890–5.
20. Johansson P, Svensson E, Alehagen U, Dahlstrom U, Jaarsma T, Brostrom A. Sleep disordered breathing, hypoxia and inflammation: associations with sickness behaviour in community dwelling elderly with and without cardiovascular disease. Sleep Breath. 2015;19:263–71.
21. Rutledge T, Reis VA, Linke SE, Greenberg BH, Mills PJ. Depression in heart failure a meta-analytic review of prevalence, intervention effects, and associations with clinical outcomes. J Am Coll Cardiol. 2006;48:1527–37.
22. Sokoreli I, de Vries JJ, Pauws SC, Steyerberg EW. Depression and anxiety as predictors of mortality among heart failure patients: systematic review and meta-analysis. Heart Fail Rev. 2016;21:49–63.
23. Woltz PC, Chapa DW, Friedmann E, Son H, Akintade B, Thomas SA. Effects of interventions on depression in heart failure: a systematic review. Heart Lung. 2012;41:469–83.
24. Conley S, Feder S, Redeker NS. The relationship between pain, fatigue, depression and functional performance in stable heart failure. Heart Lung. 2015;44:107–12.
25. Bartels MN. Fatigue in cardiopulmonary disease. Phys Med Rehabil Clin N Am. 2009;20:389–404.
26. Celli BR, Cote CG, Marin JM, Casanova C, Montes O, Mendez RA, Pinto PV, Cabral HJ. The body-mass index, airflow obstruction, dyspnea, and exercise capacity index in chronic obstructive pulmonary disease 1. N Engl J Med. 2004;350:1005–12.
27. Oga T, Nishimura K, Tsukino M, Sato S, Hajiro T. Analysis of the factors related to mortality in chronic obstructive pulmonary disease: role of exercise capacity and health status. Am J Respir Crit Care Med. 2003;167:544–9.
28. McGavin CR, Gupta SP, Lloyd EL, McHardy GJ. Physical rehabilitation for the chronic bronchitic: results of a controlled trial of exercises in the home. Thorax. 1977;32:307–11.
29. Geertsma A, van der BW, de Boer WJ, TenVergert EM. Survival with and without lung transplantation. Transplant Proc. 1997;29:630–1.
30. Martinez FJ, Chang A. Surgical therapy for chronic obstructive pulmonary disease. Semin Respir Crit Care Med. 2005;26:167–91.
31. Jarad NA, Sequeiros IM, Patel P, Bristow K, Sund Z. Fatigue in cystic fibrosis: a novel prospective study investigating subjective and objective factors associated with fatigue. Chron Respir Dis. 2012;9:241–9.
32. Brooks CM, Richards JM Jr, Bailey WC, Martin B, Windsor RA, Soong SJ. Subjective symptomatology of asthma in an outpatient population. Psychosom Med. 1989;51:102–8.
33. Small SP, Lamb M. Measurement of fatigue in chronic obstructive pulmonary disease and in asthma. Int J Nurs Stud. 2000;37:127–33.
34. Gosselink R, Troosters T, Decramer M. Peripheral muscle weakness contributes to exercise limitation in COPD. Am J Respir Crit Care Med. 1996;153:976–80.
35. Mahler DA, Harver A. A factor analysis of dyspnea ratings, respiratory muscle strength, and lung function in patients with chronic obstructive pulmonary disease. Am Rev Respir Dis. 1992;145:467–70.
36. Guilleminault C, Cummiskey J, Motta J. Chronic obstructive airflow disease and sleep studies. Am Rev Respir Dis. 1980;122:397–406.
37. Sharafkhaneh A, Jayaraman G, Kaleekal T, Sharafkhaneh H, Hirshkowitz M. Sleep disorders and their management in patients with COPD. Ther Adv Respir Dis. 2009;3:309–18.
38. Davies L, Angus RM, Calverley PM. Oral corticosteroids in patients admitted to hospital with exacerbations of chronic obstructive pulmonary disease: a prospective randomised controlled trial. Lancet. 1999;354:456–60.
39. Rich A. Corticosteroids and chronic obstructive pulmonary disease in the nursing home. J Am Med Dir Assoc. 2005;6:S68–74.
40. Gift AG, Shepard CE. Fatigue and other symptoms in patients with chronic obstructive pulmonary disease: do women and men differ? J Obstet Gynecol Neonatal Nurs. 1999;28:201–8.

41. Theander K, Unosson M. Fatigue in patients with chronic obstructive pulmonary disease. J Adv Nurs. 2004;45:172–7.
42. Baltzan MA, Scott AS, Wolkove N, Bailes S, Bernard S, Bourbeau J, Maltais F. Fatigue in COPD: prevalence and effect on outcomes in pulmonary rehabilitation. Chron Respir Dis. 2011;8:119–28.
43. Theander K, Jakobsson P, Torstensson O, Unosson M. Severity of fatigue is related to functional limitation and health in patients with chronic obstructive pulmonary disease. Int J Nurs Pract. 2008;14:455–62.
44. Al shair K, Muellerova H, Yorke J, Rennard SI, Wouters EF, Hanania NA, Sharafkhaneh A, Vestbo J. Examining fatigue in COPD: development, validity and reliability of a modified version of FACIT-F scale. Health Qual Life Outcomes. 2012;10:100.
45. Hanania NA, Mullerova H, Locantore NW, Vestbo J, Watkins ML, Wouters EF, Rennard SI, Sharafkhaneh A. Determinants of depression in the ECLIPSE chronic obstructive pulmonary disease cohort. Am J Respir Crit Care Med. 2011;183:604–11.
46. Baghai-Ravary R, Quint JK, Goldring JJ, Hurst JR, Donaldson GC, Wedzicha JA. Determinants and impact of fatigue in patients with chronic obstructive pulmonary disease. Respir Med. 2009;103:216–23.
47. Landbo C, Prescott E, Lange P, Vestbo J, Almdal TP. Prognostic value of nutritional status in chronic obstructive pulmonary disease. Am J Respir Crit Care Med. 1999;160:1856–61.
48. Flenley DC. Sleep in chronic obstructive lung disease. Clin Chest Med. 1985,6.651–61.
49. George CF, Bayliff CD. Management of insomnia in patients with chronic obstructive pulmonary disease. Drugs. 2003;63:379–87.
50. Klink M, Quan SF. Prevalence of reported sleep disturbances in a general adult population and their relationship to obstructive airways diseases. Chest. 1987;91:540–6.
51. Chaouat A, Weitzenblum E, Krieger J, Ifoundza T, Oswald M, Kessler R. Association of chronic obstructive pulmonary disease and sleep apnea syndrome. Am J Respir Crit Care Med. 1995;151:82–6.
52. Gorroll AH, May LA, Mulley AG. Office evaluation and management of the adult patient. 6th ed. Philadelphia: JB Lippincott; 2009.
53. Global Initiative for Chronic Obstructive Lung Disease. Global strategy for the diagnosis, management, and prevention of chronic obstructive pulmonary disease; 2011. 2013. 5-21-2014. Ref Type: Online Source.
54. Qaseem A, Wilt TJ, Weinberger SE, Hanania NA, Criner G, van der Molen T, Marciniuk DD, Denberg T, Schunemann H, Wedzicha W, et al. Diagnosis and management of stable chronic obstructive pulmonary disease: a clinical practice guideline update from the American College of Physicians, American College of Chest Physicians, American Thoracic Society, and European Respiratory Society. Ann Intern Med. 2011;155:179–91.
55. Calverley PM, Anderson JA, Celli B, Ferguson GT, Jenkins C, Jones PW, Yates JC, Vestbo J. Salmeterol and fluticasone propionate and survival in chronic obstructive pulmonary disease. N Engl J Med. 2007;356:775–89.
56. Tarpy SP, Celli BR. Long-term oxygen therapy. N Engl J Med. 1995;333:710–4.
57. Weiner P, Magadle R, Berar-Yanay N, Davidovich A, Weiner M. The cumulative effect of long-acting bronchodilators, exercise, and inspiratory muscle training on the perception of dyspnea in patients with advanced COPD. Chest. 2000;118:672–8.
58. Troosters T, Casaburi R, Gosselink R, Decramer M. Pulmonary rehabilitation in chronic obstructive pulmonary disease. Am J Respir Crit Care Med. 2005;172:19–38.
59. Ries AL, Bauldoff GS, Carlin BW, Casaburi R, Emery CF, Mahler DA, Make B, Rochester CL, Zuwallack R, Herrerias C. Pulmonary rehabilitation: joint ACCP/AACVPR evidence-based clinical practice guidelines. Chest. 2007;131:4S–42S.
60. Puhan MA, Scharplatz M, Troosters T, Steurer J. Respiratory rehabilitation after acute exacerbation of COPD may reduce risk for readmission and mortality – a systematic review. Respir Res. 2005;6:54.

Chapter 13
Fatigue Management in the Hospital

Garrett Bird and Philip Alapat

Managing fatigue among the varied groups that comprise a hospital workforce requires an understanding of their specific needs and duties. The main groups at risk of fatigue significant enough to impact patient care are physicians in training, nurses, and practicing physicians. Physicians in training are the most studied group of hospital practitioners with respect to sleep deprivation and the attendant fatigue. Some hospitals are staffed mostly by physicians in training, and the need for 24 h patient care in the hospital setting creates longer than usual work schedules. Physicians in training are also less experienced than practicing physicians and have both educational and work goals to attain. Recent modifications have decreased continuous hours spent in the hospital but the 24 h need for patient care will continue to limit the sleep time available to physicians in training. In some hospitals, the rigors of internship and residency are considered a "rite of passage" similar to hazing of pledges to a fraternity or sorority [1]. Long hours in the hospital, required study time, and personal and social activities all increase the risk of sleep deprivation.

Sleep deprivation has severe effects on many areas which can adversely affect physician performance including cognition, mood, immunity, performance of tasks, interpersonal relationships, and judgment [2–6]. Moderate to severe sleep deprivation produces impairments in cognitive and motor performance equivalent to a blood alcohol content of 0.1% [7]. Residents' daytime sleepiness in both baseline and post-call conditions are near or below levels associated with clinical sleep disorders [8]. Sleep-deprived physicians miss more radiology findings [9], miss impor-

G. Bird, MD, CM
Department of Pulmonary, Critical Care, Sleep, Steward Health Care,
West Jordan, UT, USA

P. Alapat, MD (✉)
Department of Medicine – Pulmonary/Critical Care/Sleep, Baylor College of Medicine,
Houston, TX, USA
e-mail: palapat@bcm.edu

© Springer Science+Business Media, LLC, part of Springer Nature 2018
A. Sharafkhaneh, M. Hirshkowitz (eds.), *Fatigue Management*,
https://doi.org/10.1007/978-1-4939-8607-1_13

tant vital sign changes [10, 11], make more mistakes in the performance of simulated surgeries [12, 13], have greater psychological impairment, and use more sedatives [14, 15]. Even having a "black cloud" (a perceived increase in work due to random variation) can be related to the amount of sleep deprivation [16]. Physicians may perform slightly better than nonphysicians in the setting of sleep deprivation, which is touted as a reason to exempt physicians from fatigue management protocols. However, this finding is likely due to compensatory mechanisms from adaptation to chronic sleep deprivation, and the small difference is not significant [17]. Medical errors are estimated to take between 44,000 and 98,000 lives each year, and many are felt to be preventable [18]. Total resident work hours correlate with reported stress and hours of sleep per week [19]. Managing fatigue of physicians in training is necessary to prevent potentially deadly medical errors [20].

Dr. Baldwin from the Accreditation Council for Graduate Medical Education (ACGME), Rush Medical College, Chicago, Illinois, has published several studies about resident sleep habits and performance. In summary, doctors who average less than 5 h of sleep a night make more medical mistakes, are more likely to be involved in a traffic accident, and are more likely to be involved in a lawsuit or have a serious conflict with the nursing staff. Doctors who average less than 5 h of sleep a night are also less satisfied with their work, feel more impaired, have a higher stress rating, and are more likely to feel belittled or humiliated at work [19, 21].

Work is not the only goal of physicians in training—they must also attain educational milestones to advance in their careers. Whether they meet educational goals can also be determined by how well systems in the hospital manage their fatigue. When physicians in training are subject to sleep deprivation, they perform poorly on educational tasks. For example, family practice residents with one night of sleep deprivation immediately prior to the exam performed worse on their in-training exam scores [22]. This decrease in performance was equivalent to a year of training. Obstetrics-Gynecology residents with a night float and a monitored 75 h work week improved in-training exam scores [23].

Physicians in training serve a dual role that places them at an immediate conflict with the systems in place to protect their training time, education, and sleep. They need appropriate training and experience with patients to hone their skills. They perform duties in the hospital while receiving an education about their chosen field through on-the-job training, lectures, research, and other scholarly activities. At the same time there are patient care responsibilities, which must be performed to fulfill obligations to the hospital system. Hospitals need to provide 24 h care to patients with complicated medical histories and severe acute medical problems. Physicians in training are monitored and educated by their residency or fellowship training programs, but they are utilized by hospitals and clinics run by administrators whose primary concern often is patient throughput. Physicians in training are considered by some hospital administrators as an expendable resource. One New York hospital administrator stated "Many people think that interns and residents are putting in time chiefly to meet their educational requirements. In my administrative capacity that is of no concern. I have to look at these people as resources—resources that we use to deliver services at a reasonable cost. I'll tell you truthfully, in my book they are just cheap labor. With no effective union to back them, the fiscally wise procedure is for us to have them work as many hours as possible" [24]. The discrepancy between expectations of patient care by administrators and appropriate balancing of education and patient care by the training programs requires some compromise. Motivating change in physicians in training schedules to combat fatigue must focus on the benefits to both patient care and educational goals.

When the hospital has a steady number of patients, staffing schedules can be mutually agreed upon by the residency training program, and the hospital and residents can be "protected" and kept to within their required duty hours. Problems can arise when an increased number of patients are admitted to the hospital, e.g., during an influenza outbreak, after a natural disaster, or due to an increase in the population served by the hospital residents have to compensate and care for these patients. The hospital cannot hire more residents, and the residency program cannot refuse to help the hospital. These types of situations are, fortunately, the exception rather than the rule—but any perturbations to this system can lead to taxing work schedules and increased risk for sleep deprivation.

Even during times of a "stable" hospital census, lack of available physicians in a particular field can lead to increased resident hours, decreased sleep time, and increased sleep deprivation. Surgeons in training have perhaps the most extreme schedules. In 2003, surgical residents worked a mean of 105 h a week [25]. This was almost 15 years after the Bell Commission cited sleep deprivation among house officers as a major cause of the death of a young woman in New York, and the suggested duty hours per week was decreased from 100 to 80 [26, 27].

The studies on surgeons in training and sleep deprivation have given mixed results likely due to the inability to "normalize" work schedules for research. For example, residents on 1:2 call schedule with less than 4 h of sleep per 24 h period over several weeks showed no difference in cognition, discernment, visual and auditory vigilance, or rapid eye-hand coordination on a battery of tests performed daily [28]. This extremely aggressive call schedule led to significant overall sleep debt, so testing after one night of "normal" sleep preceded by a 24 h call was unlikely to show difference in any measured parameters due to the chronic sleep deprivation effects. Surgeons may also underreport symptoms and effects of sleep deprivation. Surgeons self-reported less emotional stress, alcohol usage, and drug usage than other residents despite a more rigorous call schedule [29]. Sleep-deprived surgeons also reported no difference in postoperative complications [30–32]. Surgeons also reported no difference in their in-training exams from sleep deprivation [33]. Surgeons did however have significantly less satisfaction when working every other night on call [34] and reported declining educational experiences and potential declines in clinical care [35]. Obstetric residents overwhelmingly wanted fewer nights on call despite the potential to limit surgical experiences [36]. Clinically, surgeons showed increased rates of tachycardia and an elevated white blood cell count when sleep deprived [37]. Objectively, sleep-deprived surgeons in training are reported to make 20% more mistakes and perform 14% slower on laparoscopic simulations [38, 39].

                                                                G. Bird and P. Alapat

The focus in academic hospitals has been on limiting duty hours which increase sleep time. The major concern is whether the required sign-out or changeovers will lead to a lower quality of care for patients system wide due to a lack of continuity [40]. From the available research on large groups, limiting duty hours does not appear to significantly compromise patient care. Following the ACGME implementation work limit rules from July 1, 2003, Dr. Volpp et al., with a retrospective study of 1.2 million patients, showed a small decrease in short-term mortality of high-risk medicine patients with no change in surgical patients [41, 42]. The Volpp group, in 2009, then found no significant difference in mortality or "rescue" rates for high-risk medical or surgical patients [43]. The largest study to date, including 8.5 million Medicare beneficiaries from both teaching-intensive and less teaching-intensive hospitals before and after the July 1, 2003, duty hours change, showed no difference in all-cause 30-day mortality [44]. Other large retrospective studies have shown no difference in hospital stays [45] or readmission rates [46]. Increasing available sleep time may improve job satisfaction, improve neurocognitive function, reduce impairment, and reduce fatigue among physicians in training [7, 8].

Prudence dictates that hospitals and residency training programs create policies and procedures that are in keeping with ACGME or American Osteopathic Association (AOA) requirements. The 2011 ACGME duty hours standard revision [47], which were in effect from July 1, 2011 to June 31, 2017, included some important changes to their 2003 requirements (Table 13.1). While the total duty hours, 80 per week averaged over 4 weeks, remained the same for most residents, the 2011 requirements include new limits on continuous duty hours. Instead of 24 h plus 6 additional hours to "transfer care" and complete any needed work, first-year graduates were given 16 h plus 4 additional hours to complete their care plans, while all senior residents (second year of training and above) were allowed 24 h followed by 4 additional hours. There was a provision to allow residents to follow a single patient beyond prescribed duty hours for required continuity for a severely ill or unstable patient, academic importance of the events transpiring, or humanistic attention to the needs of a patient or family—but this was delineated as a rare exception. Emergency department (ED) trainees were not permitted more than 12 continuous hours and no more than 60 h per week in the ER, and no more than 72 h total per week.

The most recent ACGME revision, which took effect July 1, 2017 [49], removed the terms "duty hours," "duty periods," and "duty" and replaced them with "clinical experience and education," "clinical and educational work," and "work hours." In its most dramatic change, the 2017 Core Program Requirements removed any reference to graduate year or specialty and made the duty hours consistent for all trainees. All trainees, regardless of specialty or year of training have to adhere to the new standards which include a maximum of 24 h continuous duty followed by 4 h to "transfer care" or for educational opportunities. This removed the reduced duty hours for PGY 1 and ED trainees that were mandated in 2011. In addition to these changes, "at home" clinical work now has to be counted as equivalent to "in hospital" duty hours. Trainees, in the new standards, were given the possibility to "voluntarily" remain on duty for a unique case or educational opportunity, as long as they maintained the 80

Table 13.1 ACGME 2003 compared to ACGME 2011, 2017 and AOA 2011, 2018 work hours standards

Standard	July 2003 ACGME Standards [48]	July 2011 and 2017 ACGME Standards [47, 49]	July 2011 and 2018 AOA Standards [50, 51]
Work week duty limit	80 h per week (averaged over 4 weeks)	80 h per week (averaged over 4 weeks)	2011/2018: 80 h per week (averaged over 4 weeks)
Rest periods	"Adequate rest between duty periods"	2011: PGY2+: strategic napping, especially after 16 h of continuous duty and between the hours of 10:00 p.m. and 8:00 a.m., is strongly suggested 2017: During off-duty hours, sleep should be a priority	2011/2018: At the trainee's request, the training institution must provide comfortable sleep facilities to trainees who are too fatigued at shift conclusion to safely drive 2018: Program must provide transportation (i.e "cab fare" if the trainee is too fatigued to drive
Continuous time on the job	24 h plus 6 h for continuity of care, 30 h total	2011: PGY1: no more than 16 continuous hours on duty Maximum additional 4 h to "transfer care" PGY2+: no more than 24 h continuous hours on duty Maximum additional 4 h to "transfer care" *Residents are allowed to follow a single patient beyond prescribed duty hours for required continuity for a severely ill or unstable patient, academic importance of the events transpiring, or humanistic attention to the needs of a patient or family ER: while on duty in the emergency department, residents may not work longer than 12 continuous scheduled hours. A resident should not work more than 60 scheduled hours per week Seeing patients in the emergency department and no more than 72 duty hours per week [47] 2017: all residents maximum of 24 continuous hours on duty and maximum additional 4 h to "transfer care" with rare exceptions. Home-based work counts towards all other duty hour rules	2011/2018: No more than 24 h continuous hours on duty Maximum additional 4 h to "transfer care" ER: no longer than 12 h shifts with no more than 30 additional minutes allowed for transfer of care 2018: In cases where a trainee is engaged in patient responsibility which cannot be interrupted at the duty hour limits, additional coverage shall be assigned as soon as possible by the attending staff to relieve the trainee involved. Patient care responsibility is not precluded by the duty hours policy

(continued)

Table 13.1 (continued)

Standard	July 2003 ACGME Standards [48]	July 2011 and 2017 ACGME Standards [47, 49]	July 2011 and 2018 AOA Standards [50, 51]
Days off	1 day out of 7 free from all duties (averaged over 4 weeks)	2011/2017:1 day out of 7 free from all duties (averaged over 4 weeks). No "home-call" allowed for days off	2011/2018 One 48 h period off on alternate weeks or at least one 24 h period off each week 2018: No home call allowed during days off
Call	No more than once every three nights (1:3), averaged over 4 weeks	2011/2017: No more than once every three nights (1:3), averaged over 4 weeks The frequency of at-home call is not subject to the every-third-night limitation but must satisfy the requirement for 1-day-in-7 free of duty, when averaged over 4 weeks	2011/2018: No more than once every three nights (1:3), averaged over 4 weeks Home call does not count in the 1:3 rule but any time spent returning to the hospital must be included in the 80 h maximum limit
Moonlighting	Only moonlighting done in the "sponsoring institution" counts toward the 80 h limit External moonlighting should not interfere with the education of the resident	2011/2017: PGY1: no moonlighting allowed *PGY2+: all moonlighting (internal and external) counts toward the 80 h work week	2011/2018: No moonlighting Others: moonlighting must be counted toward the 80 h work week
Time between shifts	Should have 10 h between shifts and all on-call duties	2011: PGY-1 and "intermediate" residents should have 10 h and must have 8 h free of duty between scheduled duty periods Residents in the final years of education [as defined by the review committee] must be prepared to enter the unsupervised practice of medicine and care for patients over irregular or extended periods 2017: all residents must have 14 hours free from service after 24 hours of call	2011/2018: Upon conclusion of a 20–24 h duty shift, trainees shall have a minimum of 12 h off before being required to be on duty or on call again Upon completing a duty period of at least 12 but less than 20 h, a minimum period of 10 h off must be provided

Standard	July 2003 ACGME Standards [48]	July 2011 and 2017 ACGME Standards [47, 49]	July 2011 and 2018 AOA Standards [50, 51]
Night float	No guidelines	2011: No more than six nights in a row 2017: The maximum number of consecutive weeks of night float, and maximum number of months of night float per year may be further specified by the Review Committee	2011: No guidelines 2018: Can use ACGME Standards
Exceptions	A review committee may grant exceptions for up to 10% or a maximum of 88 h to individual programs based on a sound educational rationale	2011/2017: A review committee may grant exceptions for up to 10% or a maximum of 88 h to individual programs based on a sound educational rationale	2011: No guidelines 2018: Can use ACGME Standards

h per week total. Residents were specifically encouraged to prioritize sleep during their off-duty hours but the 2017 Standards removed specific rest periods or sleep requirements.

The American Osteopathic Association (AOA) 2011 Basic Standards [50] were similar to the ACGME Duty Hours Standards of 2011 and, when updated in 2018, the AOA specifically allowed programs to choose either the 2018 AOA Standards or the 2017 ACGME Core Requirements work hours rules in their programs. The other major differences in the AOA 2018 guidelines included maintaining a separate rule for Emergency Medicine trainees hours, requiring programs to pay for transportation costs for fatigued trainees, allowing some exceptions to the 24 h plus 4 h rule and preventing home call on days off.

"Moonlighting," the practice of working after-hours for supplemental income was previously only counted toward duty hours if it was performed in the trainees program—so-called "internal" moonlighting. A trainee could work at outside facilities doing "external" moonlighting without reporting that time to their home program. Now both internal and external moonlighting needs to be monitored, and the hours at both sites count toward the 80 h work week limit.

Hospitals have been forced to create new systems to allow compliance with previous requirements which now need to be reevaluated to ensure compliance with the new rules. These modifications include night float systems where a resident or intern works a night shift to allow other residents time to go home or nap and protected cross-coverage time for sleeping. Night float is now limited in ACGME programs to 6 days in a row. Some hospitals have limited the number admissions to the teaching service and been forced to employ additional practicing physicians to take the overflow. Some training programs have hired additional physician extenders (medical assistants, nurse practitioners, nurse/physician assistants, etc.) or pushed advanced fellows to take more clinical responsibilities and have less time for research in order to make up for the reduced work hours of junior physicians in training. These changes come with their own potential risks and benefits. Each hospital or clinic will have to evaluate whether to hire additional help, decrease provided patient care, or increase the workload on more senior trainees.

The limitation in intern (PGY1) duty hours is estimated to cost the system a significant amount of money nationwide. The ACGME recently released mathematical models that assumed their 2011 reduction in resident work hours would lead to an increase in the cost to the system of $380,766,262 nationwide (in 2008 dollars). The revised policy would be cost-saving for society if it reduced preventable adverse events by 2.4% and cost-saving for major teaching hospitals if it reduced preventable adverse events by 10.9% [52].

Improving resident work hours may have other positive benefits for patients. The Veterans Hospital in Minnesota found that using a schedule designed to reduce sleep deprivation reduced the length of stay (10.9 vs 9.3 days) and the number of laboratory tests ordered per patient (24.0 vs 19.0) for patients cared for under the new work schedule compared with those cared for under the traditional work schedule. Resident physicians also committed fewer medication errors under the new work schedule (16.9 vs 12.0 per 100 patients discharged) [53].

The 80 h work week has already been shown to improve the mood of physicians [54] while not increasing attending responsibilities or decreasing admissions to medical school [55]. During the time spent in the hospital, further modifications to the schedule may improve sleep deprivation among residents. A small study at the University of Chicago, Chicago, Illinois, showed that providing residents with a nap period at night reduced their post-call and overall fatigue and increased their sleep time at night [56].

Provision of protected time for sleep may not always improve total sleep time. Interns on a 36 h call day with protected time for sleep, via cross coverage, were found to have significant chronic sleep deprivation which was relatively unaffected by sleep obtained in the hospital. This was due to the "protected time" being used for clinical duties and not for additional sleep as planned [57]. Some have proposed increasing the length of residency programs [58] or using pharmacologic enhancement [59], but these options are likely to be unpopular with residents and fellows [60].

Other interventions may improve the fatigue and sleepiness reported by residents in training. Residents need to be taught to "plan the night" to avoid unnecessary interruptions. Emergencies do occur, but many calls or pages are related to more mundane issues that are not time sensitive. The resident can pick a specified time after the nursing change of shift to address all concerns that arise during the sign-out process. Nurses should also be told to avoid calls for non-urgent issues until the morning when the staffing by physicians is more robust. Residents should then communicate with the nursing staff about when they plan to take a nap during the night shift and when they plan to be available for orders, questions, and other urgent nursing issues. The morning staff also needs to be proactive in seeking out the nurses as soon as they finish their sign-out to address these issues. This method provides a better working environment for both parties. At Stanford, discussion between surgical residents and nursing staff at a predetermined time to address issues that were non-emergent led to fewer interruptions in overnight sleep. This started by creating an environment where non-emergent issues were collated into a single phone call, via a notebook system, and calls were avoided, unless emergent, during a 4 h block. This "cooperative system" improved the work environment and provided additional time for sleep or study [61]. When residents plan ahead and give guidelines to the nursing staff, expectations are clear to both parties: nurses are able to provide excellent service without having to call the resident at inopportune times, and residents are not called several times for small issues when one call with many issues would suffice.

Managing fatigue in physicians in training comes down to limiting hours on duty while providing an adequate educational experience. Fatigue management among resident physicians should use the provided guidelines from the AOA and ACGME as a foundation and then build specific programs that work in their local practice. Due to the possibility of losing accreditation for residency programs from noncompliance, these guidelines should be adhered to strictly.

The ACGME and AOM recommendations for work-hour restrictions on residents in training have a positive effect on the residents' mood, sense of well-being, and performance while not compromising patient care when global scheduling modifications are made. Hospital administrators need to work closely with residency training programs to build schedules and support mechanisms so that patient care is not affected. The management of fatigue in these individuals will require a multi-faceted approach. Creating better sign-out and paging processes, decreasing hours spent in the hospital and teaching time management skills to physicians in training will improve their experience in training and positively impact patient care.

Though there are currently no national guidelines regarding limits to duty hours for healthcare workers other than physicians in training, efforts at determining and implementing work-hour limits are being debated [62]. Nurses are affected by sleep deprivation and the consequent fatigue for a variety of reasons many of which overlap with physicians in training. As previously mentioned, hospitals, and their patients, have 24 h service needs—many of which are directly addressed by the nursing staff. Shifts are often added when large numbers of patients are admitted, making planning around a fixed schedule difficult. Nurses who care for dependents at home are also at increased risk of sleep deprivation due to additional family responsibilities [63]. Ironically, night nurses are tasked with creating a peaceful environment for the patient to get restful sleep which adds to their responsibilities [64–68]. Nurses do not have duty hour reporting requirements like physicians in training, and they can choose to work back-to-back shifts whenever desired without the oversight of a regulatory committee like the ACGME.

Sleep deprivation can usually be counteracted by limiting the number of weekly hours nurses are allowed to work. Unfortunately this solution assumes they only work at a single institution and do not "moonlight" at other facilities. In a recent Brazilian study, 31.5% of the nursing staff (including nursing aides and administrators) worked two jobs [69]. Brazilian nurses with two jobs also spent more time sleeping while on service [70]. Nurses may also prefer to work fewer days with longer shifts without understanding the potential adverse effects.

Sleep deprivation among nurses is important to consider; however, another consideration related to working night shifts and rotating shifts is shift work sleep disorder (SWSD). Nurses choose to work the night shift because the pay is often higher [71]. SWSD consists of symptoms of insomnia or excessive sleepiness that occur in relation to work schedules that are not compatible with the individual's circadian rhythm. Thus, SWSD can contribute an additional component of sleepiness to an already sleep-deprived healthcare worker. While nursing errors increase with nurse fatigue [72], one of the most dangerous aspects of SWSD among nurses is the high incidence of automobile accidents or near misses on travel to and from the workplace [71, 73].

Limits to work hours must be placed by the hospital administration and nursing coordinators to prevent inadvertent sleep deprivation among nurses from extensive and/or continuous shifts. Educating nurses about the ill effects of excessive consecutive work hours should also be undertaken.

Changing the shift schedule to improve nursing fatigue can be difficult. Shift work scheduling has many possible permutations. In one English study, over 122 different style of shift schedule plans were found in the major English and Wales hospitals (>400 beds) [74].

Many studies have found less satisfaction, and more fatigue, with a backward-rotating shift (going from mornings to night then to afternoons). Many hospitals work on a 12 h shift system which increases nursing fatigue [75] despite evidence showing that shift duration of 12 h or greater is the single most important determinant of nurse fatigue [76, 77].

Recent studies have shown pronounced negative results of shift work on nurses. A 1995 study by Marziale et al. found that rapidly rotating shifts led to significant irritability and both physical and mental fatigue [78]. A Japanese study in 1996 by Matsumoto et al. of 152 nurses on rotating shifts found nurses had the most difficulty after the first night shift—and they were more likely to take sleep-inducing drugs. It has also been noted that older nurses had more fatigue and dysregulation of sleep than younger nurses on the same schedule [79, 80]. Particularly in nurses over the age of 40, this dysregulation adversely impacted patient care by causing decreased attention to detail and inability to recognize small changes in patient physiology potentially leading to medical errors [81]. However, another study using only self-reported information, from Japan, showed no significant difference in "near miss" errors among nurses on day, evening, and night shifts [82]. Nurses working shifts greater than 12.5 h are at significantly increased risk of experiencing decreased vigilance on the job, suffering an occupational injury, or making a medical error [62]. Interestingly, long-term health of nurses working night shifts may also suffer with increased risk for breast cancer, endometrial cancer, and cardiovascular morbidity and mortality [83].

Specific training and management of nurses to help them cope with the fatigue caused by night nursing has been suggested for over 30 years [84]. More recently, it has been suggested that sleep education and training of nurses should begin at the undergraduate level and continue throughout a nurse's career [85]. The difficulty arises in determining what education is most effective. Different end points are used in the available research, namely, fatigue and job satisfaction—with the goal of avoiding "burnout." The most reasonable solutions include specific changes to the schedules and making changes to the workload at night. Using a more traditional 8 h schedule will likely decrease nurse fatigue; however, the effects of increased patient hand-overs have not been conclusively evaluated. Computerized schedules, which set up targets within algorithmic parameters to avoid backward-rotating schedules, allow days off, and minimized consecutive work hours seem to be better than hand-created schedules [86]. Maximizing weekends off also improves job satisfaction [87]. Allowing flexibility for "night owls" and "morning larks" to build their own schedules may also negate some of the fatigue inducing effects of a single rigid schedule [88]. Limiting night work responsibilities to tasks that can only be completed at night has also been suggested [89] along with helping nurses to avoid "indirect" patient care responsibilities [90]. Documenting information in multiple locations; completing logs, checklists, and collecting data; traveling to equipment, supply, and utility rooms; and entering and reviewing orders are the most commonly reported indirect patient care responsibilities [29]. Based on the previous information about aging nurses and sleep dysregulation, allowing older nurses to preferentially have the day shift is another possible solution.

Preventing fatigue among nurses will decrease burnout, improve satisfaction of nurses, and, hopefully, translate into better care for patients. Hospital administrators must therefore be actively involved in creating schedules that minimize extended hours, limit moonlighting, and focus on education of the nursing staff to increase their awareness of the dangers of sleep deprivation and SWSD. Specific recommendations must be provided to supervisors responsible for schedules and shift responsibilities. Overall, changing the predominant 12 h shift based schedules to 8 h shifts and limiting the number of total shifts per week, including at other facilities, is most likely to improve sleep quality and decrease fatigue among nurses.

Another group of individuals at risk for sleep deprivation and fatigue in the hospital setting is physicians in practice. This group comprises three distinct subgroups: academic physicians, hospital-affiliated physicians, and hospital-employed physicians. While employed physicians and affiliated physicians are primarily responsible for the care and management of patients with or without physician extenders, academic physicians must also teach and supervise physicians in training. The differences in these groups make it difficult to create guidelines regarding sleep deprivation and fatigue management. Additionally different practice sites like large inner-city hospitals, private surgical facilities, and rural hospitals vary greatly in their number of patients and requirements for coverage. Fatigue management among practicing physicians must focus on educating the physicians about the dangers of inadequate sleep to both their personal and professional lives as well as their satisfaction with their jobs. Unfortunately the research into this all important group is limited.

Surgeons, as mentioned earlier, can have very long hours with limited recovery time due to the rigors of the job [91]. A recent matched retrospective cohort study showed that procedures performed at night by surgeons that had worked the previous night without a 6 h break in between had a higher rate of complications. Among these attending physicians (86 surgeons and 134 obstetricians/gynecologists) who had been in the hospital performing another procedure involving adult patients for at least part of the preceding night (12 a.m.–6 a.m.), there was a significant increase in complication rates in procedures performed the following day or "post nighttime." Complications occurred in 82 of 1317 post nighttime procedures with sleep opportunities of 6 h or less (6.2%) versus 19 of 559 post nighttime procedures with sleep opportunities of more than 6 h (3.4%) (odds ratio, 1.72; 95% CI, 1.02–2.89). The most impressive part of this blinded study was that the controls were the physicians themselves performing the same procedure (up to five other times) with a full night free from surgery prior [92].

The data are mixed for other subspecialties. Among anesthesiologists performing epidural catheter placement, sleep deprivation showed no significant change in either performance or complications [93]. In another study, perceived sleep deprivation among Finnish anesthesiologists correlated well with burnout and on-the-job stress [94].

Emergency room physicians have also provided some helpful information regarding fatigue and its effect on physicians in practice. Their 24/7 rotating shifts and limitless permutations of shift combinations provides an excellent milieu for research. Considering that emergency department (ED) physicians report working fewer hours [91] than many other acute care specialties, these data may actually represent a group of relatively mildly sleep-deprived physicians. Night shift ED physicians show decreased speed of intubation, vigilance reaction times, and subjective alertness [95]. When coupled with small amounts of alcohol, sleep deprivation correlated with an increased number of road accidents for ED physicians in an Italian study [96]. It is felt that reducing ED physicians' fatigue will decrease burnout and improve patient care, but there are no conclusive randomized control studies [97].

Unlike in residency programs, there is limited guidance from the American Medical Association (AMA) for physicians in practice despite a recent Institute of Medicine report detailing fatigue as a major cause of errors leading to in-hospital mortality [98]. The AMA recently adopted guidelines for nighttime lighting for all jobs requiring 24/7 coverage—but has no specific policy for fatigue management which applies to physicians in practice [99]. The lack of specific guidelines and recommendations from the AMA means individual hospitals must adopt programs which promote adequate sleep and limit fatigue among physicians. The varied practice styles, job requirements, and training of physicians mean that one-size-fits-all policies are likely to be poorly received [100]. On the other hand, allowing physicians to practice without any guidelines is not appropriate either [101]. Limiting sleepless nights and continuous duty hours will likely lead to improved patient care and job satisfaction.

The best policies for fatigue management in this group will employ education and recommendations similar to those discussed for physicians in training. Educating practicing physicians about the benefits to their patients and to themselves with adequate fatigue management is likely the best way to change their practices.

Other healthcare workers such as respiratory therapists, hospital administrators, and ancillary hospital staff are also at risk of fatigue associated with sleep deprivation and SWSD; however, there is very little research conducted in these groups. The research and recommendations made for physicians in training, nurses, and physicians in practice can likely be extended to these individuals.

Medical care in the hospital setting requires continuous attention by a variety of individuals which can lead to concerns regarding excessive fatigue compromising quality of patient care. Some amount of fatigue is likely to be present; however, appropriate planning and education for these various groups can promote a LESS fatigued, LESS sleepy state ultimately leading to better patient care.

References

1. Whetsell JF. Changing the law, changing the culture: rethinking the "sleepy resident" problem. Ann Health Law. 2003;12(1):23–73. Table of contents.
2. Goel N, Rao H, Durmer JS, Dinges DF. Neurocognitive consequences of sleep deprivation. Semin Neurol. 2009;29(4):320–39.

3. Durmer JS, Dinges DF. Neurocognitive consequences of sleep deprivation. Semin Neurol. 2005;25(1):117–29.
4. Papp KK, Stoller EP, Sage P, Aikens JE, Owens J, Avidan A, et al. The effects of sleep loss and fatigue on resident-physicians: a multi-institutional, mixed-method study. Acad Med. 2004;79(5):394–406.
5. Everson CA. Clinical assessment of blood leukocytes, serum cytokines, and serum immuno-globulins as responses to sleep deprivation in laboratory rats. Am J Physiol Regul Integr Comp Physiol. 2005;289(4):R1054–63.
6. Rose M, Manser T, Ware JC. Effects of call on sleep and mood in internal medicine residents. Behav Sleep Med. 2008;6(2):75–88.
7. Williamson AM, Feyer AM. Moderate sleep deprivation produces impairments in cognitive and motor performance equivalent to legally prescribed levels of alcohol intoxication. Occup Environ Med. 2000;57(10):649–55.
8. Howard SK, Gaba DM, Rosekind MR, Zarcone VP. The risks and implications of excessive daytime sleepiness in resident physicians. Acad Med. 2002;77(10):1019–25.
9. Mann FA, Danz PL. The night stalker effect: quality improvements with a dedicated night-call rotation. Investig Radiol. 1993;28(1):92–6.
10. Denisco RA, Drummond JN, Gravenstein JS. The effect of fatigue on the performance of a simulated anesthetic monitoring task. J Clin Monit. 1987;3(1):22–4.
11. Sharpe R, Koval V, Ronco JJ, Qayumi K, Dodek P, Wong H, et al. The impact of prolonged continuous wakefulness on resident clinical performance in the intensive care unit: a patient simulator study. Crit Care Med. 2010;38(3):766–70.
12. Eastridge BJ, Hamilton EC, O'Keefe GE, Rege RV, Valentine RJ, Jones DJ, et al. Effect of sleep deprivation on the performance of simulated laparoscopic surgical skill. Am J Surg. 2003;186(2):169–74.
13. Jakubowicz DM, Price EM, Glassman HJ, Gallagher AJ, Mandava N, Ralph WP, et al. Effects of a twenty-four hour call period on resident performance during simulated endoscopic sinus surgery in an accreditation council for graduate medical education-compliant training pro-gram. Laryngoscope. 2005;115(1):143–6.
14. Hurwitz TA, Beiser M, Nichol H, Patrick L, Kozak J. Impaired interns and residents. Can J Psychiatr. 1987;32(3):165–9.
15. Handel DA, Raja A, Lindsell CJ. The use of sleep aids among emergency medicine residents: a web based survey. BMC Health Serv Res. 2006;6:136.
16. Tanz RR, Charrow J. Black clouds. Work load, sleep, and resident reputation. Am J Dis Child. 1993;147(5):579–84.
17. Philibert I. Sleep loss and performance in residents and nonphysicians: a meta-analytic exami-nation. Sleep. 2005;28(11):1392–402.
18. Kohn LT, Corrigan J, Donaldson MS. To err is human: building a safer health system. Washington, D.C.: National Academy Press; 2000.
19. Baldwin DC Jr, Daugherty SR, Tsai R, Scotti MJ Jr. A national survey of residents' self-reported work hours: thinking beyond specialty. Acad Med. 2003;78(11):1154–63.
20. Kramer M. Sleep loss in resident physicians: the cause of medical errors? Front Neurol. 2010;1:128.
21. Baldwin DC Jr, Daugherty SR. Sleep deprivation and fatigue in residency training: results of a national survey of first- and second-year residents. Sleep. 2004;27(2):217–23.
22. Jacques CH, Lynch JC, Samkoff JS. The effects of sleep loss on cognitive performance of resident physicians. J Fam Pract. 1990;30(2):223–9.
23. Carey JC, Fishburne JI. A method to limit working hours and reduce sleep deprivation in an obstetrics and gynecology residency program. Obstet Gynecol. 1989;74(4):668–72.
24. Coren S. Sleep thieves: an eye-opening exploration into the science and mysteries of sleep. New York, NY: Free Press; 1996.
25. Whang EE, Perez A, Ito H, Mello MM, Ashley SW, Zinner MJ. Work hours reform: percep-tions and desires of contemporary surgical residents. J Am Coll Surg. 2003;197(4):624–30.
26. Asch DA, Parker RM. The Libby Zion case. One step forward or two steps backward? N Engl J Med. 1988;318(12):771–5.

27. Holzman IR, Barnett SH. The bell commission: ethical implications for the training of physicians. Mt Sinai J Med. 2000;67(2):136–9.
28. Deaconson TF, O'Hair DP, Levy MF, Lee MB, Schueneman AL, Codon RE. Sleep deprivation and resident performance. JAMA. 1988;260(12):1721–7.
29. Bunch WH, Dvonch VM, Storr CL, Baldwin DC Jr, Hughes PH. The stresses of the surgical residency. J Surg Res. 1992;53(3):268–71.
30. Haynes DF, Schwedler M, Dyslin DC, Rice JC, Kerstein MD. Are postoperative complications related to resident sleep deprivation? South Med J. 1995;88(3):283–9.
31. Ellman PI, Kron IL, Alvis JS, Tache-Leon C, Maxey TS, Reece TB, et al. Acute sleep deprivation in the thoracic surgical resident does not affect operative outcomes. Ann Thorac Surg. 2005;80(1):60–4. Discussion 4-5.
32. Yaghoubian A, Kaji AH, Putnam B, de Virgilio C. Trauma surgery performed by "sleep deprived" residents: are outcomes affected? J Surg Educ. 2010;67(6):449–51.
33. Minion D, Plymale M, Donnelly M, Endean E. The effect of prior night call status on the American Board of Surgery in-training examination scores: eight years of data from a single institution. J Surg Educ. 2007;64(6):416–9.
34. Sawyer RG, Tribble CG, Newberg DS, Pruett TL, Minasi JS. Intern call schedules and their relationship to sleep, operating room participation, stress, and satisfaction. Surgery. 1999;126(2):337–42.
35. Mittal V, Salem M, Tyburski J, Brocato J, Lloyd L, Silva Y, et al. Residents' working hours in a consortium-wide surgical education program. Am Surg. 2004;70(2):127–31. Discussion 31.
36. Defoe DM, Power ML, Holzman GB, Carpentieri A, Schulkin J. Long hours and little sleep: work schedules of residents in obstetrics and gynecology. Obstet Gynecol. 2001;97(6):1015–8.
37. Tendulkar AP, Victorino GP, Chong TJ, Bullard MK, Liu TH, Harken AH. Quantification of surgical resident stress "on call". J Am Coll Surg. 2005;201(4):560–4.
38. Taffinder NJ, McManus IC, Gul Y, Russell RC, Darzi A. Effect of sleep deprivation on surgeons' dexterity on laparoscopy simulator. Lancet. 1998;352(9135):1191.
39. Grantcharov TP, Bardram L, Funch-Jensen P, Rosenberg J. Laparoscopic performance after one night on call in a surgical department: prospective study. BMJ. 2001;323(7323):1222–3.
40. Fletcher KE, Saint S, Mangrulkar RS. Balancing continuity of care with residents' limited work hours: defining the implications. Acad Med. 2005;80(1):39–43.
41. Fletcher KE, Davis SQ, Underwood W, Mangrulkar RS, McMahon LF Jr, Saint S. Systematic review: effects of resident work hours on patient safety. Ann Intern Med. 2004;141(11):851–7.
42. Volpp KG, Rosen AK, Rosenbaum PR, Romano PS, Even-Shoshan O, Canamucio A, et al. Mortality among patients in VA hospitals in the first 2 years following ACGME resident duty hour reform. JAMA. 2007;298(9):984–92.
43. Volpp KG, Rosen AK, Rosenbaum PR, Romano PS, Itani KM, Bellini L, et al. Did duty hour reform lead to better outcomes among the highest risk patients? J Gen Intern Med. 2009;24(10):1149–55.
44. Volpp KG, Rosen AK, Rosenbaum PR, Romano PS, Even-Shoshan O, Wang Y, et al. Mortality among hospitalized Medicare beneficiaries in the first 2 years following ACGME resident duty hour reform. JAMA. 2007;298(9):975–83.
45. Silber JH, Rosenbaum PR, Rosen AK, Romano PS, Itani KM, Cen L, et al. Prolonged hospital stay and the resident duty hour rules of 2003. Med Care. 2009;47(12):1191–200.
46. Press MJ, Silber JH, Rosen AK, Romano PS, Itani KM, Zhu J, et al. The impact of resident duty hour reform on hospital readmission rates among Medicare beneficiaries. J Gen Intern Med. 2011;26(4):405–11.
47. The ACGME 2011 Duty Hour Standards [cited 2018 May 26]. Available from: https://www.acgme.org/Portals/0/PDFs/jgme-monograph[1].pdf.
48. Resident duty hours in the learning and working environment comparison of 2003 and 2011 standards [cited 2012 Feruary 28]. Available from: http://www.acgme.org/acWebsite/dutyHours/dh-ComparisonTable2003v2011.pdf.
49. ACGME Common Program Requirements 2017 [cited 2018 May 26]. Available from: http://www.acgme.org/Portals/0/PFAssets/ProgramRequirements/CPRs_2017-07-01.pdf.

50. AOA Basic Documents for Postdoctoral Trainings, BOT 7/2011 [accessed 2012 February 28]. No longer available: http://www.osteopathic.org/inside-aoa/Education/interns-residents/Documents/aoa-basic-document-for-postdoctoral-training.pdf.
51. The Basic Documents for Postdoctoral Training [cited 2018 May 26]. https://www.osteopathic.org/inside-aoa/accreditation/postdoctoral-training-approval/postdoctoral-training-standards/Documents/aoa-basic-document-for-postdoctoral-training.pdf.
52. Nuckols TK, Escarce JJ. Cost implications of ACGME's 2011 changes to resident duty hours and the training environment. J Gen Intern Med. 2012;27(2):241–9.
53. Gottlieb DJ, Parenti CM, Peterson CA, Lofgren RP. Effect of a change in house staff work schedule on resource utilization and patient care. Arch Intern Med. 1991;151(10):2065–70.
54. Kiernan M, Civetta J, Bartus C, Walsh S. 24 hours on-call and acute fatigue no longer worsen resident mood under the 80-hour work week regulations. Curr Surg. 2006;63(3):237–41.
55. Schenarts PJ, Anderson Schenarts KD, Rotondo MF. Myths and realities of the 80-hour work week. Curr Surg. 2006;63(4):269–74.
56. Arora V, Dunphy C, Chang VY, Ahmad F, Humphrey HJ, Meltzer D. The effects of on-duty napping on intern sleep time and fatigue. Ann Intern Med. 2006;144(11):792–8.
57. Richardson GS, Wyatt JK, Sullivan JP, Orav EJ, Ward AE, Wolf MA, et al. Objective assessment of sleep and alertness in medical house staff and the impact of protected time for sleep. Sleep. 1996;19(9):718–26.
58. Birrer R, Kozdemba D. Around the hospital in 80 hours. Resident work rules don't ease educational strain; are longer residencies an option? Healthc Leadersh Manag Rep. 2003;11(12):1–6.
59. Sugden C, Housden CR, Aggarwal R, Sahakian BJ, Darzi A. Effect of pharmacological enhancement on the cognitive and clinical psychomotor performance of sleep-deprived doctors: a randomized controlled trial. Ann Surg. 2011;255(2):222–7.
60. Czeisler CA. Wake-promoting therapeutic medications not an appropriate alternative to implementation of safer work schedules for resident physicians. Mayo Clin Proc. 2010;85(3):302–3. Author reply 3.
61. Curet MJ, McAdams TR. Improving resident work environment: evaluation of a novel cooperative program. Surgery. 2003;134(2):158–63.
62. Lockley SW, Barger LK, Ayas NT, Rothschild JM, Czeisler CA, Landrigan CP. Effects of health care provider work hours and sleep deprivation on safety and performance. Jt Comm J Qual Patient Saf. 2007;33(11 Suppl):7–18.
63. Clissold G, Smith P, Acutt B. The impact of unwaged domestic work on the duration and timing of sleep of female nurses working full-time on rotating 3-shift rosters. J Hum Ergol (Tokyo). 2001;30(1–2):345–9.
64. Hodgson LA. Why do we need sleep? Relating theory to nursing practice. J Adv Nurs. 1991;16(12):1503–10.
65. Schnelle JF, Ouslander JG, Simmons SF, Alessi CA, Gravel MD. The nighttime environment, incontinence care, and sleep disruption in nursing homes. J Am Geriatr Soc. 1993;41(9):910–4.
66. Gibson J, Grealish L. Relating palliative care principles to the promotion of undisturbed sleep in a hospice setting. Int J Palliat Nurs. 2001;7(3):140–5.
67. Tamburri LM, DiBrienza R, Zozula R, Redeker NS. Nocturnal care interactions with patients in critical care units. Am J Crit Care. 2004;13(2):102–12. Quiz 14-5.
68. Richardson A, Thompson A, Coghill E, Chambers I, Turnock C. Development and implementation of a noise reduction intervention programme: a pre- and postaudit of three hospital wards. J Clin Nurs. 2009;18(23):3316–24.
69. Fischer FM, Borges FN, Rotenberg L, Latorre Mdo R, Soares NS, Rosa PL, et al. Work ability of health care shift workers: what matters? Chronobiol Int. 2006;23(6):1165–79.
70. Ribeiro-Silva F, Rotenberg L, Soares RE, Pessanha J, Ferreira FL, Oliveira P, et al. Sleep on the job partially compensates for sleep loss in night-shift nurses. Chronobiol Int. 2006;23(6):1389–99.
71. Novak RD, Auvil-Novak SE. Focus group evaluation of night nurse shiftwork difficulties and coping strategies. Chronobiol Int. 1996;13(6):457–63.

72. Dean GE, Scott LD, Rogers AE. Infants at risk: when nurse fatigue jeopardizes quality care. Adv Neonatal Care. 2006;6(3):120–6.
73. Scott LD, Hwang WT, Rogers AE, Nysse T, Dean GE, Dinges DF. The relationship between nurse work schedules, sleep duration, and drowsy driving. Sleep. 2007;30(12):1801–7.
74. Barton J, Spelten ER, Smith LR, Totterdell PA, Folkard S. A classification of nursing and midwifery shift systems. Int J Nurs Stud. 1993;30(1):65–80.
75. Lindborg C, Davidhizar R. Is there a difference in nurse burnout on the day or night shift? Health Care Superv. 1993;11(3):47–52.
76. Pati D, Harvey TE Jr, Barach P. Relationships between exterior views and nurse stress: an exploratory examination. HERD. 2008;1(2):27–38.
77. Rogers AE. The effects of fatigue and sleepiness on nurse performance and patient safety. In: Hughes RG, editor. Patient safety and quality: an evidence-based handbook for nurses. Rockville: Agency for Healthcare Research and Quality (US); 2008. Chapter 40.
78. Marziale MH, Rozestraten RJ. Alternating shifts: mental fatigue in nurses. Rev Lat Am Enfermagem. 1995;3(1):59–78.
79. Matsumoto M, Kamata S, Naoe H, Mutoh F, Chiba S. Investigation of the actual conditions of hospital nurses working on three rotating shifts: questionnaire results of shift work schedules, feelings of sleep and fatigue, and depression. Seishin Shinkeigaku Zasshi. 1996;98(1):11–26.
80. Cooper EE. Pieces of the shortage puzzle: aging and shift work. Nurs Econ. 2003;21(2):75–9.
81. Muecke S. Effects of rotating night shifts: literature review. J Adv Nurs. 2005;50(4):433–9.
82. Seki Y, Yamazaki Y. Effects of working conditions on intravenous medication errors in a Japanese hospital. J Nurs Manag. 2006;14(2):128–39.
83. Lo SH, Lin LY, Hwang JS, Chang YY, Liau CS, Wang JD. Working the night shift causes increased vascular stress and delayed recovery in young women. Chronobiol Int. 2010;27(7):1454–68.
84. Pryde NA. Night nursing for trainees: living up to the image. Int Nurs Rev. 1987;34(3):80–3.
85. Shao MF, Chou YC, Yeh MY, Tzeng WC. Sleep quality and quality of life in female shift-working nurses. J Adv Nurs. 2010;66(7):1565–72.
86. Chen JG, Yeung TW. Hybrid expert-system approach to nurse scheduling. Comput Nurs. 1993;11(4):183–90.
87. Ruggiero JS. Health, work variables, and job satisfaction among nurses. J Nurs Adm. 2005;35(5):254–63.
88. Brooks I. The lights are bright? Debating the future of the permanent night shift. J Manag Med. 1997;11(2–3):58–70.
89. Gadbois C. Different job demands of nightshifts in hospitals. J Hum Ergol (Tokyo). 2001;30(1–2):295–300.
90. Desjardins F, Cardinal L, Belzile E, McCusker J. Reorganizing nursing work on surgical units: a time-and-motion study. Nurs Leadersh (Tor Ont). 2008;21(3):26–38.
91. Leigh JP, Tancredi D, Jerant A, Kravitz RL. Annual work hours across physician specialties. Arch Intern Med. 2011;171(13):1211–3.
92. Rothschild JM, Keohane CA, Rogers S, Gardner R, Lipsitz SR, Salzberg CA, et al. Risks of complications by attending physicians after performing nighttime procedures. JAMA. 2009;302(14):1565–72.
93. Hayter MA, Friedman Z, Katznelson R, Hanlon JG, Borges B, Naik VN. Effect of sleep deprivation on labour epidural catheter placement. Br J Anaesth. 2010;104(5):619–27.
94. Lindfors PM, Nurmi KE, Meretoja OA, Luukkonen RA, Viljanen AM, Leino TJ, et al. On-call stress among Finnish anaesthetists. Anaesthesia. 2006;61(9):856–66.
95. Smith-Coggins R, Rosekind MR, Buccino KR, Dinges DF, Moser RP. Rotating shift-work schedules: can we enhance physician adaptation to night shifts? Acad Emerg Med. 1997;4(10):951–61.
96. Di Bartolomeo S, Valent F, Marchetti R, Sbrojavacca R, Barbone F. Road traffic crashes, alcohol, meals, sleep and work hours: a case-crossover study at the emergency room of Udine, Italy. Ann Ig. 2010;22(5):401–18.

97. Nelson D. Prevention and treatment of sleep deprivation among emergency physicians. Pediatr Emerg Care. 2007;23(7):498–503. Quiz 4-5.
98. Institute of Medicine of the National Academies of Science Report. To err is human: building a safer health system. Washington, DC: National Academy Press; 2000.
99. Ama. Report 4 of the council on science and public health (A-12) light pollution: adverse health effects of nighttime lighting. 2012 June 12/2012 [cited 2018 May 26]. Available from: http://circadianlight.com/images/pdfs/newscience/American-Medical-Association-2012-Adverse-Health-Effects-of-Light-at-Night.pdf.
100. Harvey EJ. Staff surgeon competence. Can J Surg. 2011;54(1):4–6.
101. Owens JA, Veasey SC, Rosen RC. Physician, heal thyself: sleep, fatigue, and medical education. Sleep. 2001;24(5):493–5.

Chapter 14
Risk of Fatigue at Work

Zahra Banafsheh Alemohammad and Khosro Sadeghniiat-Haghighi

Fatigue could be determined as a depletion of cognitive recourses that prevents a person from performing work safely and effectively. It is a workplace hazard that affects the health and safety of both the employee and his or her colleagues. The term "fatigue" with a widespread usage in occupational medicine is a complex phenomenon definition of which is very difficult [1]. Other terms such as drowsiness and sleepiness that are often used instead of fatigue have different definitions. These are actually two different, although related, states. Sleepiness is the tendency to fall asleep, but fatigue is the body's response to deficits in subjective capacity. When physical and mental exertion exceeds current capacity, fatigue is represented by an inability to function at the desired level [2]. Workers with fatigue are more likely to experience job absenteeism than workers without fatigue [3].

Prevalence and Risk Factors of Fatigue at Work

The prevalence of fatigue is associated with various factors such as sex, age, marital, employment, and socioeconomic status [4, 5]. It is a common symptom with reported prevalence in the general population ranging from 7% to 45% [6]. In a recent study, the prevalence of fatigue was 28.9% between Chinese men aged 45 and older [5]. Fatigue is a common symptom to be consulted with general physicians (GPs) with reported prevalence of 25%. It was the main reason for consulting the GPs in 6.5% and a secondary reason in 19% [7].

Few studies reported the prevalence of fatigue in workers. In the United States, 31.0% of the male workers and 45.8% of the female workers (37.9% of all workers) reported to be fatigue at work that is associated with $101.0 billion per year in

Z. B. Alemohammad, MD · K. Sadeghniiat-Haghighi, MD (✉)
Occupational Sleep Research Center, Baharloo Hospital, Tehran University of Medical Sciences, Tehran, Iran

© Springer Science+Business Media, LLC, part of Springer Nature 2018
A. Sharafkhaneh, M. Hirshkowitz (eds.), *Fatigue Management*,
https://doi.org/10.1007/978-1-4939-8607-1_14

excess health-related lost productive time (LPT) costs to US employers. The majority of the LPT cost is due to reduced performance instead of work absenteeism [6]. At the survey among 162 short haul commercial pilots, 75% of respondents reported severe fatigue [8]. According to a review, the prevalence of fatigue in industries depending on the type of work and instruments used has been reported between 7 and 45% [1].

Several factors can contribute to development of fatigue in the workplace. According to the ACOEM Guidance Statement, fatigue risk factors in the workplace could be summarized into the following categories [9]:

1. Sleep deprivation
2. Circadian variability
3. Time awake
4. Health factors (sleep disorders, medications)
5. Environmental issues (light, noise)
6. Workload

Sleep deprivation is the most important cause of work-related and non-work-related fatigue [1]. Inadequate time for sleep could be the result of the long work hours, shift work, or working in a second job.

Working out of synchronized with the circadian rhythm or natural body clock is the second work-related risk factor of fatigue, which is the most prominent issue in the shift workers. The association between circadian polymorphisms and shift work indicated that genetic polymorphism of selected clock genes may affect the adaptation to the shift work [10].

Sleep disorders and medications may cause fatigue in workers. Sleep disorders cost employers 60 billion dollars in industrial accidents and lost productivity each year [11]. Insomnia, sleep apnea, restless legs syndrome, and narcolepsy are examples of the most prevalent sleep disorders, which should be considered to contribute to the risk of fatigue.

Workload is determined as the intensity of work demands including time on a task and complexity of the work. Physical load, environmental load, and mental load are the three aspects of the workload contributing to fatigue [1].

Biomathematical Models of Fatigue and Performance

Interaction between experimental observation and theorization can provide a broader spectrum of science in the field of biomathematical models [12]. Biomathematical fatigue modeling can incorporate sleep and performance science in fatigue risk management systems. Several fatigue models have been already developed that are fundamentally influenced by the two-process model (2 PM) of sleepiness and fatigue regulation [13]. In the Fatigue and Performance Modeling Workshop held in Seattle on June 2002, seven biomathematical models have been evaluated. Developers of these biomathematical models were invited to attend the

Workshop and complete a survey of the goals, capabilities, inputs, and outputs of their models. They concluded that the two-process model is the basic model of sleep regulation, all other models influenced by which, although they differed with regard to their goals, capabilities, and the input and output variables [13].

The two-process model has the most simplicity to predict subjective alertness [14]. The key processes in this model consist of a homeostatic process (S) and a circadian process (C).

The homeostatic process describes the decline of alertness with time awake and its recovery with time asleep. It is conceived as a simple reservoir in which alertness and performance capacity decreases either linearly or exponentially during wakefulness and increases exponentially during sleep that represents as the recuperation obtained from sleep. Regarding the homeostatic process, sleep is triggered when the sleep reservoir decreases below a certain threshold, and wakefulness is triggered when the sleep reservoir increases above a different threshold [15].

The circadian process describes the diurnal variation in alertness. The biological clock or endogenous circadian regulating system is located in the suprachiasmatic nuclei (SCN) of the hypothalamus [15]. Dr. Edgar et al. conducted an animal study on monkeys and suggested that the circadian system actively promotes wakefulness during the day more than sleep during the night [16]. There is interindividual variability in the free-running circadian rhythms in healthy adult humans [17] which are in part as a result of variability in genetic basis [18]. The most frequently measured appearance of this variability is morningness–eveningness typing or chronotype [19].

In chronic sleep restriction conditions, studies revealed slower rates of recovery than acute periods of total sleep deprivation resulted in change of the homeostatic process [20, 21]. Therefore, the two-process model has not been successful in predicting neurobehavioral performance observed under chronic sleep restriction conditions [15].

Regarding some of the limitations in two-process model, other biomathematical models were developed. Three-process model of alertness (homeostatic, circadian, and sleep inertia) has been extensively validated in many occupational settings [22] and has been extended with extra components [23].

Sleep inertia is a temporary period of reduced alertness and impaired performance in transition from sleep to wakefulness. It takes from a minute to over 2 h depending on prior sleep duration, circadian phase at awakening, and sleep stage at awakening [24]. Burke et al. conducted a study on the independent and interacting contributions of sleep inertia, sleep homeostatic, and circadian processes. Inhibitory control and selective visual attention are critical to guide and control other cognitive functions. They found that circadian rhythm affected the inhibitory control, while sleep inertia influenced on selective visual attention [25].

The magnitude of fatigue is also dependent of the nature of activities (work intensity and complexity) and time on task. These components are not considered in the basic three-process model.

The sleep, activity, fatigue, and task effectiveness (SAFTE) model predicted performance effectiveness. The system for aircrew fatigue evaluation (SAFE) model predicted the decline of alertness with time on task. SAFTE and SAFE models are developed for use in aviation, but still lack peer-reviewed validation [22]. The inter-active neurobehavioral model (INM), the circadian alertness simulator (CAS), and the fatigue audit interdyne (FAID) are the other models developed in the basis of three processes including homeostatic, circadian, and sleep inertia [22].

Fatigue models can provide information to ameliorate the health and well-being of employees and advance public safety. However, because of individual differences in responses to sleep loss and circadian rhythm, biomathematical models cannot provide information about a specific person [9]. The other limitation in the majority of these models is that they cannot cover some other modulators of fatigue such as work demand, time on task, and specific drugs (stimulants or hypnotics). Keeping in mind these limitations, for practitioners in occupational sleep medicine, fatigue and performance modeling as a developing science can guide the design of better work schedules to reduce performance errors and accidents. They can also predict the operational risk by extensions of fatigue modeling.

Fatigue Detection Techniques

Fatigue is a global concern with a complex definition which makes it difficult to be measured. There is no measuring unit or single instrument as a gold standard for fatigue measurement. Consequently, it is advantageous for practical reasons to find an alternative measurement approach, which will provide a good approximation for fatigue.

The most prominent consequence of fatigue in the workplace is deterioration of cognitive performance. Therefore, cognitive performance measurement could be utilized as an alternative measurement of fatigue [26–28]. Vigilant attention is one of the most reliable effects of fatigue [29] which is measured by the psychomotor vigilance test (PVT) [30]. PVT can assess the ability of the brain to sustain attention and respond quickly by measurements of repeated reaction times (RT) to visual or auditory stimuli [31].

In a 10 min PVT, random interstimulus interval is 2–10 s, and all responses are displayed in milliseconds. Its high sensitivity to both acute and chronic sleep restric-tion and its psychometric advantages over other neurobehavioral tests of fatigue have made the 10 min PVT as the most widely used measure of behavioral alertness [32]. A 10 min PVT has also been validated to screen for sleep apnea patients with higher risk of fatigue-related accidents [33]. It can also identify fatigue in clinical [34] and occupational settings [35].

The brief PVT (PVT-B) is a shorter-duration version of the PVT that only takes 3 min to perform. In a PVT-B, random interstimulus interval is 1–4 s. Like a 10 min PVT, it has a good sensitivity to total sleep deprivation and chronic sleep restriction [36]. PVT-B is brief enough to be accepted by the target population and to allow for repeated administration in occupational setting [31].

Adaptive-duration version of the PVT (PVT-A) is a modified PVT that stops sampling when enough information to classify PVT performance were provided by the test. Therefore, the duration of the PVT-A is variable in contrast to the fixed durations of the 10 min PVT and PVT-B. The mean test duration of the PVT-A is less than 6.5 min [37].

The Johns Drowsiness Scale (JDS) is a monitoring technology based on ocular measures like blink duration. Special glasses should be worn to measure JDS by infrared reflectance oculography. JDS has a sensitivity of 77–100% and a specificity of 85–83% in comparison with the gold standard. Therefore, it could be considered as an online indicator of drowsiness as well as changes in alertness and performance [38–40].

The percentage of eye closure (PERCLOS) is the proportion of time that the eyes are closed over a specified time interval. PERCLOS is another real-time monitoring technology and one of the most effective indicators of fatigue [41].

Heart rate variability (HRV), the variation in R-R intervals, is an indicator of autonomic nervous system function. HRV monitoring is sensitive to the effects of total sleep deprivation, and it potentially can be used to predict fatigue in workplace [42].

Besides the objective techniques mentioned above, there are several question-naires developed to measure fatigue in multiple dimensions; some of them are described below:

The Chalder Fatigue Questionnaire (CFQ) is an 11-item questionnaire with two domains of physical and mental fatigue. It was originally published in 1993 [43] and updated in 2010 [44].

The Fatigue Severity Scale (FSS), a nine-item self-report questionnaire, is the most commonly used fatigue-specific questionnaire [45] which was published in 1989 [46]. The FSS measures physical, social, and cognitive effects of fatigue.

The Piper Fatigue Scale (PFS) is a 40-item questionnaire with domains of behavioral, sensory, affective, and cognitive attributes of fatigue. It revised to the PFS-R including 22 questions [47].

The Multidimensional Assessment of Fatigue (MAF) is another revision of the PFS, including 16 questions and four domains of fatigue (severity, distress, interference in activities of daily living, and change during the previous week).

The Fatigue Associated with Depression Questionnaire (FAsD), a 13-item questionnaire, evaluates fatigue and its impact in patients with major depressive disorder. Each item is rated on a five-point scale in two domains: a six-item fatigue experience and a seven-item fatigue impact [48].

The Brief Fatigue Inventory (BFI), a nine-item questionnaire, was developed primarily for the rapid assessment of fatigue severity in cancer patients. The first three items evaluate the severity of fatigue. The following six items evaluate the grade to which fatigue has interfered with daily activities. Each item is rated on an 11-point scale from 0 to 10 for a time period of the past 24 h [49].

Future studies may facilitate developing more rapid and nonintrusive techniques to measure fatigue in the operational settings, as well as developing inexpensive instruments to measure sleep quality and quantity to conduct a personalized fatigue risk management program.

Fatigue Risk Management System

Health and well-being of the workers are key factors in safety and productivity in the workplace. Hazards may be existed in any form like physical, chemical, biological and psychosocial at workplace. A workplace, in which these hazards are well controlled, can enhance safety and productivity through worker health and well-being [9]. Fatigue is also a hazard that must be controlled in the same way as other hazards [50, 51]. More or less, everybody experiences some level of fatigue at work. However, excessive fatigue in which health and well-being of the workers are affected is an important condition that has to be managed. As fatigue recognized as an unsafe condition in the workplace, "fatigue risk management" could be defined as a comprehensive process for managing the actual fatigue risk to which an industry is exposed. In the context of safety management system (SMS), "fatigue risk management" can be developed to form a "fatigue risk management system (FRMS)" [9]. Occupational sleep physicians should implement a comprehensive FRMS, the requirements of which are a wide range of skills, backgrounds, and resources [9]. Safety risk management is one of the principal components of a SMS, in which the hazards are identified, the risks associated with those hazards are assessed, and appropriate ways to control the risk are determined.

According to the ACOEM Guidance Statement, a FRMS includes the following items:

1. Fatigue management policy
2. Fatigue risk management
3. Fatigue reporting system
4. Fatigue incident investigation
5. Fatigue management training and education
6. Sleep disorder management
7. Internal and external auditing of the FRMS

All items could be found in a SMS other than "sleep disorder management" that is unique to a FRMS [9]. Changes in sleep time because of the electric light, shift working, and other necessities of modern life have contained health and safety consequences. To mitigate these consequences, regulations have been passed to limit the working hours. Working-hour limits (hours-of-service rules) are the traditional approach to manage fatigue in the workplace [9]. However, alertness at work depends not only on working hours but also on a variety of other factors such as work intensity, work complexity, time of work relative to the circadian rhythm, and obtaining high-quality restorative sleep. Some environmental and administrative factors in the workplace can promote either alertness or fatigue [9]. Hours-of-service regulation is a single line of defense against fatigue-related error, incident, and accident that is blind to the human circadian rhythm and homeostatic drive for sleep. Therefore, many industries have decided to implement a comprehensive FRMS as an alternative to the hours-of-service approach. FRMS is a layered defense in depth that based on the evidence-based sleep science [51].

James Reason proposed the concept of "defenses in depth," the consequence of which was the Swiss cheese model (SCM). According to this model, an accident happens because of a series of defects. To prevent errors, incidents, and accidents, the most effective way is development of multiple layers of defenses like a traditional battlefield. These layers with multiple defects are as Swiss cheese slices with their many holes. A problem may pass through a hole in one layer, but in the next layer, the holes are in different places. Therefore, for an error to occur, the holes need to align in a process allowing a path through the system [52].

FRMS is a multilayer system in five levels of barriers to prevent fatigue-related accidents [53]:

- Level 1 is about providing adequate sleep opportunity. The critical question in this level is "Does a specific working time arrangements provide sufficient sleep opportunity for recovery and not have employees awake for too long?"
  There are a number of guidelines and matrix to ensure employees are provided with sufficient sleep opportunity within their schedule. This level has been addressed partially by the traditional approach (hours-of-service rules).
- Level 2 is about actual sleep obtained. At this level, the organization must confirm that adequate sleep is obtained for employees to indicate fitness for duty. The critical question that employees must ask themselves in this level is "Have I not been awake for too long to be safe for myself and my colleagues and have I had enough sleep recently?"
  Fitness for work can be determined by three simple calculations:

  1. Prior sleep in the last 24 h
  2. Prior sleep in the last 48 h
  3. Length of wakefulness from awakening to end of the work

- Level 3 is about detecting behavioral symptoms of fatigue. The critical question that employees must ask themselves in this level is "Am I expressing symptoms of fatigue? Is my colleague expressing symptoms of fatigue?"
  Because of individual differences in the sleep requirement, sleep disorders, and some idiopathic factors, two prior levels do not guarantee the safety and performance in the workplace. Tools to detect fatigue symptoms could be as simple as a subjective fatigue scale to more complex physiological monitoring. The results of these tools provide the controlling mechanism from a short rest to being relieved of duty for a period.
- Level 4 is about assessment and control of fatigue-related errors. The critical question in this level is "Was fatigue a contributing factor of any near miss or error?" Performance testing, field observations, and documented errors are some of the tools used in level four of FRMS.

- Level 5 is about assessment and control of fatigue-related incidents. The critical question in this level is "Was fatigue a contributing factor of any incident?" The systematic incident investigation with respect to the possibility of fatigue as a contributing factor should be involved in this level [1].

Any organization could monitor the effectiveness of level one to three by level four and five. The aim of these levels is to present the facts to be mentioned when FRMS is not sufficient to prevent fatigue resulting in an error or incident.

FRMS and Safety-Sensitive Works

A safety-sensitive work is one in which impaired performance could result in significant risk of damage affecting the health or safety of the employee, coworkers, customers, the public, property, or the environment [54]. The list of occupations designated as high risk or safety sensitive is too long. Whether a job can be considered as safety sensitive must be mentioned within the context of each industry and workplace.

Safety-sensitive works such as the health care, transportation, and energy industries have to be especially considered in FRMS. FRMS is also important for any organization in which individuals have extended work hours or shift work. Many safety-sensitive professions such as firefighters, police officers, and health-care providers are also shift workers with challenging schedules. Therefore, comprehensive FRMS need to be developed in these safety-sensitive professions to minimize the adverse effects associated with shift work [55].

Fatigue risk in safety-sensitive works could be managed not only by optimizing work schedules using biomathematical models but also with technologies for detecting sleepiness and fatigue [31]. According to the scientific evidence, new FRMS regulations are established to help ensure public safety across safety-sensitive positions, except for health-care workers [56]. The first organizations examined the FRMS were the road transport and aviation regulatory in Australia and New Zealand. Although the concept of FRMS has been limited to the transportation industries, there are some examples of the spread of FRMS through other activities like mining and pipeline [9]. In addition to the transportation industry, there has been a good amount of research into the effects of extended shifts and night shifts in health-care workers [56–58]. However, FRMS has not been completely implemented in this setting. Therefore, occupational and environmental medicine physicians have an important role to play in development of a fatigue risk management system. They can manage the opportunities to increase productivity, safety, and health via a comprehensive FRMS. In addition, occupational sleep medicine physicians can provide a more extensive occupational consultation by screen and treat the sleep disorders that are responsible for sleepiness and fatigue [9].

References

1. Sadeghniiat-Haghighi K, Yazdi Z. Fatigue management in the workplace. Ind Psychiatry J. 2015;24(1):12–7.
2. Akerstedt T, Wright KP Jr. Sleep loss and fatigue in shift work and shift work disorder. Sleep Med Clin. 2009;4(2):257–71.
3. Janssen N, Kant IJ, Swaen GM, Janssen PP, Schroer CA. Fatigue as a predictor of sickness absence: results from the Maastricht cohort study on fatigue at work. Occup Environ Med. 2003;60(Suppl 1):i71–6.
4. Lim SM, Chia SE. The prevalence of fatigue and associated health and safety risk factors among taxi drivers in Singapore. Singap Med J. 2015;56(2):92–7.
5. Lin WQ, Jing MJ, Tang J, Wang JJ, Zhang HS, Yuan LX, et al. Factors associated with fatigue among men aged 45 and older: a cross-sectional study. Int J Environ Res Public Health. 2015;12(9):10897–909.
6. Ricci JA, Chee E, Lorandeau AL, Berger J. Fatigue in the U.S. workforce: prevalence and implications for lost productive work time. J Occup Environ Med. 2007;49(1):1–10.
7. Cullen W, Kearney Y, Bury G. Prevalence of fatigue in general practice. Ir J Med Sci. 2002;171(1):10–2.
8. Jackson CA, Earl L. Prevalence of fatigue among commercial pilots. Occup Med (Lond). 2006;56(4):263–8.
9. Lerman SE, Eskin E, Flower DJ, George EC, Gerson B, Hartenbaum N, et al. Fatigue risk management in the workplace. J Occup Environ Med. 2012;54(2):231–58.
10. Reszka E, Peplonska B, Wieczorek E, Sobala W, Bukowska A, Gromadzinska J, et al. Rotating night shift work and polymorphism of genes important for the regulation of circadian rhythm. Scand J Work Environ Health. 2013;39(2):178–86.
11. Hillman DR, Murphy AS, Pezzullo L. The economic cost of sleep disorders. Sleep. 2006;29(3):299–305.
12. Van Dongen HP. Predicting sleep/wake behavior for model-based fatigue risk management. Sleep. 2010;33(2):144–5.
13. Mallis MM, Mejdal S, Nguyen TT, Dinges DF. Summary of the key features of seven bio-mathematical models of human fatigue and performance. Aviat Space Environ Med. 2004;75(3 Suppl):A4–14.
14. Borbely AA. Refining sleep homeostasis in the two-process model. J Sleep Res. 2009;18(1):1–2.
15. Goel N, Basner M, Rao H, Dinges DF. Circadian rhythms, sleep deprivation, and human performance. Prog Mol Biol Transl Sci. 2013;119:155–90.
16. Edgar DM, Dement WC, Fuller CA. Effect of SCN lesions on sleep in squirrel monkeys: evidence for opponent processes in sleep-wake regulation. J Neurosci. 1993;13(3):1065–79.
17. Smith MR, Burgess HJ, Fogg LF, Eastman CI. Racial differences in the human endogenous circadian period. PLoS One. 2009;4(6):e6014.
18. Barclay NL, Gregory AM. Quantitative genetic research on sleep: a review of normal sleep, sleep disturbances and associated emotional, behavioural, and health-related difficulties. Sleep Med Rev. 2013;17(1):29–40.
19. Baehr EK, Revelle W, Eastman CI. Individual differences in the phase and amplitude of the human circadian temperature rhythm: with an emphasis on morningness-eveningness. J Sleep Res. 2000;9(2):117–27.
20. Van Dongen HP, Maislin G, Mullington JM, Dinges DF. The cumulative cost of additional wakefulness: dose-response effects on neurobehavioral functions and sleep physiology from chronic sleep restriction and total sleep deprivation. Sleep. 2003;26(2):117–26.
21. Johnson ML, Belenky G, Redmond DP, Thorne DR, Williams JD, Hursh SR, et al. Modulating the homeostatic process to predict performance during chronic sleep restriction. Aviat Space Environ Med. 2004;75(3 Suppl):A141–6.

22. Ingre M, Van Leeuwen W, Klemets T, Ullvetter C, Hough S, Kecklund G, et al. Validating and extending the three process model of alertness in airline operations. PLoS One. 2014;9(10):e108679.
23. Akerstedt T, Ingre M, Kecklund G, Folkard S, Axelsson J. Accounting for partial sleep deprivation and cumulative sleepiness in the three-process model of alertness regulation. Chronobiol Int. 2008;25(2):309–19.
24. Santhi N, Groeger JA, Archer SN, Gimenez M, Schlangen LJ, Dijk DJ. Morning sleep inertia in alertness and performance: effect of cognitive domain and white light conditions. PLoS One. 2013;8(11):e79688.
25. Burke TM, Scheer FA, Ronda JM, Czeisler CA, Wright KP Jr. Sleep inertia, sleep homeostatic and circadian influences on higher-order cognitive functions. J Sleep Res. 2015;24(4):364–71.
26. Goel N, Rao H, Durmer JS, Dinges DF. Neurocognitive consequences of sleep deprivation. Semin Neurol. 2009;29(4):320–39.
27. Banks S, Dinges DF. Behavioral and physiological consequences of sleep restriction. J Clin Sleep Med. 2007;3(5):519–28.
28. Van Dongen HP, Vitellaro KM, Dinges DF. Individual differences in adult human sleep and wakefulness: leitmotif for a research agenda. Sleep. 2005;28(4):479–96.
29. Lim J, Dinges DF. A meta-analysis of the impact of short-term sleep deprivation on cognitive variables. Psychol Bull. 2010;136(3):375–89.
30. Lim J, Dinges DF. Sleep deprivation and vigilant attention. Ann N Y Acad Sci. 2008;1129:305–22.
31. Abe T, Mollicone D, Basner M, Dinges DF. Sleepiness and safety: where biology needs technology. Sleep Biol Rhythms. 2014;12(2):74–84.
32. Basner M, Dinges DF. Maximizing sensitivity of the psychomotor vigilance test (PVT) to sleep loss. Sleep. 2011;34(5):581–91.
33. Zhang C, Varvarigou V, Parks PD, Gautam S, Bueno AV, Malhotra A, et al. Psychomotor vigilance testing of professional drivers in the occupational health clinic: a potential objective screen for daytime sleepiness. J Occup Environ Med. 2012;54(3):296–302.
34. Sunwoo BY, Jackson N, Maislin G, Gurubhagavatula I, George CF, Pack AI. Reliability of a single objective measure in assessing sleepiness. Sleep. 2012;35(1):149–58.
35. Gander P, Millar M, Webster C, Merry A. Sleep loss and performance of anaesthesia trainees and specialists. Chronobiol Int. 2008;25(6):1077–91.
36. Basner M, Mollicone D, Dinges DF. Validity and sensitivity of a brief psychomotor vigilance test (PVT-B) to total and partial sleep deprivation. Acta Astronaut. 2011;69(11–12):949–59.
37. Basner M, Dinges DF. An adaptive-duration version of the PVT accurately tracks changes in psychomotor vigilance induced by sleep restriction. Sleep. 2012;35(2):193–202.
38. Wilkinson VE, Jackson ML, Westlake J, Stevens B, Barnes M, Swann P, et al. The accuracy of eyelid movement parameters for drowsiness detection. J Clin Sleep Med. 2013;9(12):1315–24.
39. Ftouni S, Rahman SA, Crowley KE, Anderson C, Rajaratnam SM, Lockley SW. Temporal dynamics of ocular indicators of sleepiness across sleep restriction. J Biol Rhythm. 2013;28(6):412–24.
40. Anderson C, Chang AM, Sullivan JP, Ronda JM, Czeisler CA. Assessment of drowsiness based on ocular parameters detected by infrared reflectance oculography. J Clin Sleep Med. 2013;9(9):907–20, 20A–20B.
41. Abe T, Nonomura T, Komada Y, Asaoka S, Sasai T, Ueno A, et al. Detecting deteriorated vigilance using percentage of eyelid closure time during behavioral maintenance of wakefulness tests. Int J Psychophysiol. 2011;82(3):269–74.
42. Chua EC, Tan WQ, Yeo SC, Lau P, Lee I, Mien IH, et al. Heart rate variability can be used to estimate sleepiness-related decrements in psychomotor vigilance during total sleep deprivation. Sleep. 2012;35(3):325–34.
43. Chalder T, Berelowitz G, Pawlikowska T, Watts L, Wessely S, Wright D, et al. Development of a fatigue scale. J Psychosom Res. 1993;37(2):147–53.

44. Cella M, Chalder T. Measuring fatigue in clinical and community settings. J Psychosom Res. 2010;69(1):17–22.
45. Hjollund NH, Andersen JH, Bech P. Assessment of fatigue in chronic disease: a bibliographic study of fatigue measurement scales. Health Qual Life Outcomes. 2007;5:12.
46. Krupp LB, LaRocca NG, Muir-Nash J, Steinberg AD. The fatigue severity scale. Application to patients with multiple sclerosis and systemic lupus erythematosus. Arch Neurol. 1989;46(10):1121–3.
47. Piper BF, Dibble SL, Dodd MJ, Weiss MC, Slaughter RE, Paul SM. The revised piper fatigue scale: psychometric evaluation in women with breast cancer. Oncol Nurs Forum. 1998;25(4):677–84.
48. Matza LS, Murray LT, Phillips GA, Konechnik TJ, Dennehy EB, Bush EN, et al. Qualitative research on fatigue associated with depression: content validity of the fatigue associated with depression questionnaire (FAsD-V2). Patient. 2015;8(5):433–43.
49. Mendoza TR, Wang XS, Cleeland CS, Morrissey M, Johnson BA, Wendt JK, et al. The rapid assessment of fatigue severity in cancer patients: use of the brief fatigue inventory. Cancer. 1999;85(5):1186–96.
50. Arlinghaus A, Lombardi DA, Courtney TK, Christiani DC, Folkard S, Perry MJ. The effect of rest breaks on time to injury – a study on work-related ladder-fall injuries in the United States. Scand J Work Environ Health. 2012;38(6):560–7.
51. Dawson D, McCulloch K. Managing fatigue: it's about sleep. Sleep Med Rev. 2005;9(5):365–80.
52. Reason J. Human error: models and management. BMJ. 2000;320(7237):768–70.
53. Dawson D, Chapman J, Thomas MJ. Fatigue-proofing: a new approach to reducing fatigue-related risk using the principles of error management. Sleep Med Rev. 2012;16(2):167–75.
54. Martin S. Determining fitness to work at safety-sensitive jobs. BCMJ. 2010;52(1):48–9.
55. Barger LK, Lockley SW, Rajaratnam SM, Landrigan CP. Neurobehavioral, health, and safety consequences associated with shift work in safety-sensitive professions. Curr Neurol Neurosci Rep. 2009;9(2):155–64.
56. Blum AB, Shea S, Czeisler CA, Landrigan CP, Leape L. Implementing the 2009 Institute of Medicine recommendations on resident physician work hours, supervision, and safety. Nat Sci Sleep. 2011;3:47–85.
57. Olson EJ, Drage LA, Auger RR. Sleep deprivation, physician performance, and patient safety. Chest. 2009;136(5):1389–96.
58. Czeisler CA. Medical and genetic differences in the adverse impact of sleep loss on performance: ethical considerations for the medical profession. Trans Am Clin Climatol Assoc. 2009;120:249–85.

Chapter 15
Fatigue Management

Max Hirshkowitz and Amir Sharafkhaneh

Understanding Fatigue

Definition and Characteristics

Fatigue is both a sensation (i.e., a feeling) and a factor underlying behavioral impairment. Fatigue takes various forms, including but not limited to muscle fatigue, physical fatigue, and mental fatigue. A person afflicted with fatigue generally feels a lack of energy and/or motivation. The sensation is somewhat different from drowsiness which is the desire to sleep; however, fatigue and drowsiness often occur together. Medically, fatigue is a non-specific symptom (like stress) and has a multitude of potential causes. We typically operationalize fatigue in terms of performance failure. We characterize and assess human fatigue with metrics such as slowing in the speed of responding, failure to respond (lapsing), overall performance decrement, performance errors, and fatigue-related near misses or actual accidents. Time on task represents a key parameter in fatigue assessment. The latency from the beginning of a task until performance degradation helps index fatigue severity. By analogy, in engineering, material fatigue arises when something is repeatedly

M. Hirshkowitz, PhD
Division of Public Mental Health and Population Sciences, School of Medicine, Stanford University, Stanford, CA, USA

Department of Medicine, Baylor College of Medicine, Houston, TX, USA

A. Sharafkhaneh, MD, PhD (✉)
Department of Medicine, Baylor College of Medicine, Houston, TX, USA

Medical Care Line, Michael E. DeBakey VA Medical Center, Houston, TX, USA
e-mail: amirs@bcm.edu

© Springer Science+Business Media, LLC, part of Springer Nature 2018
A. Sharafkhaneh, M. Hirshkowitz (eds.), *Fatigue Management*,
https://doi.org/10.1007/978-1-4939-8607-1_15

Table 15.1 Factors contributing to fatigue

Behavioral stressors	Physical and psychological factors	Medical and neurological factors
Poor workplace design	Lack of exercise	Acute illness
Sleep deprivation	Vitamin or mineral deficiency	Anemia
Poor sleep	Boredom	Myasthenia gravis
Work volume too high	Pregnancy	Electrolyte imbalance
Work deadlines	Bereavement	Stroke
Work is high stress in nature	Depression	Poisoning
Workplace hostility	Anxiety disorder	Drug and/or medical treatments
	Relationship problems	Thyroid disease
	Personal worries	Low testosterone

subjected to stressors eventually weakening the material to the point that it ultimately fails. This perspective can assist our understanding of human fatigue in as much as stressors reduce stamina and impair performance more rapidly. Because drowsiness is a major source of stress and shares some common attributes with fatigue, sleepiness-related accidents are generally classified as fatigue-related.

Contributors to Fatigue

Many factors can contribute to fatigue, including medical, neurological, and psychiatric conditions (discussed elsewhere in this volume). Table 15.1 lists stressors, psychological factors, and medical factors associated with fatigue, sleepiness, or both. More generally, any physiological or psychological stressors can also contribute to feelings of fatigue, performance failure, or both. For example, chronic pain can sap endurance and depressed mood can provoke inattention. However, for human performance, for individuals who are otherwise healthy, sleep quantity, quality, and timing are critical. A strong desire to sleep can be described as drowsiness—which is a different sensation from feeling fatigued. Nonetheless, when considering fatigue in terms of performance failure, drowsiness is often the underpinning of "fatigue-related accidents." If a person has a medical, neurological, or psychiatric condition, these can synergize with drowsiness and further contribute to fatigue. Furthermore, such medical, neurological, and psychiatric conditions can also contribute to fatigue by reducing sleep quality and/or quantity.

Fatigue Model and Performance Failure

In this section we will focus on a model of fatigue and how it contributes to performance failure. We begin by considering the normal processes governing alertness and drowsiness and how such modify the risk of failure during a sustained

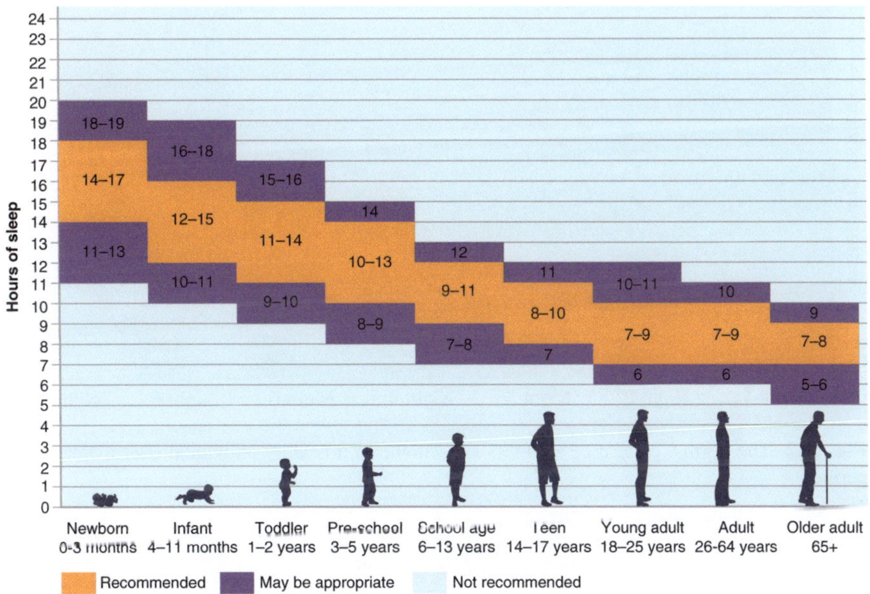

Fig. 15.1 National Sleep Foundation recommended sleep time durations across lifespan

operation. The two principle factors involved with sleep and alertness are referred to as [1] homeostatic and [2] circadian.

In its broadest sense, homeostasis is the process by which an organism attempts to maintain a certain internal balance. Sleep is one of the basic physiological drives needed for survival (along with eating and fluid intake). Sleep plays a crucial role in growth, removing toxins created by biological chemical reactions (*garbage collection*), and resupplying the body and brain with substances needed to sustain life (*material resupply*). Homeostatic levels of alertness and drowsiness vary as a function of the duration of prior sleep and the subsequent time spent awake. According to the National Sleep Foundation expert panel consensus, a working-age adult requires between 7 and 9 h of sleep nightly (see Fig. 15.1). In general, the homeostatic pressure to sleep increases as the period of wakefulness is prolonged. There is, however, a midafternoon dip in alertness, thought to be the basis for "siesta" in some cultures.

By contrast, the circadian process is the approximately (circa) 24-h daily (dias) oscillation in alertness. As diurnal animals, humans evolved to have alertness during daylight hours and sleep during darkness. The circadian rhythm in alertness helps maintain wakefulness to offset the homeostatic drive that increases over the course of a day. When the circadian wakefulness declines during darkness, the homeostatic drive to sleep asserts itself, and sleepiness ensues. Current research indicates the "off switch" for the circadian factor is controlled by the release of melatonin from the pineal gland.

Figure 15.2 illustrates the normal pattern of alertness and fatigue in a healthy, well-rested individual over the course of a week-long period. The figure shows the

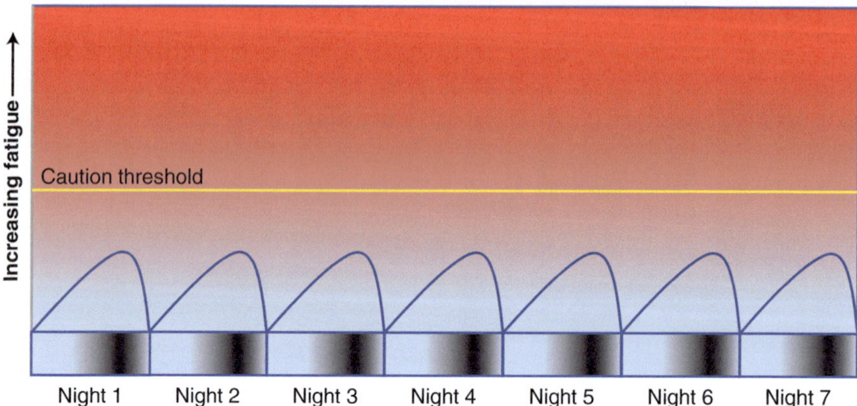

Fig. 15.2 The normal pattern of alertness and fatigue in a healthy individual over a week-long period

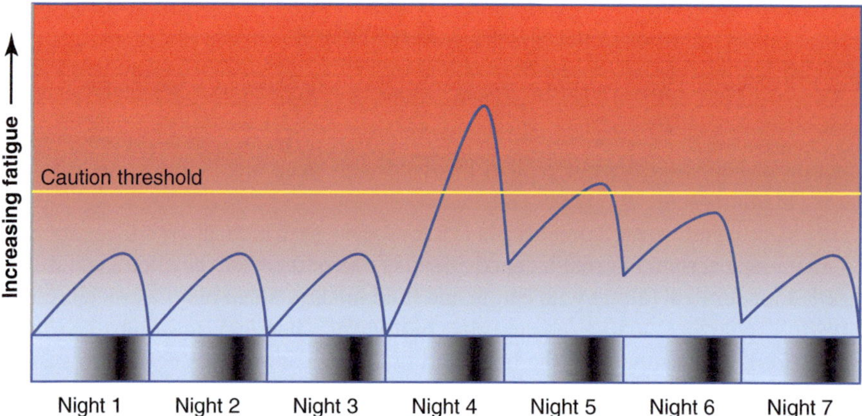

Fig. 15.3 The expected pattern of fatigue before, during, and after a night of total or severe sleep deprivation

varying degree of fatigue as the week progresses. The caution threshold indicates a point at which there is an increasing risk for performance failure. The caution threshold height can vary somewhat between individuals; however, every person has a limit. Although the actual limit is usually unknown, one should err on the side of caution. The daytime-nighttime cycle is shown at the bottom of each curve for general reference. It can be seen in the illustration that a healthy, well-rested, night-sleeping individual should remain well under the caution threshold throughout the week.

Figure 15.3 illustrates the expected pattern of fatigue provoked by a night of total or severe sleep deprivation. The graph shows the fatigue level in relationship to the caution threshold. In this illustration, the individual underwent severe sleep deprivation on night 4. Note that some spontaneous recovery occurred largely as a function of circadian factors; however, alertness did not recover sufficiently. Furthermore, as evening approached on the subsequent day, the individual was already at or approaching the caution threshold. Furthermore, recovery required several days before it reached baseline levels. Although there is some degree of individual differences between the effects of sleep loss on performance, this model provides guidance. Exceeding the caution threshold must be considered within the context of the activity performed and that activity's potential danger to self and others. A fatigued commercial airline pilot poses greater hazard than an office worker. Fatigue management has long been an issue in the transportation industry. It is not known exactly how much sleep deprivation creates an unacceptable risk to drive a vehicle, and there is currently no legal *per se* accepted for use as a surrogate. In 2016, the National Sleep Foundation conducted an expert panel review of drowsy driving and arrived at the consensus that less than 2 h of sleep in the past 24 h renders a person at too high a risk to drive, under any circumstances. This is a conservative estimate and *does not* mean that 2.5 h of sleep is enough. Some research indicates that 4 h may represent a better threshold; however, experts could not reach consensus on a 3- or 4-h minimum. What the recommendation means is that driving after less than 2 h of sleep is solidly agreed as completely inappropriate. It is hoped that subsequent research will focus on this marker and provide empirical evidence on which the recommendations can be revisited and updated.

A more insidious and widespread problem involves the increasing risk provoked by several days of partial sleep restriction. Chronic sleep deprivation is very common. Workers seeking to increase income will forgo sleep and work more hours per week. Culturally, many people proudly brag about how sleep deprived they are as evidence of their toughness and their willingness to work hard. Understaffed business contributes to the problem by needing and offering overtime pay incentives, especially at certain times of the year. In the final analysis, chronic sleep deprivation leads to poor health, lower productivity, and impaired quality of life. If you resided in a city that did not have services to perform *garbage collection* and *material resupply*, it would become unpleasant to live there pretty quickly. Figure 15.4 illus-

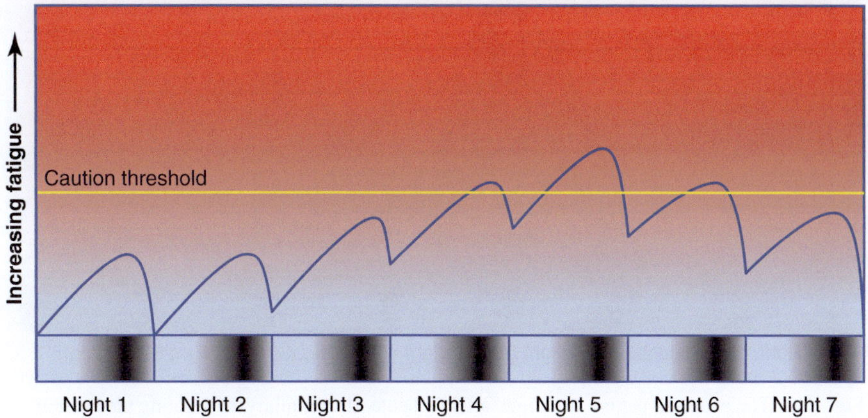

Fig. 15.4 The expected pattern of fatigue after three nights of partial sleep deprivation

trates the fatigue pattern associated with three successive nights of partial sleep deprivation. Partial sleep deprivation is considered when an individual gets less than the recommended sleep durations. The NSF recommendation is that young adults and adults should get 7–9 h of sleep nightly; however, 6 h may be appropriate for some individuals. Therefore, as a general rule, a person getting less than 6 h of sleep per night has some degree of sleep deprivation. Sleeping only 4 or 5 h per night for most people is clearly restricted sleep and unfortunately quite common.

The figure shows the expected fatigue pattern before, during, and after three successive nights of restricted sleep (nights 2, 3, and 4). It should be noted that a cascading increase in fatigue occurs and reaches the caution threshold after the second night. Fatigue exceeds the caution threshold most of the day after the third night. It also continues to exceed the caution threshold even after a recovery night of normal sleep duration.

Figure 15.5 illustrates the acute effects of a sedating medication, a 1–2-day illness or minor injury on the fatigue profile across a week. In this figure the acute problem begins on the second day and is shown as superimposed over the typical pattern. This assumes little sleep deprivation. If the acute problem also causes difficulty sleeping, one would expect the pattern to resemble Fig. 15.4 with the darkened area in this graphic superimposed.

Figure 15.6 illustrates the weekly fatigue profile expected when an individual has a stable chronic illness that characteristically is associated with fatigue (e.g., congestive heart failure). When the condition is well controlled and stable, the person may tire easily and feel fatigued for a good portion of each day; however, the level of fatigue varies. When it is at its peak each day, it may well exceed the caution threshold. The overall mean height of the blue area in the figure is proportional to the illness' severity, while the peaks and troughs vary with sleep homeostatic and circadian factors. Such individuals must avoid sleep

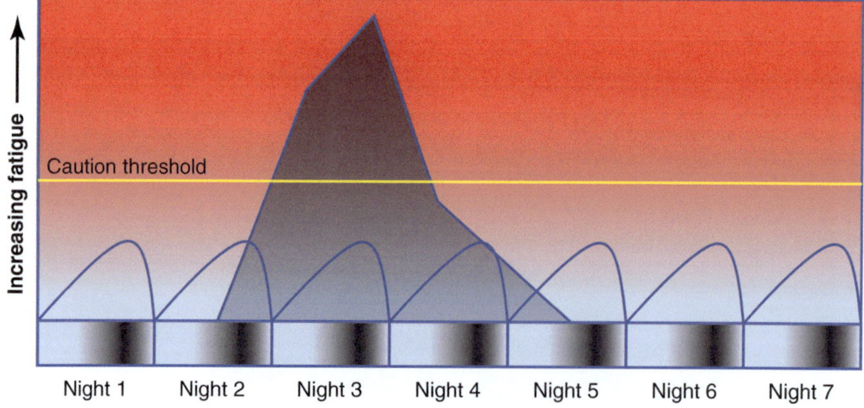

Fig. 15.5 The expected pattern of fatigue after an acute illness, injury, or sedating medication

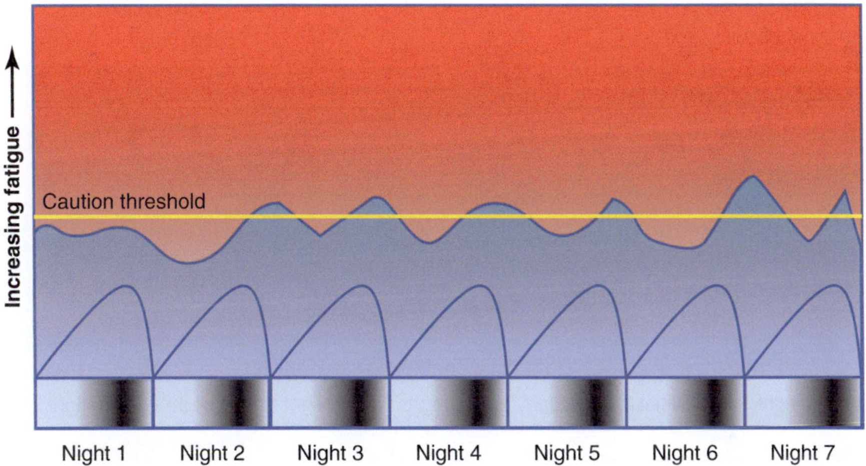

Fig. 15.6 Expected pattern of fatigue in an individual with a stable chronic medical, neurological, or psychiatric condition without sleep deprivation

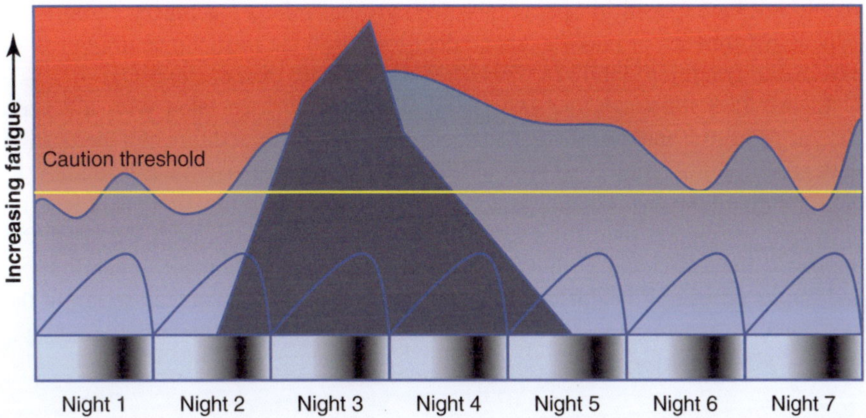

Fig. 15.7 Expected pattern of fatigue in an individual who begins taking a sedating medication or who has an acute exacerbation in an otherwise stable chronic medical, neurological, or psychiatric condition

deprivation because it will quickly and chronically impair them to a potentially hazardous extent.

Figure 15.7 illustrates the fatigue profile when an individual with a stable chronic condition has an acute exacerbation or acutely takes a sedating medication. Individuals with stable chronic conditions are often close to the caution threshold under the best of circumstances (as shown in Fig. 15.6); however, the addition of another stressor not only pushes them into an around-the-clock danger zone, the

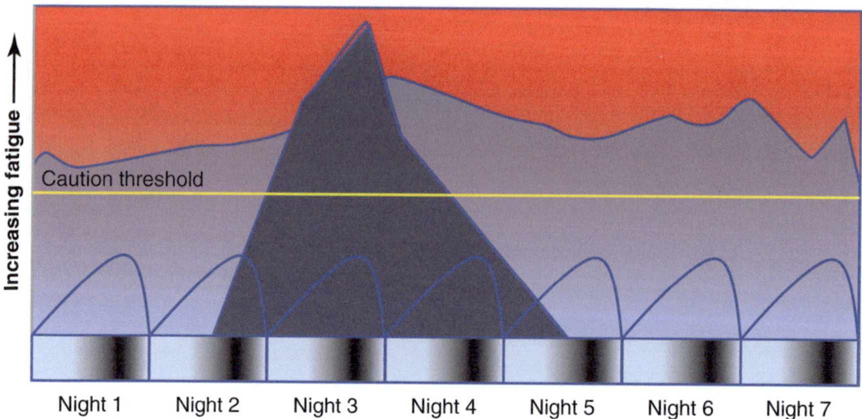

Fig. 15.8 Expected pattern of fatigue in an individual who begins taking a sedating medication or who has an acute exacerbation in an otherwise severe chronic medical, neurological, or psychiatric condition

person recovers more slowly and remains at risk much longer. Such individuals should not be engaged in operating potentially hazardous machinery, monitoring critical instruments, or making crucial decisions until the medical, neurological, or psychiatric condition stabilizes. This often takes longer than one expects.

Figure 15.8 illustrates the expected fatigue profile associated with a severe, chronic condition and the effect of an acute exacerbation or addition of a medication with sedating properties. This type of individual remains above the caution threshold throughout the day. The fatigue is so severe and unremitting; there is little or no perceived oscillation over the course of each day. In general, until the condition improves, the individual is mostly disabled. Aggressive treatment, rehabilitation, and improved overall health would be needed before this person can return to the workforce.

Reducing Performance Failure Risk

Overview

Occupational medicine often focuses on fatigue in the workplace and operational setting. By using our understanding of medicine, human factors, performance, and sleep, the goals include improving health, safety, and productivity. To improve fatigue risk management, occupational medicine's role is to screen for relevant illnesses, determine risk, recommend therapeutic interventions, and monitor outcomes. Risk reduction, however, does not end with an individual improving overall health and getting more sleep. In addition to reducing risk by taking action at a personal level, risk can be reduced by medical intervention and at an organizational level.

Martin Moore-Ede discusses the evolution of risk management system and proposes five key areas that help defend against fatigue-related incidents with particular attention to 24/7 operations [1]. Some of these defenses go beyond what an individual does to maintain good sleep and general health. Nonetheless, each area has goals, actions, and tracking metrics. The defenses include the following:

- Providing sufficient staffing (organization's responsibility)
- Providing sufficient opportunity for workers to attain adequate sleep (organization's responsibility)
- Attaining sufficient sleep (individual's responsibility)
- Providing proper and sufficient workplace environment (organization's responsibility)
- Workers having sufficient alertness (both individual's and organization's responsibility)

Reducing Risk at an Individual's Level (Good Sleep Health Practice)

Regardless of the specific underlying chemical, anatomical, physiological, and neurological roles sleep plays, sleep remains the foundation for good health. Without adequate, good quality sleep, even the best exercise and nutrition regimens will not confer good health and a desirable quality of life. The building blocks for good sleep health are:

- Adequate sleep quantity
- Good sleep quality
- Proper timing of sleep
- Absence of sleep disorders

Unfortunately, many individuals have an erroneous belief that sleep is unimportant. This belief is often supported by a negative cultural attitude toward sleep. Individuals may brag about their sleep deprivation as though it was a badge of honor. Such individuals may do so right up to the time they fall asleep while driving, have a brief alertness lapse and cause an accident, or make a sleep-related error in judgment. Being sleep deprived is nothing to be proud of… in fact it is a testimony to foolishness. Nonetheless, our capital intensive society places work and productivity above health and quality of life. It is a false value because productivity begins to decline as sleep deprivation increases.

Practices conducive to maintaining health and preventing disease fall under the heading "hygiene." As in other areas of self-care, good sleep hygiene helps prevent problems. Sleep hygiene guidelines do not work for all individuals in all situations.

However, in the absence of special circumstances, sleep hygiene recommendations represent positive health practices. The following rules are a series of Do's and Don'ts for good sleep.

Do
- Maintain regular hours of bedtime and arising.
- Maintain a regular exercise schedule.
- If you are hungry, have a *light* snack before bedtime.
- Give yourself an approximately an hour to wind down before going to bed.
- If you are preoccupied or worried about something at bedtime, write it down and deal with it in the morning.
- Keep bedroom cool.
- Keep the bedroom dark.
- Keep the bedroom quiet.

Don't
- Nap frequently and for long durations.
- Watch the clock at night to determine your insomnia's severity.
- Watch television in bed when you can't sleep.
- Eat a heavy meal before bedtime to help you sleep.
- Drink coffee in the afternoon and evening.
- Smoke a cigarette if you can't sleep.
- Use alcohol to help you sleep.
- Read in bed when you can't sleep.
- Eat in bed.
- Exercise in bed.

In principle, maintaining bedtime and arising time regularity and keeping the bedroom dark help strengthen the circadian sleep-wake cycle. Alleviating hunger, keeping the bedroom cool, winding down before bedtime, and strategies to reduce bedtime worry are all attempts to decrease autonomic (sympathetic nervous system) activation that provokes wakefulness and interferes with sleep. Similarly, ingesting caffeine and nicotine can interfere with sleep directly by stimulation. Alcohol may initially help sleep induction, but as its sedating effects wear off after several hours, withdrawal begins, and sleep becomes disturbed.

Maintaining a regular exercise program falls under the rubric of keeping fit which promotes deep, good quality sleep. Under normal circumstances, avoiding long daytime naps helps strengthen the homeostatic drive to sleep. However, if an individual has recently been sleep deprived or has reduced sleep quality (e.g., due to illness), napping may ultimately help sleep-loss recovery. Initially, after awakening from long naps, it may leave a person groggy, but overall it should reduce sleep debt. Realize that sleep hygiene recommendations were originally devised to help individuals prone to or suffering from insomnia. In such cases, avoiding napping may reduce the risk of difficulty initiating and/or maintaining sleep at night.

Finally, some of these sleep hygiene recommendations serve to strengthen the association between the bed, the bedroom, and sleep. Sleep, as an autonomic function, is amenable to conditioning. In the classic experimental demonstration of respondent conditioning, Ivan Pavlov would ring a bell and then feed his dog. Dogs salivate when they are presented with food, and by ringing a bell before feeding, the dog began associating the bell with food and ultimately would salivate when hearing the bell. By analogy, sleep is an autonomic function for which the bed acts as a cue. Therefore, to strengthen the association, it is generally recommended to use the bed primarily for sleep. Thus, eating, reading, watching television, and/or exercising in bed can be counterproductive, especially for individuals who suffer from insomnia.

Reducing Risk at a Medical Level (Optimizing Overall Health)

Fatigue is a frequent complaint in various chronic medical conditions. The fatigue could be due to the primary medical condition, associated comorbid conditions, and/or due to side effects of prescribed medications. The first approach to uncover the contributing factors to fatigue is a thorough history and physical exam. In majority of cases, the workup pinpoints potential culprits and can guide the diagnostic workup. In general, causes of fatigue due to medical illnesses can be divided into disease-specific and disease-non-specific mechanisms. Disease-non-specific mechanisms include reduced physical activity, muscle wasting, disturbed sleep, change in metabolism and nutrition, depression, and anxiety. Disease specific may work through above mechanisms or alternative mechanisms to cause fatigue. For example in a patient with advanced heart failure, reduced muscle perfusion due to low cardiac output combined with the inflammatory environment and low physical activity will result in worsening fatigue and puts the patient in a vicious cycle. In contrast, in myasthenia gravis, the involvement of neuromuscular junction results in direct power reduction at the muscle level and causes fatigue.

One other important aspect of fatigue in chronic medical conditions is the episodes of acute exacerbations. During an episode of an exacerbation, the primary involved organ fails more and results in further worsening of fatigue on top of baseline fatigue. Sometimes it may take months before the patient returns back to baseline disease status and, thus, the baseline fatigue severity.

Tables 15.2, 15.3, and 15.4 show chronic medical, neurological, or psychiatric conditions (respectively) that are associated with fatigue and recommended management strategies. In many cases, appropriate treatment and management will reduce fatigue. Interventions reviewed in this table focus on the conditions while they are stable. During acute exacerbations, the treatments are disease specific and will improve fatigue as the recovery pursues.

Table 15.5 shows various sleep disorders and therapies that may reduce fatigue. As in the prior table, the focus is on stable disease condition and interventions that can improve fatigue in that state.

Medical therapy plays an important and pivotal role in managing chronic conditions. As such, polypharmacy is very prevalent. Many of these medications may

Table 15.2 Management and expected outcomes for medical conditions contributing to fatigue

Health condition	Treatment	Prognosis
Chronic respiratory conditions like COPD [2, 3]	• Non-pharmacotherapy: pulmonary rehabilitation • Pharmacotherapy: bronchodilator, inhaled corticosteroid • Management of comorbid conditions including cardiovascular, psychiatric, and sleep disorders	Improvement in quality of life and fatigue and reduction of COPD exacerbation and hospital admission
Heart failure [4]	• Non-pharmacotherapy: cardiac rehabilitation • Pharmacotherapy: ACEI/ARB, beta-blocker, diuretics • Management of comorbid conditions including respiratory, psychiatric, and sleep disorders	Improvement in quality of life and fatigue and reduction of CHF exacerbation and hospital admission
Malignancy [5]	• Supportive care including optimizing nutritional status, preventing weight loss, and balancing rest and physical activity • Treatment of comorbid conditions like anemia and sleep disorders • Physical rehabilitation program • Self-management intervention (e.g., energy conservation and activity management) • Pharmacotherapy: antidepressant, stimulants	Improvement in quality of life and fatigue
Chronic renal disease [6]	• Management of comorbid condition like anemia (iron and erythropoiesis-stimulating agents) • Management of depression (antidepressant and CBT) • Management of mineral and bone disease (vitamin D) • Management of wasting/malnutrition • Renal replacement therapy • Management of insomnia	Improvement in disease-specific symptoms, quality of life, and fatigue
Endocrine diseases [6]	• Management of hypo- and hyperthyroidism • Management of comorbid medical condition • Management of diabetes • Management of parathyroid disorder • Management of adrenal insufficiency • Management of hypercortisolism	Improvement in disease-specific symptoms, quality of life, and fatigue
Hematological diseases [6]	• Treatment of anemia by correcting various etiology • Transfusion of RBC if indicated	Improvement in disease-specific symptoms, quality of life, and fatigue
Infectious diseases	• Infection-specific treatment of various chronic infections including HIV, HCV, and TB • Improved nutrition • Physical rehabilitation in patients with debilitation	Improvement in disease-specific symptoms, quality of life, and fatigue

Table 15.3 Management and expected outcomes for neurological conditions contributing to fatigue

Health condition	Treatment	Prognosis
Multiple sclerosis [7]	• Management of comorbid depression and sleep disorders • Stimulant like modafinil, amantadine, pemoline	Improvements in quality of life and fatigue
Parkinson's disease [8]	• Pharmacotherapy: doxepin, rasagiline, methylphenidate • Physical rehabilitation • Management of comorbid conditions including sleep and psychiatric disorders	Improvements in quality of life and fatigue
Myasthenia gravis (MG) [9]	• Pharmacotherapy of MG • Comprehensive rehabilitation program • Implement self-care techniques • Management of comorbid conditions including sleep disorders and depression	Improvements in quality of life and fatigue
ALS [10–12]	• Multidisciplinary fatigue management program including energy-saving methods, psychosocial support, and physiotherapeutic interventions • Management of comorbid depression, anemia, and hypothyroidism • Management of sleep disorders and hypoventilation • Stimulant like modafinil	Improvements in quality of life and fatigue
Post stroke [13]	• Physical rehabilitation • Mindfulness-based stress reduction • Management of associated comorbid sleep and psychiatric conditions • Vitamin replacement (limited data)	Improvements in quality of life and fatigue
Traumatic brain injury [14–17]	• Neurorehabilitation • Cognitive behavioral therapy • Management of sleep disorders • Stimulants like methylphenidate • Others: piracetam; bright blue light	Improvement in disease-specific symptoms, quality of life, and fatigue

Table 15.4 Management and expected outcomes for neurological conditions contributing to fatigue

Health condition	Treatment	Prognosis
Mood disorders [18]	Pharmacotherapy of mood disorders Management of comorbid medical and sleep disorders Cognitive behavioral therapy Graded exercise Stimulants including modafinil, armodafinil Other medications: selegiline, amantadine, pergolide	Improvement in disease-specific symptoms, quality of life, and fatigue
Anxiety disorders [18]	Pharmacotherapy of anxiety disorder Management of comorbid medical and sleep disorders Cognitive behavioral therapy Graded exercise	Improvement in disease-specific symptoms, quality of life, and fatigue
Bereavement [19, 20]	Pharmacotherapy of comorbid mood disorders Management of sleep disorders Bereavement supportive services	Improvement in disease-specific symptoms, quality of life, and fatigue

Table 15.5 Sleep disorders, treatments, and expected outcome on fatigue

Disorder	Treatment	Maintenance	Fatigue prognosis
Obstructive sleep apnea	• Effective therapy of OSA • Weight loss	Continue therapy of OSA	On rare occasion, residual sleepiness and fatigue may benefit from stimulant therapy
Central sleep apnea	• Optimization of underlying medical condition/medication causing CSA • Oxygen therapy • Trial positive airway pressure therapy	Continue the therapy	Residual fatigue due to underlying disease may continue
Restless legs syndrome	• Iron replacement if needed • Dopamine agonist	May need drug holiday if RLS symptoms return	Well controlled as long as the patient is compliant with therapy
Obesity hyperventilation syndrome	• PAP therapy • Weight loss under medical supervision • Physical rehabilitation	Continue the therapy	Well controlled as long as the patient is compliant with therapy
Narcolepsy	• Narcolepsy indicated pharmacotherapeutic and non-pharmacotherapeutic intervention	Continue the therapy	Well controlled as long as the patient is compliant with therapy

induce or worsen fatigue. Table 15.6 provides a list of medications that may cause fatigue and alternatively strategies that may improve fatigue.

Reducing Risk at an Organizational Level

Overview

In the previous sections of this chapter, we discussed reducing performance failure at the level of the individual. Except for active military service and rare circumstances where workers reside in isolated environments (e.g., aboard ships at sea), the employer or organization has little control or direct knowledge of an individual's sleep and health habits. Organizations have even less control concerning the development and course of acute and/or chronic medical conditions. Such factors are pretty much left to the individual, and he or she is expected to act in good faith and be fit for duty when arriving at the workplace. Nonetheless, there are important factors directly under the employer or organization's control, and these factors are equally, if not more, crucial for fatigue management.

Table 15.6 Medications associated with fatigue

Medication	Indication	Alternates	Notes[a]
Beta-blockers	Hypertension/heart failure	Refer to a cardiologist for therapy adjustment decisions	A systematic review did not support the notion that beta-blocker may cause fatigue
Antihypertensive medications including diuretics	Hypertension/heart failure	Refer to a cardiologist for therapy adjustment decisions; correct any electrolyte imbalance; give drug holidays	Dose -related; mainly during acute phase; chronic during treatment
Sedative/hypnotics Benzodiazepines/BZRA/ doxepin/antihistamine/ OTC medications with antihistamine	Sedative/hypnotic	CBT or reduce the dose	Dose-related; mainly during acute phase; chronic during treatment
Antiepileptics	Seizure control	Refer to a neurologist for therapy adjustment decisions	Chronic during treatment
Antipsychotics	Various psychiatric conditions	Refer to a psychiatrist for therapy adjustment decisions	Chronic during treatment
Chemotherapeutic agents	Anticancer	See cancer-related fatigue treatment recommendations	Dose-related; during acute phase and chronic during treatment
Interferons	Immunomodulatory therapy	Treat other comorbid conditions that cause fatigue Stop the medication	Mainly during acute phase

[a]Notes: Dose-related, mainly during acute phase, chronic during treatment, during withdrawal, half-life, or duration of effect

The workplace staffing and operational environment established the basic fabric and infrastructure underlying conditions contributing to or reducing fatigue-related problems and incidents. These factors are continuous and controllable. Instilling a well-considered culture of safety by example and actions goes a long way for managing fatigue-related risks. The American College of Occupational and Environmental Medicine (ACOEM) Presidential Task Force on Fatigue Risk Management Report published in the *Journal of Occupational and Environmental Medicine* (Volume 54: 2012; 231–258) provides an excellent summary of workplace fatigue risk factor management. The report describes Fatigue Risk Management Systems (FRMS), explains their necessity, and describes the key elements. The report highlights that hours-of-service regulations, while a worthwhile first step for organizational level control, fail to address many other factors associated with fatigue. Other parts of the system potentially include any or all of the following components:

- A formal written policy for fatigue management
- Training for workers and managers about dangers of fatigue and strategies to reduce such risks
- Training for workers about sleep health, sleep disorders, and other medical conditions associated with fatigue
- An ongoing effort to identify and mitigate risk and hazardous situations facing workers
- Metrics to identify possible markers related to fatigue
- A fatigue reporting system
- A fatigue-related incident investigation protocol
- Internal and external review of the system to audit outcomes and identify areas for improvement

The responsibility for several specific elements concerning fatigue management fall to the organization, these include:

- Staffing
- Scheduling
- Work environment
- Training

Staffing

Understaffing is arguably the greatest factor contributing to an organization's contribution to workplace fatigue, incidents, and accidents. A balance between workload and staffing is critical for safety. Workloads, however, can change, and organizations are compelled to maintain operations. Some workload changes are predictable and should be planned for and managed, as much as possible. Predictable workload changes include vacation scheduling, work-time training sessions, seasonal variations (e.g., package delivery during holiday season), and business at different times of day or days of the week. Unpredictable workload changes are more difficult to manage. These include worker illnesses; natural (e.g., weather) and/or man-made disasters (e.g., fires), especially for first responders and essential service providers; and sudden unexpected increases in demand or worker resignations (with long intervals to interview, vet, rehire, train, and qualify replacements). Attempting to fill the gaps with existing staff invariably leads to extending shifts and increased overtime. In the short term, such strategies may allow continued operation; however, running at "flank speed" in a long haul is inefficient, unsustainable, and hazardous. Continued reliance on double and triple shifts may also inadvertently lead to hours-of-service violations, inadequate between-shift downtime opportunity for sleep, absenteeism, and employee burnout.

Scheduling

In addition to classic 8-h day shifts, many organizations routinely used alternative schedules. 24/7 operations require night shift coverage. Alternative shifts include 12-h shifts, rotating shifts sequenced in a clockwise manner, rotating shifts sequenced in a counterclockwise manner, and variable shifts. Rotating shifts can rotate at different speeds, that is, fast rotation and slow rotation. Work shifts can affect worker's health, productivity, absenteeism, and fatigue-related problems.

Shift Time of Day

Night shifts are difficult for some workers. Our internal biological clocks respond to light, and under normal circumstances we are alert during the day and sleepy at night. It is easier to function in synch with our biological clocks than out of synch. Furthermore, it is more difficult for some individuals and easier for others. Night shift workers may chronically suffer from sleep problems even when they have the opportunity for sleep. We have seen many individuals who come home after an overnight shift and sleep soundly for about 4–5 h and then awaken. They may struggle thereafter and ultimately not be able to attain the 7–8 h of sleep needed to be fully refreshed. Thus, they begin the next night work shift already sleep deprived. This pattern may continue in a downward cycle until fatigue, illness, and/or absenteeism results. There is no simple solution to this problem; however, several strategies may help mitigate some of the difficulty. Strategies include:

- Training workers to optimize their sleep by following the Do's and Don'ts of sleep hygiene previously outlined
- Building into the workplace good ergonomic designs to reduce stress, using human factor engineering to improve alertness, and implementing systems to monitor, detect, warn, and correct potential problems (especially when accidents pose a serious hazard)
- Arranging the schedule to provide additional time between night shifts to recover from sleep loss and allowing specifically timed prophylactic napping during breaks and providing an appropriate environment for that activity

Another approach to 24/7 operational environments is to use rotating shifts. It is unclear whether this strategy is beneficial for fatigue-related issues; however, it succeeds in sharing the burden of night shift work for employees who dislike working overnight. It can be argued that some individuals can adapt to night shift work when it is consistent and becomes their norm. They develop strategies to remain shifted, protect their sleep time, and arrange their sleep environment to optimize daytime sleeping. Having to continually change their routine can be disruptive. Nonetheless, rotating shifts are used, and the rotation can proceed quickly (several days) or more slowly (weeks or months).

Shifts can rotate clockwise (progressing from morning work to afternoon work to night work) or counterclockwise (morning → night → evening). While little data support an advantage clockwise vs. counterclockwise rotation, for most individuals it is easier to make clockwise transitions. Also, clockwise rotation allows more opportunity for extra sleep at the end of one shift until the beginning of the next. Some workers use that opportunity to get some extra sleep before they essentially have to stay awake later when the next shift begins. Some research indicates that one can "stock up in advance" on sleep and subsequently maintain performance longer.

Shift Length

According to research studies, increased fatigue and fatigue-related errors occur when shifts exceed 8 h. Mathematically, the longer a fixed daily shift lasts, the less time there is between shifts. This diminished time affords less opportunity to obtain enough sleep. Consecutive 12-h shifts, with 8 h reserved for bedtime, provide an individual only 4 h to accomplish all of their activities of daily living (personal hygiene, food preparation, eating, socializing, cleaning, shopping, etc.). Consecutive double shifts (16 h) leave zero additional time; consequently, for essential activities (e.g., personal hygiene and eating) an individual must steal time from bedtime. Unexpected shift extensions can create even more chaos in a person's schedule. For example, having to pull a double shift because of another worker's absence not only upsets whatever routine the individual had for after work but also allows zero time for activities other than essentials and bedtime.

When understaffing is present, sometimes shifts are extended either at the beginning, at the end, or both. The net result is less time, and therefore less sleep opportunity, between shifts. Shift extensions can occur in a predictable (with a day or longer notice) or in an unpredictable (with only a few hours' notice). Unpredictable shift extensions, in general, are more stressful and as such contribute to performance failure above and beyond the stress of sleep deprivation. The bottom line is that the individual winds up working more than 8 of the 24 h, and this increases the risk of lapses, errors, and accidents.

Work Environment

When considering the work environment, the term ergonomics immediately comes into mind. Among other things, ergonomics focuses on designing workstations, display systems, and furniture to fit the user and the task rather than forcing the worker to adapt to operating equipment. Ergonomics has its roots in what was in the past called industrial psychology and human factor engineering. Improving comfort, ease of operation, and designing controls to help safeguard against errors reduces stress and increases productivity. For example, putting the discard command key next to the save file key on your computer would be poor ergonomic design. Stress reduction goes part of the way toward reduce fatigue and relieving musculoskeletal discomfort and disorders. For those readers with an interest in ergonomics, we strongly recommend accessing, reading, and downloading the materials posted in the following link on the National Institute for Occupational Safety and Health website: www.cdc.gov/niosh/docs/97-117/pdfs/97-117.pdf. However, an optimally designed ergonomic system, no matter how good it is, will not improve performance on a watch-keeping task if the operator falls asleep. For this reason, break times for nutrition, rest, and possibly even napping are now also considered as part of workplace ergonomic design.

Environmental sounds, for example, music, conversation, and noise, have been shown to positively affect alertness. Although noise is usually attenuated below conversational levels, some research reveals that it can improve task performance in special circumstances on certain tasks. Music has been studied more widely and appears to have a positive influence on reducing fatigue (assuming it is stimulating and not a lullaby). Conversation (i.e., spoken words) that interests the worker can improve alertness and performance as long as it is not distracting. Most drivers find talk radio can be a partially effective countermeasure for sleepiness.

Temperature and humidity in relationship to comfort can increase or reduce stress. Laboratory studies vary in their results depending on type of work being performed. Overall, warm temperatures and high humidity reduce alertness. Cognitive and vigilance task performances decline at temperatures above 82–83 degrees Fahrenheit (°F). By contrast, cold temperatures can temporarily relieve drowsiness. Motorists driving at night will often set the vehicle's air conditioning to a lower temperature in attempts to counteract fatigue. However, lowering temperature will not have a sustained effect, and the sleep is the only fully effective countermeasure for sleepiness. Environmental temperature, to optimally reduce it as acting as a stressor, should be within the comfort zone. Comfort zone varies between individuals, but 68 °F is approximately the low end for most people. According to the 1992 Health, Safety, and Welfare Regulations, 60.8 °F is the lowest recommended environmental temperature for workplaces that do not involve heavy physical activity.

Bright workplace lighting turns out to be possibly a double-edged sword. Brightly lit workplaces, particularly on the night shift, improve safety and performance. Light itself acts as a stimulant. However, sustained bright light in nighttime work environments is associated with increased health risks, presumably through neuroendocrine mechanisms. Melatonin and cortisol are suppressed by bright light. Additionally, bright light can activate autonomic nervous system mechanisms and may increase heart rate, respiration, and blood pressure. While it is difficult to disentangle nighttime light exposure from other night shift stressors (and consequences of those stressors), night shift workers have increased the risk for cancer, heart disease, hypertension, hyperglycemia, and obesity. Recent work in this area indicates neuroendocrine suppression can be mitigated by blocking the light in the blue part of the visual spectrum between the wavelengths of 460 and 480nm.

Table 15.7 Fatigue management training elements

Element	General topic	Specific and additional topics
1	Benefits of being well rested	• The hazards of fatigue
2	Adverse consequences of chronic sleep deprivation and fatigue	• Effect on physical health • Effect on mental health • Effect on relationships • Effect on life satisfaction
3	Getting adequate sleep or at least optimize it	• How much sleep is needed? • When is the best time to sleep? • What is sleep quality? • How to improve sleep?
4	Info about health in general	• Diet, exercise, and sleep are the building blocks of good health • Sleep is the foundation • Stressors and general health
5	Info about sleep and sleep disorders	• Insomnia • Sleep apnea • Shift work sleep disorder • Sleep-related movement disorders
6	Recognizing fatigue in self and others	• Difficulty concentrating • Response slowing • Performance lapses • Automatic behaviors and perseveration • Irritability • Distractibility • Eyelid drooping and eye closure • Memory lapses • Disorganized thinking • Nodding
7	Coping strategies in the workplace	• Regulating caffeine intake • Timing caffeine intake • Benefit of stretching and exercise • Benefits of social interaction
8	Coping strategies outside workplace	• Awareness • Recognition and controlling reactions • Protecting sleep time and sleep environment • Importance of planning • Avoiding pitfalls and hazards

Training

Training for both workers and managers is a critical element of any fatigue management program. The organization must embrace the importance of sleep and develop a culture that rewards good behaviors. Too often, organizations pay lip service to such issues but encourage counterproductive behaviors. A curriculum should include the topics shown on Table 15.7. The first two elements are crucial and must be convincing. Real-life examples should be provided so individuals can identify with the issues being discussed.

After enumerating and exemplifying specifics of the first two elements, the goal is to define and help employees attain the third element – getting adequate sleep.

This endeavor should be amplified by information in the fourth and fifth elements about health and illness.

The final three elements serve to educate workers about recognizing inadequate sleep in themselves and others, coping with inadequate sleep when it does occur and providing knowledge about how fatigue globally impacts their lives beyond the work environment. Being aware of sleep deprivation and fatigue on mood, anxiety, relationships, social interactions, and overall quality of life is the first step toward making changes and being able to cope with life's continual challenges.

Monitoring and Improvement

In addition to training workers and managers to recognize fatigue in themselves and others, indicator monitoring can alert organizations of potential and growing risks (see Table 15.8). These same indicators are helpful after-the-fact to determine the role of

Table 15.8 Fatigue management metrics

Metric	Specifics and notes
Scheduling (planned shifts and actual work)	• Weekly and monthly scheduled shift duration—mean, lowest, highest, percent of workforce greater than 8, 12, and 16 h (or plot a distribution) • Weekly and monthly actual hours worked—mean, lowest, highest, percent of workforce greater than 8, 12, and 16 h (or plot a distribution) • Weekly and monthly discrepancies between scheduled shift and actual hours worked—mean, lowest, highest, percent of workforce with greater than 25, 50, 75, and 100% discrepancy (or plot a distribution) • Weekly and monthly time between actual shift end and next beginning tabulated separately including days off and not including days off in between—mean, lowest, highest • Weekly and monthly number of consecutive days working—mean, lowest, highest, percent of workforce greater than 5, 7, 10, 14 (or plot a distribution
Overtime work	• Weekly and monthly overtime—mean, lowest, highest, percent of workforce greater than 4, 6, and 8 h (or plot a distribution) • Weekly and monthly number of hours' notice before overtime began—mean, lowest, highest, percent of workforce given less than 2, 12, or 24 h' notice (or plot a distribution) • Also look at how overtime is arranged… pre-shift, post-shift, on days off, using double/triple shifts, etc. • Look for outliers because overtime is seldom evenly distributed
Trend lines	• Calculate across longer periods than a week or month to find variations, and look for predictable patterns
Problem analysis for: • Absenteeism • Errors • Incidents • Accidents	• Correlated against other metrics above • Also useful for fact finding and root cause analysis findings of post hoc investigation
Productivity	• Variable depending on particular organization, workplace, and industry goals

fatigue in root cause analysis of incidents and accidents. Most of the metrics address issues surrounding staffing and scheduling. Some metrics examine central tendencies (means or averages), some examine ranges, and others provide information about distribution from normal. Differentials between shift scheduling and actual work time can be very informative along with metrics concerning overtime. How overtime or additional shifts are scheduled rounds out the staffing-scheduling approach. Specific trend lines and correlations can then be calculated. The metrics can also be correlated with adverse circumstances (absenteeism, incidents, errors, and accidents). Finally, productivity can be designated an outcome and also correlated against this assortment of measures.

In special cases where work is very hazardous (e.g., military) or public safety is critically important (e.g., commercial air travel), future fatigue management systems may include:

- Continuous monitoring of operation using equipment-specific characteristics to determine fatigue (e.g., reaction times or lapsing) during operation
- Electronic and/or video fatigue monitoring of observable (e.g., eye closures) when equipment is being monitored, operated, or driven
- Electronic and/or physiological monitoring of signs of fatigue (e.g., brain wave activity) when equipment is being monitored, operated, or driven
- Sleep-wake cycle monitoring using wearable technologies or GPS location around the clock or between shifts

Appendix Materials

Sleep Screening Questionnaire

This is a questionnaire developed at our sleep center to provide general information about an individual's sleep habits, common symptoms, and overall level of sleepiness (with a modified Epworth Sleepiness Scale). Problems identified by this questionnaire should be followed up with further interview.

Sleep Problems Checklist

This is a questionnaire developed at our sleep center to provide general information about sleep problems that can be useful for identifying specific sleep disorders. Items affirmed on the questionnaire should be followed up with further interview.

Stop-Bang Questionnaire

This is a questionnaire developed to identify obstructive sleep apnea. It has good sensitivity and specificity when administered to clinical populations and essentially tabulates risk factors for the disease.

Medical Questionnaire

This is a questionnaire developed at our sleep center to provide general information about health problems commonly related to or comorbid with sleep disorders. Items affirmed on the questionnaire should be followed up with further interview. It also queries about hospitalizations and family history.

Table 15.9 Fatigue management diagram

Evaluation of a patient referred for fatigue

- Comprehensive interview to determine the following
    a. Define patient's complaint in their own word
    b. Determine to what extent fatigue has affected the patient's life and work
    c. Review of system to determine other complaints with other body systems
    d. Obtain information on quality, quantity and sleep related symptoms
    e. Obtain information about job and work schedule and work related stressors
    f. Past medical & surgical history to determine potential contributing comorbid conditions.
    g. History of any alcohol and recreational drug use
    h. Obtain information on medication use
- Detail physical exam with special focus on neurological, cardiovascular, respiratory and musculoskeletal systems

- Create list of potential causes for fatigue
- Diagnostic tests to determine causes of fatigue according to findings from the history and physical exam: Comprehensive metabolic panel, complete blood count, echocardiography, pulmonary function test, sleep study including PSG and MSLT, actigraphy, sleep diary, urine toxicology screen
- Ask for work place environment and work schedule
- Provide safety instruction about work and driving safety as it relates to fatigue and excessive sleepiness.

Individualized recommendation

- Provide safety instruction about work and driving safety as it relates to fatigue and excessive sleepiness.
- Provide general instruction to improve sleep, diet, and regular exercise
- Make referral if any major organ problems
- Provide work related schedule improvements to reduce work related fatigue
- Plans for followup as needed

Follow up

- Interview to evaluate to what degree the recommendations are implemented and to what degree fatigue has improved
- Plan for further recommendations according to medical orders

Summary

Fatigue is a common presentation that affects quality of life and performance. It may stem from various medical, psychiatric, neurological, or recreational drug-related conditions. In addition, it can be caused by workload and sleep deprivation. Thus, workup of fatigue should include detail evaluation of various contributing factors. Table 15.9 shows a simple flowchart that can be used for this purpose. After identifying causes and contributing factors for fatigue, implementation of therapeutic intervention includes disease-specific therapies and general health and lifestyle modification including improvement in work environment.

References

1. Moore-Ede M. Evolution of fatigue risk management systems: the "Tipping Point" of employee fatigue mitigation. Circadian® White Papers. Available at: www.circadian.com/pages/157_white_papers.cfm.2009/. Accessed July 2016.
2. Lacasse Y, Goldstein R, Lasserson TJ, Martin S. Pulmonary rehabilitation for chronic obstructive pulmonary disease. Cochrane Database Syst Rev. 2006;4:CD003793.
3. Celli BR, MacNee W. Standards for the diagnosis and treatment of patients with COPD: a summary of the ATS/ERS position paper. Eur Respir J. 2004;23:932–46.
4. Yancy CW, Jessup M, Bozkurt B, Butler J, Casey DE Jr, Drazner MH, Fonarow GC, Geraci SA, Horwich T, Januzzi JL, et al. 2013 ACCF/AHA guideline for the management of heart failure: a report of the American College of Cardiology Foundation/American Heart Association Task Force on Practice Guidelines. J Am Coll Cardiol. 2013;62:e147–239.
5. Balachandran D, Faiz S, Bashoura l, Manzullo E. Cancer-related fatigue and sleep disorders. Sleep Med Clin. 2013;8:229–34.
6. Majid H, Shabbir-Moosajee M, Nadeem S. Fatigue in other medical disorders. Sleep Med Clin. 2013;8:241–53.
7. Rammohan KW, Rosenberg JH, Lynn DJ, Blumenfeld AM, Pollak CP, Nagaraja HN. Efficacy and safety of modafinil (Provigil) for the treatment of fatigue in multiple sclerosis: a two centre phase 2 study. J Neurol Neurosurg Psychiatry. 2002;72:179–83.
8. Elbers RG, Verhoef J, van Wegen EE, Berendse HW, Kwakkel G. Interventions for fatigue in Parkinson's disease. Cochrane Database Syst Rev. 2015;10:CD010925.
9. Blissitt PA. Clinical practice guideline series update. J Neurosci Nurs. 2013;45:317.
10. Kos D, Duportail M, D'hooghe M, Nagels G, Kerckhofs E. Multidisciplinary fatigue management programme in multiple sclerosis: a randomized clinical trial. Mult Scler. 2007;13:996–1003.
11. Rabkin JG, Gordon PH, McElhiney M, Rabkin R, Chew S, Mitsumoto H. Modafinil treatment of fatigue in patients with ALS: a placebo-controlled study. Muscle Nerve. 2009;39:297–303.
12. Carter GT, Weiss MD, Lou JS, Jensen MP, Abresch RT, Martin TK, Hecht TW, Han JJ, Weydt P, Kraft GH. Modafinil to treat fatigue in amyotrophic lateral sclerosis: an open label pilot study. Am J Hosp Palliat Care. 2005;22:55–9.
13. Wu S, Kutlubaev MA, Chun HY, Cowey E, Pollock A, Macleod MR, Dennis M, Keane E, Sharpe M, Mead GE. Interventions for post-stroke fatigue. Cochrane Database Syst Rev. 2015;7:CD007030.
14. Lu W, Krellman JW, Dijkers MP. Can cognitive behavioral therapy for insomnia also treat fatigue, pain, and mood symptoms in individuals with traumatic brain injury? – a multiple case report. NeuroRehabilitation. 2016;38:59–69.

15. Johansson B, Wentzel AP, Andrell P, Ronnback L, Mannheimer C. Long-term treatment with methylphenidate for fatigue after traumatic brain injury. Acta Neurol Scand. 2016;135(1):100–7.
16. Cantor JB, Ashman T, Bushnik T, Cai X, Farrell-Carnahan L, Gumber S, Hart T, Rosenthal J, Dijkers MP. Systematic review of interventions for fatigue after traumatic brain injury: a NIDRR traumatic brain injury model systems study. J Head Trauma Rehabil. 2014;29:490–7.
17. Marshall S, Bayley M, McCullagh S, Velikonja D, Berrigan L, Ouchterlony D, Weegar K. Updated clinical practice guidelines for concussion/mild traumatic brain injury and persistent symptoms. Brain Inj. 2015;29:688–700.
18. Herman J. Psychiatric disorders and fatigue. Sleep Med Clin. 2013;8:213–20.
19. Fetter KL. We grieve too: one inpatient oncology unit's interventions for recognizing and combating compassion fatigue. Clin J Oncol Nurs. 2012;16:559–61.
20. Valent P. Survival strategies: a framework for understanding secondary traumatic stress and coping in helpers. In: Figley CR, editor. Compassion fatigue. 1st ed. New York: Taylor & Francis; 1995. p. 21–50.

Index

© Springer Science+Business Media, LLC, part of Springer Nature 2018
A. Sharafkhaneh, M. Hirshkowitz (eds.), *Fatigue Management*,
https://doi.org/10.1007/978-1-4939-8607-1